Neo-/Victorian Biographilia and James Miranda Barry

Ann Heilmann

Neo-/Victorian Biographilia and James Miranda Barry

A Study in Transgender and Transgenre

palgrave
macmillan

Ann Heilmann
Cardiff University
Cardiff, UK

ISBN 978-3-319-71385-4 (hardcover) ISBN 978-3-319-71386-1 (eBook)
ISBN 978-3-030-10048-3 (softcover)
https://doi.org/10.1007/978-3-319-71386-1

Library of Congress Control Number: 2017963555

Cover illustration: Aspect, Old illustration depicting Capetown in South Africa in 1880, drawn by J. Vanione in Emil Holub's Seven Years in South Africa, published in Vienna, 1881, Shutterstock Standard Licence, image ID 80580226. Foreground: Portrait of James Barry, reproduced courtesy of Western Cape Archives and Records Service, Cape Town, South Africa (reference number M774). Design by Paul de Bruin, Limelight Design.

Printed on acid-free paper

This Palgrave Macmillan imprint is published by the registered company Springer Nature Switzerland AG.
The registered company address is: Gewerbestrasse 11, 6330 Cham, Switzerland

The original version of the book has been revised.
A Preamble has been added to recognize the existence of another James Barry (Wine merchant & Member of Legislative Assembly).
The text under acknowledgements has been amended along with the caption for Fig 2.6.
Under Chapter 2, on page 267 the notes have been revised.

Preamble

In inversion of the Barry mythos, which prototypically starts at the end, this opening seeks to trouble the beginning, the image of the middle-aged James Barry that frames my book. The 'real' James Barry, I argue in this study, cannot be reconstructed because from the very outset the historical personality disappeared into the myth and its shifting, sometimes simplistic, at other times more multi-layered representations of whatever 'James Barry' came to signify for the specific cultural, gendered and socio-political contexts of the period. A striking illustration of the submersion of documentary sources in the omnipresence of the mythos is provided by the portrait of the dignified and self-possessed Barry featured in neo-Victorian life-writing both here and elsewhere. Resident in nineteenth-century Cape Town, this James Barry is not the military surgeon who is the subject of this volume but a wine merchant and member of the Legislative Assembly at the Cape.[1] He is, however, the Barry of my imagination; the Barry who captures the historical moment of my own time. This is how I envisage Barry: fully embodied and supremely at ease with his identity. Ultimately, then, all cultural representations of Barry speak potently to the myth-making powers of neo-/Victorian biographilia.

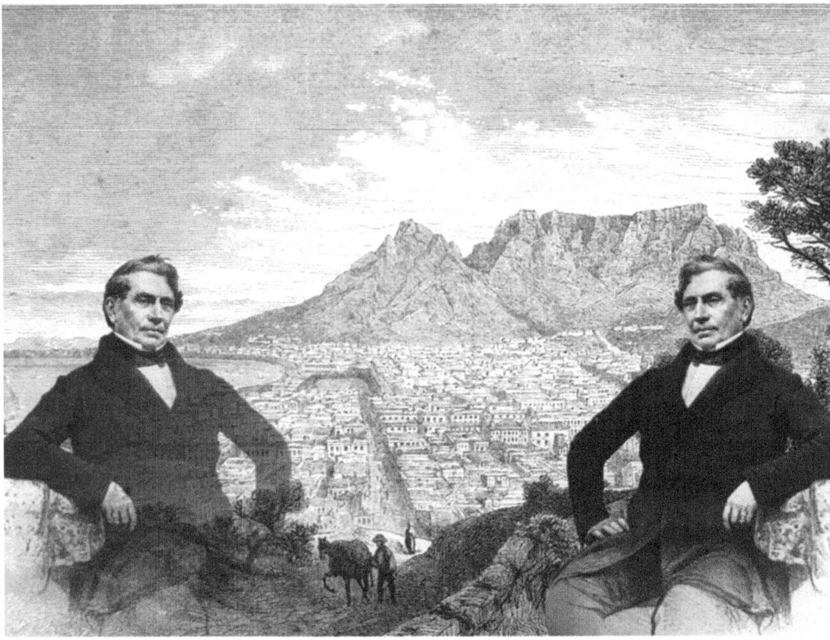

Note

1. I am grateful to David Obermayer, University Archivist, Forsyth Library, Fort Hays State University, US, for drawing my attention to the two James Barrys.

Preface

This book took shape a civilisation ago. It was 2015, and James Barry had been born into his afterlives a century and a half earlier. The British Empire had long dissolved, or so it seemed. I enjoyed my trans-European, hybrid Continental-British identity even more than Barry appears to have enjoyed his hybrid/transgender self. Having grown up in a firmly European culture, I had turned into a committed internationalist during my university years and especially my studies abroad. My elective affinities with British culture and Anglophone literatures, above all my passion for the Victorians and the first women's movement had long settled me in my second home country, where I had by then lived and worked for the longer part of my life. Academically, I had moved across several disciplines (Modern Languages, Women's Studies, English Literature) and different universities in two of the four nations of the UK as it is currently constituted. Perhaps it was this experience of straddling languages, cultures, nationalities, disciplines, and (in intellectual, imaginative ways) time periods that drew me to Barry. But it was not until 2016, when completing the first draft of my book, that I started to share Barry's sense of utter alienation and anger in the face of the enormity of the irresponsibility and dishonesty of the prevailing powers. That is when I realized that the world and values I had considered to be unassailable and self-evident had ceased to exist.

Raised in Ireland, educated in Scotland, and trained in England, Barry crossed several continents in his postings to multiple territories (the Cape Peninsula, Mauritius, the West Indies, St Helena, Malta, Corfu and Canada). In doing so, he bestowed dignity on the position of citizen of the world before this identity came to be disparaged as 'unpatriotic' and subversive in the words of a (then) unelected Prime Minister. As a medical officer of the British army, Barry operated from within, yet in his unswerving defence of the rights of Othered individuals and groups of people remained resistant to the imperial mindset, a worldview that has resurfaced with such atavistic force in our own time. When he saw indigenous female patients subjected to abuse by male hospital attendants, he appointed a black matron. Incandescent, he stepped in to stop the institutionalized brutalization of prisoners and leprosy sufferers. It was this determination to call out injustice, cruelty, corruption and professional misconduct wherever it occurred that led to his court-martial, from which he emerged fully vindicated. If he were to live today, Barry would scoff at the mindlessness (and worse) of those who want to Make Us Great Again and Take Back Control by breaking away from our nearest neighbours and our shared histories and rights cultures to return to the toxic delusions and violations of a Glorious Empire. He would lobby for sheltering children displaced by war and stand up against hate speech, refugee vilification, detention camps, night-time deportations, ethnically motivated family partition and racialized travel bans. He would be appalled by the ethical, intellectual and emotional impoverishment and rising fundamentalism at the heart of our brave new world. His life was a political statement. So is ours, and the afterworld will judge us.

Cardiff, UK
29 March 2017

Ann Heilmann

Acknowledgements

It is a convention of James Barry life-writing to refer to the irresistible allure of this extraordinary personality and story: once encountered, so the trope goes, they possess and haunt the biographilist for evermore. Barry, as I explore in this book, touches a nerve in our thinking about sex and gender. While the roots of my interest go back to my early work on Victorian feminism, in particular the New Woman and fin-de-siècle cross-dressing narratives, my entanglement with Barry himself began with Patricia Duncker's *James Miranda Barry* and the research into biographies and earlier biofictions that it inspired, resulting in a conference paper on 'Doctored Lives' in 2005. Since this coincided with a change of post, the new curriculum took over, and I did not get back to Barry until one of my PhD students devoted part of a chapter of her thesis on 'Neo-Victorian Impersonations' on the subject; I am grateful to Allison Neal for the long conversations we had, not least about the tricky question of pronouns. Another professional move inspired me to return to my expanding Barry archive in 2012 for a plenary lecture at a workshop on 'Gender, Genre and Identity'; this focused my attention on the conceptual connections between Barry's gender crossing and the genre crossings of Barry life-writing. By then I knew the subject deserved further development, but again other demands and commitments intervened. That is why, when I started preparing a keynote in 2015, I decided that this time I would write the article before the actual paper – and ended up with 18,000 words. When following the conference I presented my work-in-progress to colleagues, hoping for advice on how to condense the over-long essay, the unanimous suggestion was to extend it into a short book. In the drafting process, as more and more source material caught my notice, this project grew into the current monograph. It is tempting to conjure up parallels with Barry himself: maybe that's how it all started, as a temporary adventure, and then it became the life. But that, of course, would mean indulging in the representational self-constructions of biographiliacs that this study seeks to investigate.

Writing this book became an adventure – and like an adventure it was beset with difficulties, predominantly those that pertain to mystery tales. For just as Barry remains elusive as a personality, so does some of the early source material. *Madeline's Mystery* (1882), Mary Braddon's single-volume edition of Ebenezer Rogers's rambling three-decker *A Modern Sphinx* (1881), proved particularly hard to track down, until, with the aid of Janine Hatter and the Mary Braddon Society, I found one of two extant library copies at the Harry Ransom Center (which kindly sent me the novel in digitized format). An even greater mystery arose around George Edwin Marvell's story 'The Mystery of the Kapok Doctor', published in the *Cape Times Christmas Annual* of 1904, an issue that is not held in the British Library and that a worldwide inter-library loan search failed to discover; thanks to Mark Llewellyn it was subsequently located in the National Library of South Africa. Following the complex histories of publishing houses on their journey of regrouping, merging and being absorbed into one another made the permissions process in some cases a detective story in its own right. Final complications involved tracing the whereabouts of the one portrait I knew my book could not forego because it features a serenely self-assured man at the culmination point of his professional success. When later struggling to find the best design for my cover, I realized that representing the subject (and subject matter) was not quite as 'straight' as I had imagined. Many thanks go to Megen de Bruin-Molé for recommending Paul de Bruin, Limelight Design, who made the trans/formation possible. Paul arrived at the 'perfect' representational play on this book's reflections of (and on) the cultural processes of inflecting Barry's story through the pictorial traces of the material body and this body's performances. The idea was to depict a man eminently comfortable in his body against a Cape Town and Table Mountain background, while at the same time visualizing the tropes of Barry life-writing in the doubling and mirrored ghosting of the figure of the transcender – hence the opening illustration to this book. Ironically, this Barry was a namesake; I thank David Obermayer, University Archivist, Forsyth Library, Fort Hays State University, US for this information.

Countless further individuals not mentioned above and also institutions assisted me in researching and writing this book. I want to begin by thanking Cardiff University and the School of English, Communication and Philosophy for sabbatical leave awarded for the autumn semester of 2015–16, when a first part-draft of the book was written. In addition to the regular staff research budget the School's Strategic Research and Research Innovation funds offered generous support for conferences, engagement opportunities, archival trips, digital resource acquisition and permissions and reproductions arrangements across a number of years. Of the many people who made this book possible I am most grateful to my colleagues at Cardiff who gave invaluable hands-on advice on the initial draft-in-progress – Sophie Coulombeau, Jane Moore, Becky Munford – and who read, copy-edited and provided comprehensive feedback on later incarnations of the full manuscript: Catherine Butler, Holly Furneaux and Martin Willis. Their comments ranged from Dickens's potential involvement in the composition of the first biostory to women in trousers and from Laqueur's one and two-sex theories and nineteenth-century science to trans narratives. I also benefited tremendously from the wide-ranging support of colleagues from further afield – Linda Anderson, Kate Mitchell and Nathalie Saudo-Welby – who all read the manuscript and offered enormously helpful suggestions; many thanks in particular to Nathalie for her astute comments and assistance with translations from the French. Neil Badmington and Damian Walford Davies inspired me by example to experiment with creative openings and to cultivate the aesthetics of style; any shortcomings are my responsibility only. Jenny Hulin expertly handled incoming research admin to shield me from work flows in the most intense period of finalizing the book. Warm thanks go to Angela V. John for her serendipiditous rediscovery of a 1988 article that alerted me in the final revision stage to Jean Binnie's 1988 biodrama *Colours*, a play that would otherwise have escaped my notice. Mel Kohlke was a constant wellspring of information generously shared and vibrant stimulus for exchange of ideas on neo-Victorian life-writing; her essay-collection on *Neo-Victorian Biofiction* (co-edited with Christian Gutleben in the Brill imprint) is much-awaited. Rachel Carroll's excellent book on *Transgender and the Literary Imagination* (Edinburgh University Press) was completed just in time for me to consult it during the proofing stage of mine; I am grateful to Rachel and the publisher for giving me access to the manuscript. Equally, thanks go to Kirsti Bohata for drawing my attention to Kate Milsom's *No Man's Land* exhibition, which includes a (2017) creative re-imagination of James Barry (Martin Tinney Gallery, Cardiff, 28 February to 24 March 2018, http://www.artwales.com/exhibition-mtg-en.php?locationID=263). Another source of boundless inspiration were those greats of Victorian women's writing and historical gender studies, Elaine Showalter and Margaret Stetz – blazing examples of the indivisibility of highest-level research and teaching, collegiality and human kindness. I am also deeply grateful to my undergraduate, postgraduate and PhD students, past and present, for always grounding me when nervous excitement threatened to get the better of me: Megen de Bruin-Molé, Daný van Dam, Katherine Mansfield, Karen Power and Akira Suwa. Now academic or librarian colleagues, Catherine Han and Bronwen Blatchford tracked down details of drama manuscripts and related material for me, while Valerie Goulden drew my attention to a Facebook clip of Barry, and Eden Day prompted me to think about shadow femininities in Victorian literature, a concept that can be applied to constructions of Barry's dual gender identity across Barry biographilia. The enthusiasm and creative-analytical talents of successive cohorts of students contributing to my modules on 'Gender and Monstrosity: Late Victorian to Neo-Victorian' and 'Neo-Victorian Metatextualities' kept my passion for neo-Victorianism alive and opened up new critical and imaginative avenues. Further inspiration came from Patricia Duncker (herself one of the key figures to energize Barry life-writing) and her always conference-rousing, passion-inciting keynotes, not to mention her general generosity and kindness in personal exchange. Thanks are also due to Chris Balme for clarifying *Commedia dell'Arte* contexts; to Martin Dubois and Marco Graziosi for advising on a Barry cartoon that has been (mis)attributed to Edward Lear; to novelist Faysal Mikdadi for email conversations on autobiographiction; to David James, Monique Rooney, Martin Goodman, Catherine McNamara for drawing my attention to trans memoirs, criticism and the activities of *Gendered Intelligence*; to Jana Funke and Jen Grove, themselves engaged in a fascinating project on 'Rethinking Sexuality', for sharing and discussing Barry biographilia; and to Tomos Owen for bringing to my notice Derrida's exploration of the apocalyptic interplay of beginnings and endings. I am hugely indebted to the anonymous Palgrave reader and to Ben Doyle, Eva Hodgkin, Camille Davies and the publisher's production team.

The following libraries, archives and professional staff generously supported this project with their holdings and expertise: the subject librarians, Document Supply and Special Collections staff, Cardiff Arts and Social Sciences Library, Helen D'artillac-Brill, Andrew Blackmore, Bronwen

Blatchford, Alison Harvey, Stephanie Mauritz, Jackie Roach, Erica Swain; Jill Sullivan, Bristol Theatre Collection (who very kindly granted access out of opening times); Bill Emery and Sue Waterhouse (Customer Services) and Lisa Kenny (News Reference Team) at the British Library; Maria Victoria Fernandez (Public Services Intern) at the Harry Ransom Center, University of Texas at Austin; Rob McIntosh (Curator, Archives and Library), Museum of Military Medicine; Eleanor Johnson Ward (Record Copying Department) at the National Archives, Kew; Ulrike Hogg, Lynsey Halliday and Sally Harrower at the National Library of Scotland, Edinburgh; Harry Nkadimgeng, Legal Deposit Coordinator, South Africa; Antenie Carston (Head of Repographics and Digital Services), Melanie Geystyn (Principal Librarian, Special Collection) and Ronel Rogers (Librarian) at the National Library of South Africa, Cape Town Campus; Kate Bowe and Eve Watson (Head of Archives) at the RSA (which houses some of James Barry RA's finest paintings and prints); Dominika Chanerley at the Science Photo Library; Claire McKentrick at the Scottish Theatre Archive, Glasgow University Library; the licensing team at Shutterstock; Richard Keenen (Bespoke Archive Digitisation Ltd) and Peter Judge at the Wellcome Library; Marisa Bronkhurst and Erika Le Roux at Western Cape Archives and Records Service, Cape Town, South Africa.

Warm thanks are also owing to friends and fellow academics – citizens of the world all of them – for inviting me to deliver keynotes, plenary and guest lectures and involving me in workshop and paper contributions to the following research events, listed in chronological order: 'Doctored lives: James Miranda Barry in twentieth and twenty-first-century fiction and biography', paper given at 'The Twentieth Century and the Victorians' conference, Leeds Centre for Victorian Studies, Leeds Trinity University, July 2005; 'Gender, genre and neo-Victorian impurities: James Miranda Barry in biography and biofiction', plenary delivered at the AHRC-funded Genre Research Network workshop conference on 'Gender, Genre and Identity', organised by Natasha Rulyova, University of Birmingham, November 2012; 'Re/Tracing James Miranda Barry in neo-Victorian biographilia: Performances in gender/genre hybridity', keynote delivered at the 'Material Traces of the Past in Contemporary Literature' conference, organized by Rosario Arias at the University of Málaga, May 2015; 'From James Barry to Mary Braddon: Writing gender imposture and *Madeline's Mystery* (1882)', keynote address, 'From Brontë to Bloomsbury III: Reassessing Women's Writing from the 1880s and 1890s' conference organized by Carolyn Oulton, International Centre for Victorian Women

Writers, Canterbury Christ Church University, July 2016; 'James Miranda Barry and neo-Victorian biodrama', paper delivered in panel 11 (5), on 'Modern Literature' organized by Anne Varty and Warwick Gould, IAUPE annual conference, Institute of English Studies, London, July 2016; a masterclass and guest lecture on 'Writing games with Doctor James: James Miranda Barry in neo-Victorian life-writing' at the invitation of Lucy Neave and Kate Mitchell, Research School of the Humanities and the Creative Arts, Australian National University, Canberra, Australia, November 2016; 'Performance games with Dr. James: Remediating historical transgender and the case of James Barry', a guest lecture coordinated by Maria Delgado and Kate Pitt at the Royal Central School of Speech and Drama, University of London, March 2017; 'Cross-dressing and/in life-writing: Transgender, transgenre and the case of James Miranda Barry', keynote address, 'Cross-Dressing in Fact and Fiction: Norms, Bodies, Identities' conference organized by Catherine Delyfer, University of Toulouse, France, April 2017; 'Writing the nineteenth-century cross-dresser: James Miranda Barry in life-writing', invited paper delivered at the 'Writing Women's Lives: Past and Present Perspectives' workshop organized by June Purvis at University of Portsmouth, June 2017; 'Trans/*form*ations in gender and genre: James Miranda Barry in neo-Victorian life-writing', guest lecture invited by Steffanie Brusberg-Kiermeier, University of Hildesheim, Germany, June 2017; 'Consuming historical transgender: James Miranda Barry', contribution to 'Consuming Gender' symposium organized by Akira Suwa under the aegis of Assuming Gender at Cardiff University, July 2017; '"A Mystery Still" (1867): Victorian transgender and *All the Year Round*'s foundation myth of James Miranda Barry', paper presented at the 'Victorians Unbound: Connections and Intersections' annual BAVS conference organized by Claudia Capancioni and Alice Crossley at Bishop Grosseteste University, Lincoln, in August 2017; '"Tell me your secret, Doctor James": Gender-crossing, life-writing and James Barry', keynote delivered at the biennial conference on English Studies, themed 'From Queen Anne to Queen Victoria. Readings in eighteenth and nineteenth-century British literature and culture', organized by Grażyna Bystydzieńska at the University of Warsaw, Poland, September 2017. I enjoyed the lively audiences of these events and am grateful for the plentiful ideas stimulated by conference discussion.

A number of colleagues and organisations offered engagement opportunities with the wider public, such as a short talk on 'Transgender, sexology and the nineteenth century' and contribution to a panel discussion following a screening of *The Danish Girl*, at a 'Tinted Lens' event curated by Katie Featherstone, Chapter Arts Centre, Cardiff (National Cinema for Wales) in collaboration with the British Film Institute (film hub Wales), in January 2016. This was followed by a learning and discussion session on James Barry and 'Transgender in historical perspective' in a strand on 'Inheriting Liberation' organized by Debi Withers at the 'World Emergenc(i)es' event at Bristol Community Centre in June 2016.

Permission was kindly granted by Katriona Gilmore, Gilmore & Roberts, for the reproduction of lines from the lyric 'Doctor James', *The Innocent Left,* released by Navigator Records, 2012; and by playwright David McKail (Frederic Mohr) for use of quotations from his unpublished work held at the National Library of Scotland, Edinburgh and the Scottish Theatre Archive, Glasgow and for quoting from email correspondence. I am also grateful to the following organisations that granted me permission to reproduce the illustrations and appendices in this book: the British Library; the Museum of Military Medicine, Keogh Barracks, Ash Vale, Aldershot; the National Library of South Africa, Cape Town Campus; Western Cape Archives and Records Service, South Africa; Patrick Gabler of Rothfos & Gabler. The book cover illustrations are reproduced courtesy of the following publishers: Claire Weatherhead, Bloomsbury Publishing; Peter London, Harper Collins; Helen Bradbury and Annette Fuhrmeister, The History Press; Ilona Chavasse, Oneworld Publications; Ann Porter and Sofia Wennerstrom, Penguin/Random House and Penguin Random House LLC Permissions Department; Alia McKellar, Profile Books; Holly Doll, Red Deer Press. For further details of permissions see the List of Figures and the captions underneath the illustrations. The author and publishers have made every effort to contact copyright and permission holders of images reproduced in this book. If there has been any oversight, we would welcome correspondence from relevant parties so that correction can be made to future editions.

Finally, my greatest debt, more than ever, is to my most important reader and co-author of many projects, Mark Llewellyn. This book could not have been written without his always warm and generous support. And last not least, the 'Heavenly Twins' of Oakfield, Angelica and Diavolo, deserve recognition for never giving up on calling me to bed during extended nightshifts and for always settling on my lap and purring at the right time.

Contents

List of Figures

CHAPTER 1

Writing Barry – Writing Gender/Genre Crossing: An Introduction

If for a single instant … I could imagine I have lost sight of the character of a gentleman I should have spared this or any other tribunal the task of investigating my conduct.

James Barry, closing speech, court martial at St. Helena (1836)[1]

[T]he woman who performed the last offices … said Dr. Barry was a female and that I was a pretty Doctor not to know this … [She] seemed to think that she had become acquainted with a great secret and wished to be paid for keeping it. I informed her that all Dr. Barry's relatives were dead, and that it was no secret of mine, and that my own impression was that Dr. Barry was a hermaphrodite. – But whether Dr. Barry was male, female or hermaphrodite I do not know …

Staff Surgeon McKinnon to the Registrar General of Somerset House (1865)[2]

I start from the premise … that trans is good to think with: that we can use the transgender experience … as a lens through which to think in new and fruitful ways about the fluidity of [other] identifications.

Rogers Brubaker, *trans* (2016)[3]

[L]ocated on the border between historiography and literature, fact and fiction, … biofictions show a pronounced tendency to cross boundaries and to blur genre distinctions.

Ansgar Nünning, 'Fictional Metabiographies and Metaautobiographies' (2005)[4]

A. Heilmann, *Neo-/Victorian Biographilia and James Miranda Barry*, https://doi.org/10.1007/978-3-319-71386-1_1

His end marked the beginning of James Miranda Barry. A mythos was born, literally and literarily, from the reverberations of Barry's death. Delivering Barry into cultural reincarnation, that death raised (and continues to raise) pointed questions about gender, identity and representation that render the historical character at the centre of the myth, and the cultural production that has sustained it, an exemplary model for reflecting on the complex border crossings between historiography and literature, fact and fiction that are performed by neo-Victorianism and by life-writing, the two genres that in their combined form and in their specific interpellation of James Barry are key to this book. If neo-Victorian life-writing is about the resurrection of the 'ex-centric' nineteenth-century subject so that we can discover versions of ourselves in the mirror of the re-invented past that leads to our imagined future, this resurrection finds particular resonance in the afterlives of James Barry.[5] Self-identified officer and gentleman, yet returned in death to the 'truths' of an ostensibly female body, Barry also speaks powerfully to twenty-first-century concerns around transgender. The precise nature of the interaction between these coordinates within the medium of life-writing – James 'Miranda' Barry, trans/gender, neo-Victorianism – constitute the central axes around which this study is organized.

Straddling and crossing the fields of Victorian to neo-Victorian studies and grounded in feminist and gender criticism, this book seeks to undertake a comprehensive conceptualization of neo-Victorian life-writing, or 'biographilia', through analysis of the later-Victorian to neo-Victorian remediation of a spectacular case of transgender. The cultural response to Victorian gender crossing, refracted as it is in biography, biofiction and biodrama, can, I contend, serve to illuminate the genre paradigms of neo-historical life-writing. My approach is focused on reading neo-Victorian life-writing through the lens of the cultural construction and representation of James Barry (1789–1865), senior colonial medical officer of the British army from 1816 to 1859. A pioneer of sanitary science and medical reform whose preventative measures anticipated Florence Nightingale's by over three decades, Barry attained the highest rank in his profession, that of Inspector General.[6] Known for his pugnacious, iconoclastic personality during his lifetime, he became the object of intense speculation after his death in 1865 when rumours arose about his sex. These followed a visit to Staff-Surgeon David Reid McKinnon (a doctor long acquainted with Barry who had tended to him in his last illness) by the charwoman who had laid out the body.[7] With only one testimony to lay claim to physical evidence of Barry's bodily condition, and with his female birth identity not confirmed until the latter twentieth century,[8] Barry's 'real' sex, gender identity and life circumstances have in the intervening one and a half centuries prompted considerable interest among life-writers, novelists and playwrights.

The cultural appeal of the 'enigma' represented by a prominent figure of medical and gender history has, at the time of writing, inspired four biographies, five biodramas, four short stories, seven bionovels (including one in the French medium), a folk-song lyric, and several radio and TV broadcasts.[9] Two movie biopics are at different stages of planning and development.[10] The proliferation of critical-creative texts and productions that, from the Victorian to the contemporary period, have sought to re-imagine Barry's life, ranging across the spectrum from literary fiction and experimental stage drama to popular culture, is remarkable. What is particularly striking about the cultural dissemination of the 'Barry mythos' is that the historical personality in question was not a prominent writer or artist with an oeuvre that has wide visibility and yet enjoys a measure of the 'medial framework' otherwise reserved for what Laura Savu calls the 'author fiction' of Shakespeare, Austen, Dickens, the Brontës or Wilde.[11] If the figure of Barry touches a cultural nerve, this is evidently because his story of crossing is intrinsic to Victorian, twentieth-century and contemporary interrogations of the sex/gender/sexuality/identity 'conundrum'.[12]

My key rationale for using James Barry as a case study to interrogate neo-/Victorian biographilia is that Barry is paradigmatic of the category of instability because of the very uncertainty of any certainty about his story of gender variance. The resulting *gender fluidity* of cultural representations of Barry, I argue, affords an exemplary model for the *genre fluidity* of neo-Victorian life-writing. The Barry story helps to illuminate the resisting category of 'trans*'; like Halberstam's asterisk, it too opens itself up to a plurality of readings 'organized around but not confined to forms of gender variance'; by so doing, it 'modif[ies] the meaning of transitivity by refusing to situate transition in relation to a destination, a final form, a specific shape, or an established configuration of desire and identity'.[13] In specifically seeking to tease out the intersectionality of gender and genre in the construction of the cultural memory of Barry, I build on recent queer and feminist narratology,[14] in particular Monique Rooney's argument that the passer acts as a figure of representational instability: 'The passer cannot exist without a reader who only temporarily engages in passing and is therefore able to disavow his/her part in the crossing. Caught in a mediating role, the passer is a marker of representational transience and is thus a pivotal figure for thinking about figuration and narration'. As a consequence, the 'representation of passing has historically operated as a kind of metanarrative, a reading of reading'.[15] It is this metanarrative about the genre crossings involved in writing and reading the gender crosser that is at the heart of my book. The best illustration of how neo-Victorian life-writing operates is furnished by drawing on an historical figure who features across biography, biofiction and biodrama from the Victorian through to the contemporary period, and who features both as a boundary transgressor *and* as a boundary marker.

Without doubt a considerable part of the fascination that has ensured Barry a place in the cultural imagination derives from the unknowability of his 'true' bodily condition in the absence of any 'hard' evidence (in the form of a post-mortem or DNA examination) and, since the discovery of his birth name, of his 'real' gender identity: was Barry a woman who disguised herself to lead the life of her choice, an intersex individual, a transman?[16] How conclusive in terms of Barry's sense of self/selves across time is documentary evidence of his original identity? As Marjorie Garber argues with reference to Barry's older contemporary, the Chevalier d'Éon, the most pressing question arising from historical cases is 'the relativity of "proof". According to what canons? Dictated by what exigencies? With what ideological concerns in view: medical, political, social, sexual, erotic?'[17] And, one might add, on the basis of what erratic data? Even Barry's gravestone with his incorrectly recorded date of death testifies to the instability of the subject.[18] Just as the desire for neo-Victorian fiction and life writing is fed by our knowledge of the irretrievability of the Victorian past, so it is the unattainability and forever speculative nature of any enquiry into Barry – precisely the mystery that 'Doctor James' will not yield up – that has kept the subject of Barry alive.[19]

There is an element of the spectral to the Barry myth, a cultural haunting visualized in the anecdote of the phantom 'young officer in Georgian uniform' reputed to walk the woods in the vicinity of Cape Town that the co-authors of the first biodrama and third novel reference as the source of their interest in Barry and a catalyst for their work: 'The moment I saw that haunting figure …I wanted to trace her life.'[20] In the twenty-first century, which has seen increased momentum in the production of biographilia, Barry's story continues to exert a ghostly allure. At the end of her 2002 biography, Rachel Holmes invokes the Barry narrative as a quest across the centuries: 'Dr James Barry has haunted me, but will continue to wander the pathways of our imagination, in search of the spirit of an age, now or in the future, that can accommodate his difference.'[21] Barry as a revenant: Terry Castle's apparitional lesbian here transmutes into the shadowy, only ever partially materializing and therefore eternally irresistible figure of the transman.[22] Ghosting is, as Jack/Judith Halberstam notes, one of mainstream culture's containment strategies to make transgender both visible and invisible at one and the same time.[23] My argument, then, revolves around the ways in which Victorian to contemporary life-writing transgenders – or, conversely, spectralizes transgender by heteronormalizing – the persona of James Barry. Given contemporary conceptualization of transgender as an umbrella category, this concept will be the framework for discussion of Barry's gender variance.[24]

That the questions about gender and especially transgender that Barry's story raises are closely connected to present-day concerns is signalled by the vibrancy of recent cultural and political debate. Transgender studies as an academic discipline and a catalyst for community and international activism was established in the 1990s; the twenty-first century has seen the 'mainstreaming' of transgender in wider culture.[25] This is evidenced in exhibitions on transgender history[26] and the rise of non-binarity in the use of gender-neutral titles and pronouns, including legal documents[27]; in legislation like the UK's Gender Recognition Act of 2004,[28] the House of Commons and Women and Equality Committee's 2016 'Transgender Equality' report;[29] and the decision, in 2013, to remove transgender from the Diagnostic and Statistical Manual of Mental Disorders.[30] A regular feature in news provision,[31] transgender has prompted widespread cultural interest in memoirs, novels and biopics about genderqueer identities and gender-reassignment/confirmation.[32] Beyond the mainstream appeal of transgender celebrity culture,[33] a broader public is now engaging with questions around intersexuality[34] and transgender children and family life[35] while also being attentive to high-profile court cases.[36] These concerns are addressed in institutional cultures through the implementation of transgender policies[37] and public and institutional responses to alt-right endeavour to reverse Equality and Diversity legislation such as the attempt to enforce a transgender ban on the US military.[38] Barry speaks to twenty-first-century awareness of gender variance, non-binarism and what Stephen Whittle calls our 'cultural obsession' with all matters 'trans' as much as the woman warrior in male garb did to twentieth-century feminisms and the swashbuckling heroine to the Victorians in the age of female educational, professional and political campaigns.[39]

As a gender passer (making the best of gender binarity) who in posthumous representation becomes a gender crosser (transgressor against gender normativity), Barry presents an epistemic challenge to late-twentieth and twenty-first-century thought about transgender (the psychological and experiential grounds for his change of gender and potentially shifting sense of identity over time will remain forever speculative). Barry's case can thus serve to highlight our own blindspots and ongoing 'gender trouble'. For that an historical individual with a female birth and male adult identity should to this day predominantly, and insistently, be figured as a woman indicates that *historical* trans identity is far from being 'mainstreamed', and also, perhaps, that we devote more attention to transwomen than transmen.[40] Is this because transfemininity is more of a threat: to heteronormativity since it disturbs the commodification of the female body as an object of (straight) sexual consumption; to feminism because it calls into question the key premise that women are subjected to oppression and violence globally because of their innate bodily difference from men? (In approaching James Barry's representation in life-writing through the combined lens of feminism and transgender, this study seeks to contribute to the bridging of the troubled waters between these two liberation discourses, arguing for inclusiveness in political and cultural practice.)[41] As Rogers Brubaker points out, transwomen 'face more intensive policing than their female-to-male counterparts.'[42] Is transfemininity both more challenging and more stereotypically 'sexy' than transmasculinity? Or is society less concerned with transmen because they started their journey as girls or women and their gender migration is rationalized as the desire to appropriate the economically and socially 'dominant' identity position?

Beyond heteronormative contexts, the complexities of Barry's life also go some way towards illustrating tensions in transgender studies, as pinpointed by Katrina Roen, between the respective politics of passing and crossing, of adopting 'either/or' or 'both/neither' identities.[43] Placed in his historical background, Barry's gender performance cuts across both positions. In his determination to protect himself against exposure (when gravely ill, he issued instructions for his body to be buried in his clothes without examination), the historical Barry was, in Kate Bornstein's terms, a 'gender defender', an upholder of the sex/gender system.[44] (Given historical conditions and his choice of career, it is of course questionable how he could have acted otherwise; the constraints to which the socially more privileged Chevalier d'Éon was subjected offers a good illustration of the dangers of crossing).[45] In Brubaker's more recent, less value-laden terms, Barry's life offers an historical angle on the 'trans of migration': 'moving from one established sex/gender category to another'.[46] At the same time, Barry's spectacular over-performance of both masculinity *and* femininity mark him out as one of Bornstein's 'gender outlaws' (seeking 'every opportunity of making himself conspicuous', Barry sported 'the longest sword and spurs he could obtain', while displaying the voice, diminutive size and habits of a 'woman').[47] Brubaker's model refers to this as the 'trans of between': 'defining oneself with reference to the two established categories, without belonging entirely or unambiguously to either one'. (Brubaker's third position, 'trans of beyond', which transcends the gender binary through deliberate resistance to categorization, was adopted by the Chevalier d'Éon and is played out in postmodern biofictional representations of Barry such as Patricia Duncker's).[48] The particular challenge Barry posed with a gender performance that mixed gender stereotypes will be considered in the third chapter's discussion of Barry caricatures.

Passer and crosser, 'trans-migrant' and 'trans-betweener', gender changer and gender challenger at once: from a twenty-first-century perspective Barry can convincingly be placed in a transgender context.[49] The question that this book investigates, however, is not so much whether Barry was 'actually' a transgender individual as, rather, what complexities arise from applying – or withholding – contemporary identity categories to historical subjects and how this translates to biographical, biofictional and biodramatic constructions of the figure under review. For, as this study will illustrate, the majority of texts across the 150 year time period covered (1865–2016) cast Barry as a cross-dressing *woman* rather than a transman. That this is also the case in recent textual production runs counter to contemporary developments in postmodern studies, where, as Halberstam notes, 'the transgender body has emerged as futurity itself, a kind of heroic fulfillment of postmodern promises of gender flexibility'.[50] The frequency of references in my book to Barry's 'masquerade', 'impersonation' and 'imposture' serves to reflect this representation of femininity in disguise embracing masculinity as performance. The emphasis of most biographilic works is on the protagonist's *process* of enacting and in the act imperceptibly *'becoming'* rather than 'being' James Barry. Even though in many of these texts Barry remains essentially (or remains essentialized as) a woman, the attention paid to processes of transformation resonates with contemporary transgender theory and experience: as Virginia Goldner observes, transgenderism constitutes not 'another gender *position* (a kind of "third sex")' but, rather, 'a novel gender *stance*, one that constitutes gender as a process rather than a thing in itself, a gerund, rather than a noun or adjective, a permanent state of becoming, rather than a finished product.'[51] At the level of text and form, the enactment of trans/gender performance gradually turning into trans/formation is carried into effect with the props, screens and costume changes of biographilia.

As a genre that itself draws on performative acts to stage the formative experiences of its subject, biographilia – and its inflections of life-writing – offers an apt medium for interrogating the representation of historical gender variance in cultural discourse. Brought to prominence in Cora Kaplan's study of (neo-) *Victoriana*, the term biographilia has been used to refer to the contemporary appeal of the interconnecting genres of biography and biofiction (the standard descriptor for biographical fiction). In my conceptualization, biographilia, in the singular, serves as an umbrella category for fictional(ized) life-writing in a wider sense, and in the plural designates biographilic works; in both contexts the term is applied more broadly to extend beyond biography and biofiction to biodrama.[52] Though usually neglected in discussions of life-writing, biodrama accords with Hermione Lee's definition of 'different ways of telling a life-story – memoir, autobiography, biography, diary, letters, autobiographical fiction'.[53] Materially invested as it is in the performance of selves, biodrama lends itself with particular force to an examination of neo-Victorian constructions of Victorian explorations of gender, identity and subversion. Indeed, as Beth Palmer and Benjamin Poore observe, 'the stage brings the neo-Victorian concern with the instability of identity into even sharper focus.'[54] At the same time, the 'play with … double-consciousness' inherent to any self-reflective neo-Victorian text – the fact that both author and reader are aware of the historical context serving a mirror function in making us think about the present moment – finds its most distinct resonance in neo-Victorian stage performance.[55]

This is specifically the case for biodrama. As Poore notes, biodrama adds a further layer to neo-Victorianism's 'double vision' of reflecting on contemporary society through the voices of the past by drawing our attention to the metadramatic relationship between actor and role, thereby both problematizing and 'historicizing the performance event'.[56] This book contends that the interplay between the theatrical staging of a 'real' life story, the *mise-en-scène* of gender imposture and/or gender variance, and the historical Barry's sartorial, behavioral and writerly performances point to the wider connections that can be traced between neo-Victorian biographilia's negotiation of genre conventions and Barry's breaching of normative sex/gender codes.[57] The instability of gender that is constitutive of this figure and 'his'/'her'/'their' representation serves the purpose of investigating the instability of the genre of neo-Victorian life-writing. Barry's gender crossing, I posit, is represented in forms that are marked by genre crossing; *transgender* thus finds its most typical expression in *transgenre*.

In following Rogers Brubaker's call to 'think with' trans[58] and scrutinizing the complex interconnections between transgender and transgenre in biographical, biofictional and biodramatic representations of James Barry's gender crossing, this study extends and adds a Victorian/neo-Victorian angle to the work of transgender scholars like Jay Prosser. Prosser has defined 'trans- or intergeneric' parameters of contemporary transsexual autobiography, a form frequently invested with or dressed as fiction and as such situated 'as [much] between genres as its subject is between genders'.[59] Autobiography's doubling of voices (of enunciating subject and subject of enunciation; of narrating and narrated I) correlates with the split between sex and gender identity in transgender narrative. The ability to perform the autobiographical act convincingly toward a listener/reader is the precondition for transgender recognition: 'to be diagnosed as transsexual', Prosser reminds us, an individual 'must recount a transsexual autobiography'.[60] Autobiography and transsexuality thus 'mirror each other'; and '[l]ike two mirrors [they] are themselves caught up in an inter-reflective dynamic, resembling, reassembling, and articulating each other.'[61] The intersecting articulations and mirror effects of transgender and life-writing are key to this book's examination of Victorian and neo-Victorian biographilia.

A form that thrives on the crossing of boundaries (between fact and fiction, reconstruction and fabrication, claims to authenticity and metatextual simulation), neo-Victorian life-writing, this study argues, draws inspiration from nineteenth-century gender transgression for its own performance of genre breaching. Narratives of Barry's sexual border crossing illustrate the textual boundary blurring that Ansgar Nünning (in one of my opening epigraphs) identifies as integral to (postmodern) biofiction and, by implication, other forms of biographilia. As Marjorie Garber argues, 'the figure of the transvestite ... *opens up the whole question of the relationship of the aesthetic to the existential.*'[62] If the fundamental question the crosser invokes about the relationship of the aesthetic and the existential, performance and identity entails a 'critique of the possibility of "representation" itself',[63] neo-Victorian biographilia equally manifests and effects a crisis of representation.

It is this representational crisis that *Neo-/Victorian Biographilia and James Miranda Barry* seeks to address by scrutinizing how textual and sexual forms of hybridization intersect in the construction of the historical and yet always imaginary and invented figure of gender subversion. The parameters and paratextualities of this (self-)fabrication will be examined in more detail in the following section, before attention is turned to a conceptualization of neo-Victorian life writing. In my discussion of gender/genre hybridities, I draw on Robert J. C. Young's exposition of hybridization's 'double logic' of 'making difference into sameness, so that it becomes impossible for the eye to detect the hybridity' of the parts that have been forged together, and of 'severing a single object into two, turning sameness into difference'.[64] This is reflected in the fusion of, for example, biofictional and biographical modes into one single work of life-writing that is, nonetheless, categorized as belonging only to one of these forms (separation). The same 'both/and' dynamic applies to the trans subject's construction as 'Other' within the gender binary (cartoons of James Barry always accentuate the 'odd' conjunction of disparate elements; see Fig. 3.6), even though the predominant gender identity that Barry is assigned in Victorian and neo-Victorian biographilia is that of a woman. Barry himself contributed to this ontological and epistemological instability in his self-representation.

(Self-)Representations: Gender, Genre and Transgression

Even in name and age Barry presents a baffling case of representational ambiguity. His name was purloined posthumously from the idiosyncratic and quarrelsome Irish history painter and Royal Academician James Barry (1741–1806) whom mid-twentieth-century biographical scholarship established as his uncle,[65] and with whom he shared a number of personal traits. As Barry's first biographer, Isobel Rae, put it, 'both were small of stature, had fiery tempers and quick brains, and were noted as brilliant conversationalists.'[66] But Barry's name also carries echoes of an earlier unruly namesake, the Jacobite conspirator James Barry, fourth earl of Barrymore (1667–1748).[67] No connection exists, and yet the resonances between the names have prompted biographilic speculation about Barry's high-born origins and family relations in which 'Barrymore' features as aristocratic progenitor or villainous spouse.[68]

Barry's middle name is equally volatile. Borrowed from his Venezuelan republican mentor, General Sebastián Francisco de Miranda, it also invokes Barry's gender variance. But while Barry devoted an entire page of his M.D. dissertation to a dedication to Miranda and his 'paternal care', his signature on extant letters reads, simply, 'James Barry'.[69] James 'Miranda' Barry is a biographilic device, in the title of my book as elsewhere: the gender duality of the names is a knowing wink by contemporary authors

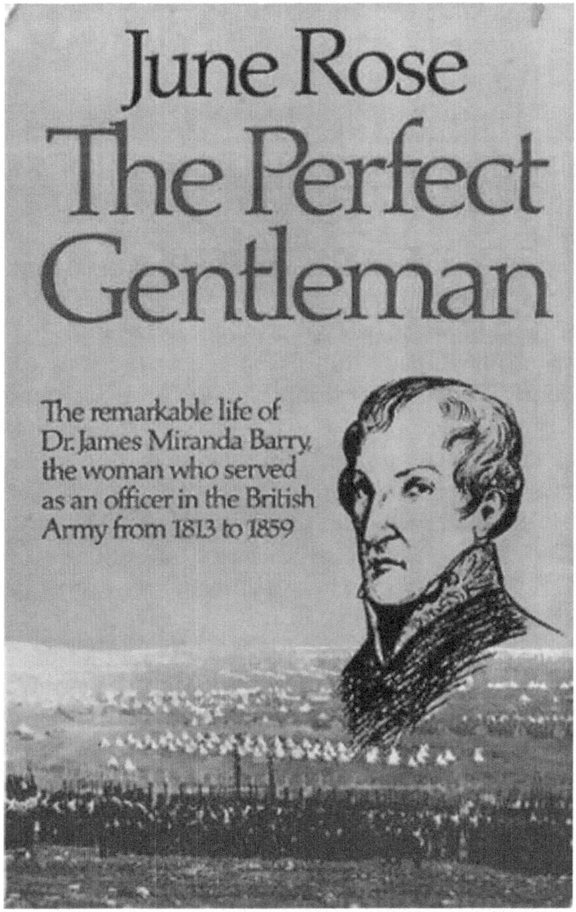

Fig. 1.1 Cover of June Rose's biography *The Perfect Gentleman* (London: Hutchinson, 1977), reproduced by permission of Random House Group Ltd

to contemporary readers, not a tongue-in-cheek act of veiling and unveiling on the part of Barry himself. This is reflected paratextually in the cover illustration of June Rose's biography (Fig. 1.1). The visual immediacy of Barry's androgynous profile, combined with the textual play with *female* **masculinity** in the author/title section (*June Rose*: The perfect **gentleman**) draws our attention to Barry's cross-gender performance, highlighted in the subtitle in his composite name and echoed in the subsequent description: '**Dr James** *Miranda* Barry, the *woman* who served as an **officer** in the British **Army**'.

If the play with Barry's transgender name points to our own game with his gender impersonation, his shifting age was his own invention. In the words of Elizabeth Longford, Barry's elusiveness is epitomized by his 'three different dates of birth, several suggestions for fathers, two possible mothers'.[70] Until Barry's original identity was discovered, his deliberately misleading account of having 'entered the Army as a Medical Officer [in 1813] under the age of fourteen' led to 1799 being recorded as his year of birth.[71] Since Barry registered at Edinburgh University in 1809, this would have made him barely ten at the start of his medical studies. Evidently, in an act of double imposture, Barry passed himself off as younger in order to pass for male. What is perhaps most baffling is that such an extraordinary level of academic precocity should have been taken at face value, even in our own time, as if the ability to cross gender simultaneously entailed the power to transcend age.[72] Another frequently cited date, 1795, also originates from Barry himself: at his army examination in 1813 the age he gave was eighteen.[73] His most probable year of birth has been traced to 1789 instead.[74] However much writers and critics have aspired to establish a precise, evidential frame of references (even to the point of identifying, to the day, the '*actual* date of … transformation' from girl to boy),[75] in gender, age, body and ethnicity Barry defied – and continues to defy – the desire to stabilize this most elusive of personalities. This is also reflected in his geographical fluidity: Irish-born, he studied medicine in Scotland and, after a short training and apprenticeship period in London and Portsmouth, spent the remainder of his life crossing seas and continents in the service of the British Crown. So frequent and varied were his postings that he has been placed in locations he never visited.[76]

Occupying a third space between male and female, Celtic (Irish/Scottish) and English, colonial and insubordinately reformist, Regency and Victorian identities, the 'real' James Barry does not exist, any more than does the 'faithful' biographical, biofictional or biodramatic rendering of a life or the 'true' neo-Victorian reconstruction of the Victorian period and of Victorian subjectivities. Instead of the authentic, what Barry represents and how he is represented invariably pinpoints the speculative and the performative: reflections and refractions in the glass of genre. Just as

'James Miranda Barry', as a subject of cultural enquiry, comes into being, and remains in view, in the act of crossing gender, so neo-Victorian life-writing constitutes itself through similar acts of border transgression. This cultural history explores the triangulation of subversive performance by reading the representational politics of Barry's gender acts as illustrative both of biographilic processes of self-fabrication and of the broader neo-Victorian project of counterfeiting the Victorian. The resisting nature of the figure under investigation, James Barry, is embodied in hybrid forms and genres.

The textual-visual exploration of this hybridity as illustrated by the cover of Rose's biography has a counterpoint in Barry's subject constitution as 'the perfect gentleman'. That Barry self-identified as male and as a member of his professional class is demonstrated by his response to his court-martial in November 1836, in which he stood accused (and was 'fully and honorably acquit[ted]' on 7 December 1836) of the charge of 'conduct unbecoming to an officer and gentleman'.[77] As his closing speech at the trial made plain, Rachel Holmes notes, '[n]ot to be a gentleman was unthinkable to him'.[78] But if Barry conceived of himself as a (gentle)man, what has preoccupied biographers, fiction writers and playwrights as well as cultural and medical commentators and critics is in what sense he was also a 'woman': a matter that raises axiomatic questions about the interfaces between, or radical dissociation, of sex, gender and performance. For, as Garber pertinently asks in her discussion of the case, 'what does it mean to say that "he" was *really* "she"? If a person lives his or her life consistently under a gender identity different from that revealed by anatomical inspection after death, what is the force of that reality?'[79] Barry exemplifies Judith Butler's much-cited proposition that '[g]ender is the repeated stylization of the body, a set of repeated acts within a highly rigid regulatory frame that congeal over time to produce the appearance of substance, of a natural sort of being'.[80] Just as there is never anything authentic about either gender or sex in that both are continually constructed and deconstructed through multiple and shifting performances, so too 'James Barry' constituted himself through repeated acts of performance within strictly demarcated regulatory regimes (the university, the military, medical and colonial hierarchies) that his insurgent spirit and odd (queer) personality always exploded.

Performance is key to biographilia's play with authenticity through subversion. The reinvention of an historical character like Barry whose sense of identity remains paradigmatically unresolved offers authors multiple opportunities for engaging with and breaching conventions and expectations both of gender and of genre. This book, then, examines how the representation of Barry's uncertain gender has been negotiated in the unstable and hybrid genre of neo-/Victorian (Victorian to neo-Victorian) life-writing. While the factual James Barry has attracted interest in gender, transgender and queer studies,[81] social history,[82] the history of medicine,[83] popular culture[84] and the media,[85] and while postmodern works by Patricia Duncker and Sebastian Barry have received a measure of critical attention,[86] this is the first study to draw together Victorian, modern and contemporary biofictional, biographical and biodramatic configurations of the subject. By combining a comparative analysis that pays attention to the paradigms of the broad corpus of biographilia that constitutes the 'Barry archive' (as discussed in Chapter 2) with focused consideration of the generically and conceptually most significant texts, this book provides the first fully comprehensive examination of the Barry mythos. It seeks to offer a new conceptualization of the genre of neo-Victorian biographilia in light of the (para)textual constructions of 'James Miranda Barry' from his death in 1865 through to 2016, the publication date of the most recent biography. My primary concern is with how Victorian, modern and twentieth to twenty-first-century fiction writers, dramatists and biographers conceptualize, endeavour to stabilize or, by contrast, amplify the unstable gender identity of an historical character, working as they do from within Victorian and neo-Victorian life-writing, a genre that in and by itself is defined by boundary transgression. This will involve investigating how biographilic works negotiate the interplay of sex and gender in their depiction of Barry and that of a broader selection of characters.

Throughout, my approach is premised on the fundamental affinity between the performance, and subversion, of gender and that of genre. This is explored further in the next section's discussion of neo-Victorian biographilia. Here, too, parallels arise between gender and genre taxonomies. Jacques Derrida and Avital Ronell's emphasis on genre as a category that is constitutive of participation rather than belonging, of 'taking part in without being [fully] part of, without having [complete] membership,' offers a productive analogy between Barry's passing and crossing of gender and the impersonations and genre crossings enacted by Victorian and neo-Victorian life writing.[87]

META/TEXTUAL IMPERSONATIONS: NEO-VICTORIAN BIOGRAPHILIA

A major contention of this book is that the story of Barry's gender transgression speaks to the cross-boundary experimentation of genre.

Genre theorists maintain that a desire for transgression is inherent to genre because its imposition of a regulatory regime invites infringement of its rules. In 'The Law of Genre' Derrida and Ronell posit the 'principle of contamination, a law of impurity, a parasitical economy' as the prime denominator of genre: 'as soon as genre announces itself, one must respect a norm, one must not cross a line of demarcation, one must not risk impurity, anomaly, or monstrosity.' But what, they ask, 'if there were, lodged within the heart of the law itself, a law of impurity or a principle of contamination? And suppose the condition for the possibility of the law were the *a priori* of a counter-law, an axiom of the impossibility that would confound its sense, order, and reason?'[88] It is therefore only by the disruption of its tenets, in particular the crossing of generic parameters, that a taxonomy of genre can be established. Genre is thus defined by the breaching of genre boundaries.

A similar point is made by Hayden White, who sees genre as being marked by '[m]ixture, hybridity, epicenity, promiscuity'.[89] Generic hybridity, 'promiscuity' and intermixing are prominent traits of neo-Victorianism in its broadest conception. Twentieth and twenty-first-century culture as it engages creatively with the Victorian has embraced multiplying forms: fiction, poetry, drama; radio, screen and TV production; visual and material cultures such as photography, museum exhibition practice, graphic and performance art, steampunk, and the multi-medial mashup.[90] These forms can take a variety of inflections (life-writing, Gothic, sensation, crime and detection, costume, heritage, to name a few), focusing on a range of often interrelated key themes (gender and sexuality; race, ethnicity and the history of empire; class and family relations; trauma and madness; science and medicine vs religion and spiritualism). Scholarly approaches to neo-Victorianism (the cultural remediation, adaptation, re-imagination of the Victorian/s) are equally heterogeneous, extending as they do from postmodernist historiography and metafiction[91] to nostalgia, cultural memory, adaptation and trauma studies,[92] from the exploration of science[93] to spectrality and ventriloquism,[94] and from feminist and postcolonial[95] to global conceptualizations of the long nineteenth century beyond specifically Victorian contexts.[96]

This critical diversity notwithstanding, Nadine Boehm-Schnitker and Susanne Gruss argue that the vibrancy of new forms of neo-Victorianism 'calls for newly calibrated tools of analysis' with which to investigate the category 'as a symptom of a contemporary literature and culture which more strongly integrates questions of ethics, reconsiders the author, allows the referent to become visible again behind the veil of material signifiers.'[97] This interplay of author and referent in the context of the ethics and aesthetics of an 'old' but newly conceptualized form of neo-Victorianism – biographilia – is pivotal to my study. Life-writing holds particular significance for neo-Victorianism, not least because it constitutes its original form. For although the starting point of neo-Victorianism is usually dated to the rise of postmodernism in the 1960s and the publication of Jean Rhys's *Wide Sargasso Sea* (1966) and John Fowles's *The French Lieutenant's Woman* (1969), it was the earlier, immediately post-Victorian period of the modernists that saw the emergence of neo-Victorianism in the form of biographilia: Lytton Strachey's revisionary biographies *Eminent Victorians* (1918) and *Queen Victoria* (1922), Virginia Woolf's biocomedy *Freshwater* (1923/1935) and bionovel *Flush* (1933). These early texts manifest, in satirical mode, the genre blurring displayed in later neo-Victorian life-writing.

A key premise of my approach is that the instability and multiplicity of neo-Victorianisms are typified in the interconnecting sub-genres of neo-Victorian life writing. The fluidity of categories is most prominent in biography and biofiction. In postmodernist criticism in particular, Hayden White notes, biography has become conceptualized as a prime exemplar of the 'real simulacrum' or 'fake authentic'.[98] No longer merely impure and promiscuous, the genre is distinguished by its oxymoronic strategy of advancing truth claims by having recourse to novelistic devices. As Leon Edel famously put it in his 1978 manifesto, 'Biography is a work on the imagination – the imagination of form and style and narrative. … It should be narrated as if it were a story'; though a biographer 'always knows less about his characters than a novelist', this means that 'often a biographer must be even more skillful in craft than a novelist.'[99] In its terminological espousal of hybridity and its self-advertisement as factually grounded fiction, biofiction ironically constitutes a less self-divided, if anything more 'credible' genre than biography.[100] 'Who is the more real, the Milly Threale of *The Wings of the Dove* or the Henry James of Leon Edel's biography?', Joanna Scott, herself the author of a novel on the Viennese painter Egon Schiele, muses in her contribution to a 2016 special issue of *a/b: Auto/*

Biography Studies on 'Biofictions'. At its most accomplished, Scott suggests, biography blurs into fiction:

> If I did not know better, I would call Peter Gay's Sigmund Freud and Hermione Lee's Virginia Woolf both fictional characters. … The territories of fiction and history are demarcated by a border that is jagged, maybe even porous … Biography gives actual lives a fictional tinge, and fiction gives invented lives an uncanny presence.[101]

Writing in the same issue, biographer and biographical novelist Jay Parini similarly posits that the dead are most compellingly brought back to life by the invention of the real.[102] Biofiction thus appears more 'authentic' than either biography or the novel, which may be one of the reasons for its popularity; it is in its fusion with, rather than, as Michael Lackey contends, in juxtaposition to neo-historicism that it has 'become one of the most dominant literary forms in recent years.'[103] By 'highlighting the tension between biography and fiction, as well as marking the overlap between them', Cora Kaplan observes, biofiction 'references a more essentialised and embodied element of identity' than the novel (since it deals with an historical subject as opposed to an invented character), while drawing attention to the fictionalization processes at work in biographical writing.[104] In its playful juggling with notions of authenticity and fakery, its 'generic self-reflexivity', revisionary impetus and focus on epistemology, biofiction might, then, be considered the 'ur-form' of neo-Victorianism: the genre that, through historically informed reinvention, seeks to reconstruct the Victorian in the contemporary imagination. The 'bi-temporality' that obtains from engaging with the past to offer a commentary on the present connects biofiction with neo-Victorianism, while the 'alternative relations to time and space' that are thus opened up also establish points of contact with the queer temporalities of transgender identity.[105]

The proximity of biofiction and biography has led scholars to consider sub-categories that place more explicit emphasis on the blurring of the two genres. Building on Ina Schabert's discussion of fictional biography (the traditional designation for 'novels on historical individuals'), Ansgar Nünning has proposed a complex model of five different types of biofiction. 'Documentary fictional biographies' place attention on historical facts, while 'realist fictional biographies' foreground the plot. More inventive than the latter, 'revisionist fictional biographies' are concerned with 'revis[ing] both the content of the biographical record and the conventions of biographical fiction', but they do not 'foreground either the process of biographic reconstruction or the fictionality of the text'. This is the province of the last two types, 'biographic metafiction' and 'fictional metabiography', forms that Nünning does not clearly differentiate.[106] Biographic metafiction, fictional metabiography and, in Eckart Voigts's terms (also adopted by Nünning), 'metabiographical fiction' is fiction 'concerned with the recording of history and the problems of biography'.[107] In focusing on the 'process of historical reconstruction', and in shifting 'the emphasis from the mere writing, or rewriting, of an historical individual's life to the epistemological and methodological problems involved in any attempt at life-writing itself', Nünning argues, such biofictions display a 'metabiographical self-consciousness' that 'foregrounds the paradoxical relation between life and writing which the ... term "biography" tries to conceal'.[108]

Nünning's and Voigts's categories are related to Linda Hutcheon's 'historiographic metafiction', that is, intensely self-reflexive novels that play with historiography in order to 'problematize the very possibility of historical knowledge.'[109] Hutcheon's concept remains the most substantially theorized and widely adopted of the three. The metatextual and postmodernist inflection of these terms arguably makes them less suitable for the broader temporal and generic framework of the corpus considered in this book, which includes texts from the Victorian to the neo-Victorian periods across a wide spectrum ranging from the popular to the postmodern. In addition, Nünning's 'fictional metabiography' is not the most straightforward of terms and appears to establish a closer connection of the form to biography than to fiction. 'Biofiction' has the advantage of simplicity, pointing as it does to the dynamic interplay between biographical and novelistic genres while highlighting the latter. For this reason, while Nünning's model will be considered with reference to the contemporary texts discussed in Chapter 4, the term biofiction will be used as a primary concept for novelistic and short story explorations of James Barry. Marie-Luise Kohlke's insightful differentiation of biofiction into three different strands ('celebrity biofiction', 'biofiction of marginalised subjects' and 'appropriated biofiction') will be examined as a conceptual framework for the analysis of Barry foundation myths in Chapter 3.[110]

Two final terms relevant to this study are 'heterobiography' and 'biografiction'. 'Heterobiography' neatly signals duality in form, but its autobiographical inflection – in Lucia Boldrini's classification, 'fictional autobiographies of historical characters' or 'autobiographies of others' –

has little direct bearing on Barry biographilia since autobiofiction (fiction that mimics autobiography) is represented with primarily one novel, which, alongside biodrama, is inspected in relation to Boldrini's concept in Chapter 4.[111] More suitably complementary to biofiction, 'biografic-tion', coined by Max Saunders in his excellent book on modernist autobiography, *Self-Impression*, emphasizes the fictionalizing strategies of biography and will be used to contextualize the discussion of Barry biographies in Chapters 3 and 4. 'Biografiction' is adapted from 'autobiografiction' (fiction-inflected autobiography) or, in novelist Faysal Mikdadi's terms, 'autobiographiction'. The variants in spelling are indicative of the different emphases that may be placed on each of the constituent elements of a composite genre situated at the interface between autobiography and fiction, and whose fluid position may find expression in shifting use of first and third-person narration.[112] As Saunders points out, 'autobiografiction' has been referenced in postmodernist scholarship since the 1990s, but its first usage can be traced back to the early twentieth century.[113] Similarly to Kohlke, Saunders distinguishes between three different modes of biografiction: 'pseudo-biography' (which 'fictionalizes with serious intent, to provide convincing impressions of authentic life-writing'), 'mock-biography' (which 'fakes life-writing for satiric or parodic purposes') and 'meta-biographic fiction' (fiction that features biographers as protagonists).[114] Barry life-writing straddles these categories (the latter in adapted form, in the shape of the fiction-inflected authorial self-performances of biographers).

If biography, biofiction and biodrama overlap in their performative project of counterfeiting lives, the inherently slippery category of gender offers significant further scope for neo-Victorian games-playing. Thus an historical subject's gender transgression may be co-opted to queer or, as the case might be, unqueer and heteronormalize biographilic exploration. Oscar Wilde is a prominent example, having inspired a plethora of biofictional gender/genre experiments, from Peter Ackroyd's sophisticated stylistic pastiche through Gyles Brandreth's murder mysteries to Floortje Zwigtman's Dutch-language Adrian Mayfield trilogy of Young Adult coming-out novels.[115] What interests me here is what specifically ethical issues might arise from our contemporary fascination with uncovering the sexual secrets, so obsessively guarded (or sensationally exposed) during their lifetimes, of eminent Victorians; prominent examples that spring to mind are Dickens and Ruskin.[116] In other words, to what extent do the acts of writing and reading biographilia represent 'a form of scopophilia –

the desire to know forbidden secrets as instanced in the desire to look – an illicit intrusion on the living subject and a somewhat more macabre activity in relation to the dead'?[117] Kaplan's reference to the subversive pleasures involved in life-writing invokes Janet Malcolm's memorable comparison of the biographer to a burglar and the reader to a voyeur, 'tiptoeing down the corridor together, to stand in front of the bedroom door and try to peep through the keyhole'.[118] This image resonates with that of the prowling 'publishing scoundrel' in Henry James's *The Aspern Papers* (1888), itself a biofictional *mise-en-scène* of biographical grave robbing that, in its reflection on late-Victorian prurient interest in the sex lives of the Romantics, anticipates the neo-Victorian preoccupation with the 'Other Victorians'.[119] Dubbed the 'New Orientalism' by Kohlke, and invested with a necrophilic edge by Kaplan, what does our desire to examine contemporary libidinalities through the inverted mirror of the nineteenth century suggest about our relationship with the past?[120] Helen Davies has drawn attention to the 'ethical stakes at play' in neo-Victorian ventriloquism of Victorian voices: 'There can be no dialogue, no exchange, only neo-Victorianism talking to itself.'[121] As the following chapters seek to establish, however, neo-Victorian biographilia are markedly always also engaging with the Victorian foundation texts that gave rise to the Barry mythos.

Passing Reflections and Structures

This book is organized into five chapters that seek to provide insight into the cultural history and key parameters of the texts constitutive of what I term the 'Barry archive' (Chapters 1 and 2) before shifting attention to the foundation stories that have sustained and shaped the mythos (Chapter 3). The fourth chapter focuses on contemporary and postmodernist remediations, and the concluding discussion of the 'trans/formations' of the Barry mythos probes the wider applicability of key ideas and structures by giving consideration to two additional literary examples of nineteenth-century transgender identity.

Chapter 2, which in allusion to the echo effect in Barry biographilia takes its title from the refrain of Gilmore & Roberts's 2012 lyric, 'Tell me your secret Doctor James', begins with an examination of what is known about the historical figure of Barry and then turns to the textual corpus, considering the 'writing games' of Barry biographilia. Scrutiny of the representational strategies of these texts, including their construction of

Barry's gender identity, necessarily entails attending to the language choices involved in any discussion of James Barry. For, as Rachel Holmes points out, the 'telling of James Barry's story is a struggle with pronouns'.[122] The question of what pronoun/s to use is manifestly bound up with the act of (re/trans)gendering the figure of Barry. The sexual/textual strategies that underpin the shifting representation of James Barry and his/her gender identity are investigated in the final section of this chapter.

Chapter 3 explores the central paradigms of the Barry story that have shaped biographilic approaches. This involves interrogating the Victorian foundation myth that originated with the first biofiction, 'A Mystery Still', and its inflection in late-Victorian cultural discourse. The reverberations of this tale echo into the twenty-first century. What can the afterlives of the original myth tell us about the sexual and textual politics of modern and contemporary representations of Barry? What insights might a closer understanding of the different refractions of the Barry mythos provide more generally into neo-Victorian biographilia? In considering the narrative strategies adopted by Victorian and post-Victorian authors, critical attention will be paid to different strands in biofictional writing as proposed by Kohlke. This serves to probe the various functions the myth may have fulfilled, from feeding popular interest in the uncovering of hidden lives through reclaiming women's or transgender history to engaging readers and spectators in a metatextual game with gender and performance.

In a second part the chapter inspects three central tropes of the Barry mythos. Like twentieth-century and contemporary accounts of transgender, Barry biographilia draws on the script of 'self-discovery, self-transformation, and self-realization'.[123] As Brubaker has pointed out, transgender memoirs typically 'begin with a divided self, in a condition of pain, suffering and alienation; ... pass through crises or critical turning points on the way; and ... culminate in the overcoming of alienation and the affirmation of the true self'.[124] Barry life-writing, too, is shaped by different phases and transitions, represented in plot structures that perform the purpose of what Hermione Lee calls 'bodily relics'[125]: mnemonic symbols that mark defining moments or 'critical turning points' in the construction and figuration of Barry's body and gender. The first of these is the mirror. If the reflection in the looking glass dramatizes the process of Barry's subject constitution, the experience of 'becoming James', it also acts as a signifier of gender duality. Here the protagonist's sartorial gender performance is first tested. The agency conferred at the intradiegetic level by the looking glass as a catalyst of self-construction and self-reflection has its extradiegetic counterpoint in Barry portraiture. How do the caricature, the portrait, the photograph operate in biographilia in sustaining the myth or offering alternative angles on Barry's self-presentation? A second trope of the Barry mythos is the duel: this is where the newly constructed self meets the other, where masculinity is performed and undercut, where desire can be encoded in ritualized acts that involve physical exchange, but also where the reconstituted body is always at risk of penetration and exposure. The third constitutive element of Barry biographilia is the bedroom: a space of possibility for the exploration of bodily encounters, the bed can become the locus of crossed sexual desire. As a site of unconsciousness in sleep, illness and death, it also marks the scene of detection.

If the third chapter focuses on the key determinants of the Barry mythos, Chapter 4, on performances, scrutinizes the *mise-en-scène* of this mythos by examining how texts stage themselves in staging Barry staging gender. How is Barry's gender performance reflected in the performative acts of contemporary and specifically postmodernist biography, biodrama and biofiction? Among the questions to be considered is in what ways Barry's subversion of gender codes might affect an author's choice and negotiation of genre and genre blurring. How does biodrama, for example, represent what Kit Brennan terms the 'Two-Faced' ontology of the category transgressor?[126] In seeking to fill in the gaps in history and gauge the inner life of the individual, how does Barry biography draw on narrative conventions? Max Saunders's concept of auto/biografiction offers a productive context for examining the interpenetration of autobiography, autobiodrama, biography and biofiction. Finally, in novelistic explorations, does Barry as a subject defy treatment by the classic realist narrative? To what extent does a heteronormative genre like romance become queered in the process of seeking to feminize a transgender character? Is sensation fiction a 'natural home' for Barry's story? In the effort to capture the instability of the Barry figure, how do neo-Victorian and postmodern forms of life-writing enact the instability of genre? This instability of Barry representations across the range of cultural remediations will be investigated in the next chapter.

If the complex interconnection of depictions of (trans)gender and narrative configurations of (trans)genre is a framing principle of this book, so is the relationship of textual and pictorial expressions of material culture as separate yet intersecting forms of representation. My methodology throughout is grounded in the recognition of the centrality of visual imagery to the construction of the Barry mythos. As Julia Thomas emphasizes, Victorian illustration was typically neither supplementary to nor a simple instance of the 'medial transposition' of a text: 'There is always a semantic gap between the illustration and the text because they are different modes of representation, a difference that is often exposed at the very moment that the illustration seems most faithfully to depict what the text inscribes'.[127] This point can be extended to neo-Victorian illustration as a mode of Barry biographilia. It is, Thomas points out, the 'combination of word and image that ... generates meanings, meanings that are bound up in cultural values and ideologies'.[128] As subsequent chapters seek to demonstrate, pictorial enactments of Barry's gender acts across the time period under investigation play a substantial and indeed constitutive part in the cultural remediation in biographilia of the historical transgender subject. This is also the case for other products of material culture such as song; the next chapter starts with consideration of a recent example, Katriona Gilmore's lyric 'Doctor James'.

CHAPTER 2

'Tell Me Your Secret, Doctor James': A Cultural History of James Barry

> [W]e have here all the elements of a first-rate novel. What an interesting autobiography it might have made! Was it an early folly that led her to find too late that men betray, and did she embrace the army to soothe her melancholy, or with the hope of meeting and shooting her betrayer?
>
> 'A Female Medical Combatant', *Medical Times and Gazette* (26 August 1865)[1]

Trained in medicine joined the army
Joined the army to make your name
You cursed and swore the worst of all, a ladies' man they claim…
Your voice was high and they called you names
You fought two duels and you won them both, put them all to shame
Tell me your secret Doctor James

Katriona Gilmore, Gilmore & Roberts, 'Doctor James', *The Innocent Left* (2012)[2]

> The concept of remediation is highly pertinent to cultural memory studies. Just as there is no cultural memory prior to mediation there is no mediation without remediation; all representations of the past draw on available media technologies, on existent media products, on patterns of representation and medial aesthetics … [N]o historical document and certainly no memorial document is thinkable without earlier acts of mediation
>
> Astrid Erll and Ann Rigney, 'Cultural Memory and its Dynamics' (2009)[3]

A. Heilmann, *Neo-/Victorian Biographilia and James Miranda Barry*, https://doi.org/10.1007/978-3-319-71386-1_2

This chapter begins with two instances of the cultural memorialization of James Barry, a century and a half apart, connected by the 'medial aesthetics' of two different technologies: one among the first periodical press responses, the other one of the most recent representations in the medium of popular music culture. Published a bare month after Barry's death, 'A Female Medical Combatant' constitutes an early remediation of the cultural memory that was then in the process of being constructed by reading Barry's story through the lens of a prior news report, *Saunders's News-Letter*, the text of which is incorporated into the piece. In ironic reflection of Astrid Erll and Ann Rigney's comments (in the third epigraph above) about the synergy of cultural memory and remediation, it is difficult to trace the original text, while its remediation is freely accessible. Whereas the neo-Victorian example addresses Barry himself in invocation of a fictional dialogue with the nineteenth century that seeks to shed light on the unresolved questions of the past, the *Medical Times and Gazette* encourages the Victorian reader to envision dramatic back stories that turn Barry's life into the stuff of fiction.

Faced with the conundrum of the female man, the Victorian concern, it appears, was to refeminize 'her' mind to match the 'facts' of the body by constructing a romantic tale of love betrayed and revenged (was this what the duel referenced in a later section of the article was about?): a darker nineteenth-century version of the Shakespearean heroine in breeches crossed with the Amazonian woman warrior. This portrait still resonated with the early twentieth century: Colonel Nathaniel John Crawford Rutherford's patchwork story-article 'Dr. James Barry' of 1939 invokes the same tropes (the lovelorn maiden who follows the object of her undeclared desire to the battlefield) and adds the feminist to the mix (slighted, the girl vows revenge, turning into an 'inveterate man-hater … an enemy of the male sex').[4] This script, as Jack Halberstam has noted, seeks to stabilize or trivialize gender subversion by casting the 'masculine woman … as the outcome of failed femininity, or as the result of pathetic and unsuccessful male mimicry.'[5] By contrast, the twenty-first-century memorial imagination remediates Barry (in inflection of the earliest story, 'A Mystery Still') as 'Doctor James', a professional of ambiguous gender who performs old-style masculinity (a gent successful with the ladies who is at the same time ever ready to engage in ritualistic exchange between men), perhaps to counterbalance his perceived femininity; an individual whose difference continues to pose a challenge; a gender transgressor of a kind.[6]

While Katriona Gilmore's lyric ends with the disclosure of Barry's female body and the narrator's appropriation of his story ('I'm telling your secret, Doctor James'), it may be tempting to infer from the juxtaposition of the epigraphs on the opening page that the gender choices embraced by biographilic works are determined by the respective time period: if Barry was a cross-dressing woman to the Victorians, we might expect him to be more often cast as a gender-variant individual today. Whether this is borne out by what I call the Barry archive, the corpus of biographilia that spans texts from the Victorian to the contemporary period, will be the subject of this chapter. What are the specific dynamics that result from the interplay of gender and genre when Victorian and neo-Victorian biography, biofiction and biodrama select as their nucleus of enquiry a figure as perplexing as James Barry? To explore this question in depth, it is important first to establish the ostensible 'facts' that frame the textual constructions and remediations of what has been perceived to be a near-inscrutable personality: the 'creature of shadowed origin' that playwright Sebastian Barry invokes in *Whistling Psyche* (2004).[7]

A 'Creature of Shadowed Origin': In Search of James Barry

Following biographers Isobel Rae and June Rose's lead, the original identity of James Barry was traced by art historian William Pressly and urologist H.M. du Preez to that of Margaret Bulkley, born most probably in 1789 in Cork, the elder of two daughters of Irish greengrocers Jeremiah and Mary Anne Bulkley.[8] When bankruptcy led to the break-up of the family, Mary Anne sought the assistance of her estranged brother, the London-based history painter James Barry.[9] A highly gifted if difficult man who counted Edmund Burke among his supporters but whose irritable temper, exacerbated by some form of mental illness, had resulted in his expulsion from the Royal Academy, Barry failed to act on his sister's overtures, but on his death in 1806 she obtained joint possession of his estate with her brother Redmond.[10] She also made the acquaintance of her brother's friends, in particular David Steuart Erskine, 11th Earl of Buchan and General Francisco de Miranda, who would assume an important role in her daughter's life. This, however, did not resolve the female Bulkleys' financial straits, for some time after Barry's death Margaret made enquiries for a post, presumably as a governess or companion, in a lady's household in Camden town. That she did not relish the idea of such feminine service may be inferred from her frustration about women's lack of opportunities, as expressed in an 1808 letter to her brother, whom she took to task for his apparent inability to make a success of his man's estate: 'Was I not a girl I would be a Soldier!'[11]

It is tempting to see the nineteen-year-old Margaret as a risk-taker and adventurer in the making. Born in a year of revolution and tired of the social disabilities of femininity, was she drawn to a life of action, even danger, in foreign locations? The contemporary popularity of tales about swashbuckling women in male disguise who had braved physical hardship and distinguished themselves in military action may have provided inspiration and encouragement for her own assumption of a male identity. The autobiographies of the female soldiers Christian Davies and Hannah Snell ('James Grey') had been published in 1740 and 1750 respectively.[12] Other women of a distinctly 'masculine spirit and make', albeit of more doubtful morals, were the seventeenth-century highway robber Moll Cut-Purse (Mary Frith) and the eighteenth-century women pirates Mary Read and Anne Bonney, discussed in Daniel Defoe's *General History of the Pyrates* (1724) and James Caulfield's *Portraits, Memoirs and Characters of Remarkable Persons* (1794).[13] Some of these books may have been available to Margaret in the private libraries of her mentors after her uncle's death.[14] Another female cross-dresser much closer in time to Margaret (and her mother's namesake), Mary Anne Talbot, had served on board a battleship in the guise of 'John Taylor' before revealing her identity in 1793; her *Life and Surprising Adventures* were issued in 1809, the year of Margaret's transformation into the medical student James Barry.[15]

Barry biographilia tend to emphasize the role of powerful men who, keen to launch a social experiment, steered the girl into masculinity and a military career; but Margaret's letter to her brother evinces an active desire for change.[16] Michael du Preez cites documents by Mary Anne and Margaret Bulkley's solicitor Daniel Reardon that record Margaret's change of identity in November 1809, a week before s/he enrolled as a medical student at Edinburgh University.[17] Edinburgh was at the forefront of medical research and had no formal minimum age requirement, which helped sustain Barry's impersonation: he had to appear more youthful than he was in order to be accepted as male.[18] One of Barry's fellow-students who took up his studies (of divinity) at the same time was Thomas Carlyle; given their versatility and breadth of interests, their paths may have crossed (Carlyle would be offered the rectorship of the university the year of Barry's death).[19] Later accounts recall a hard-working student who kept himself at a distance, lodged with his 'aunt', attracted the other students' mirth for covering himself up in a 'long surtout' instead of donning more fashionable attire, and who could not be taught to box.[20] Following the revelations after Barry's death, former fellow-student John Jobson admitted to being 'much astonished', for, 'although he remembered [Barry's] womanly traits, they had never caused him to have the slightest suspicion of her sex.'[21]

The ruse of assuming a younger age paid off but came with its own difficulties. When in his third year Barry wanted to register for his final examination, concerns were raised about his 'extreme youth', and it was only at the intervention of his patron, the Earl of Buchan, that he was permitted to proceed.[22] Graduating with a thesis on the femoral hernia, Barry addressed his examiners with an epigraph that, while ostensibly playing on his youth, subtly hinted at his gender subversion: 'Do not consider whether what I say is a young man speaking, but whether my discourse with you is that of a man of understanding.'[23] The mask of the 'young man' here conceals (even as, to the modern reader who has the benefit of hindsight, it alludes to) the 'young woman' who seeks acknowledgement from the older male professoriate. Barry's appeal to be recognized for his knowledge rather than any difference in body found an inadvertently ironic riposte two centuries later in Edinburgh University honouring Barry with the unveiling of a plaque that qualifies his professional accomplishment (a 'pioneering army surgeon') with reference to his sex, as the first woman to graduate from the institution.[24] Where Barry had wanted his sex to disappear in the wealth of his learning, it is this very sex that continues to be invoked as the primary marker of his attainment, implying that Barry's achievements were so extraordinary because he was 'really' (only) a 'woman'.

Alongside pre-eminent medical tutors like Sir Astley Cooper, James Hamilton and others, Barry had inspirational and influential mentors in three of his uncle's friends. Involved in editing the posthumous *Works of James Barry* (1809), these were the scholars Edward Fryer, the Scottish Lord Buchan and the charismatic Venezuelan revolutionary General Miranda (with whom Barry was to share the experience of crossing nations).[25] Although it is a matter of conjecture whether all three men were aware of Barry's change of gender, they were all ardent supporters of female education and (in Miranda's case) republican politics. Miranda and Buchan enabled access to their scholarly libraries and introduced Barry to the lifestyle of a gentleman; Buchan additionally sought out further mentors, such as Robert Anderson, who provided free lodgings and coached Barry in Latin and the classics.[26]

If Buchan became a port of call during and after Barry's studies, Miranda appears to have acted as the most colourful role model. Born in 1750 in Caracas to a Venezuelan mother and a father from a distinguished Spanish family, Miranda had served in the Spanish and revolutionary French armies. His 'extraordinary blend of charm' issued from a personality that exuded charisma yet also boasted an enormous sense of self-importance, overbearing 'haughtiness, and ...an independence of mind that verged on insubordination': a conjunction of character traits that proved highly irritating to figures of authority. As a result Miranda was variously charged with and even arrested for misdemeanours that failed to be substantiated (an experience that would find multiple echoes in his adoptive son's career). A dandy and inveterate womanizer as well as an exceptionally well-read thinker, he had travelled widely in the United States, Europe and Russia, where he was a lover of Empress Catherine and countless other women, generally 'display[ing] a truly astonishing variety of sexual and intellectual appetites'; 'in that order', as his biographer Robert Harvey notes. After he settled in London in 1789 (the year of Margaret Bulkley's birth), his home became a centre for South American dissidents. Having thrown himself into the French revolutionary cause, he had been singled out for a French baronetcy in 1792, had met Napoleon but come under royalist suspicion and narrowly escaped the guillotine not once, but twice. By the time he met Barry, Miranda had become engrossed in schemes for Venezuelan liberation, for which he was seeking assistance from the British and American governments; to further his plans, he left for Caracas in 1810. His imprisonment in Spain in 1812 thwarted any hopes Barry may have had to join him at the end of his studies.[27] After Miranda's and Buchan's deaths in 1816 and 1829, the Dukes of Beaufort, the family of Barry's Cape employer, Lord Charles Somerset, and later Charles's brother Fitzroy, Lord Raglan, provided a base during visits to Britain and offered support against the many enemies Barry made throughout his professional life. Lord Raglan repeatedly interceded on Barry's behalf. With the support of these men, Barry embarked on a formidable medical career that spanned half a century and crossed several continents.

Following graduation and spells as 'Pupil Dresser' in St Thomas and Guy's in London and 'Hospital Assistant' at Plymouth, Barry was posted to what was then the Cape Colony in South Africa in 1816 as Assistant

Staff Surgeon of the Army.[28] Shortly after his arrival, having cured one of his employer's daughters (Georgina) and Lord Charles Somerset himself of a dangerous illness, in the latter case so grave that it was believed to be life-threatening by the Cape's chief medical practitioners, Barry was additionally assigned senior civil positions, first as personal physician of the Governor and, from 1822 to 1825, as Colonial Medical Inspector.[29] In 1826 he became one of the first surgeons in the world to conduct (under pre-anaesthetic conditions) a successful Caesarian section survived by both mother and child (the boy, James Barry Munnik, named after him at his request, was born the very day Barry would die thirty-nine years later).[30] Appointed Staff Surgeon in Mauritius in 1828, Jamaica in 1831, and the Windward and Leeward Islands in 1838, Barry held the post of Principal Medical Officer in St Helena in 1836 and Malta in 1846 before rising to Deputy Inspector General of Hospitals in Corfu in 1851. His last appointment in 1858 was as Local Inspector and then Inspector General of Hospitals in Montreal, Canada: a very different and considerably less hospitable climate than the tropical islands where he had spent so much of his life.[31] In 1859 ill health and his 'uncontrollable temperament', as perceived by his military superiors, forced him into retirement and a return to London, where he died in 1865 in a dysentery epidemic.[32]

Though Barry acceded to the highest rank in his profession, his fierce promotion of sanitary conditions in medical practice, staunch commitment to the professionalization of trades related to medicine and unflagging advocacy of the humane treatment of minority groups – hospital patients, prisoners, leprosy sufferers, slaves, prostitutes, the insane – in conjunction with his resolute exposure of corruption and combative, high-handed response to bureaucracy and officialdom frequently placed him at variance with authority.[33] During his years at the Cape, he incurred the wrath of countless officials for implementing sweeping reforms to the culture of neglect and abuse that prevailed in the provincial asylum, prison institutions and leper colony. He upset social and racial hegemonies when he demanded that 'the parties [suffering from leprosy] must be considered not as Convicts but as Unfortunate' and caused outrage when approaching black prisoners directly about their ailments, prompting one exasperated prison official to exclaim: 'Why ask Blacks when Christians are present to answer?'[34] Throughout his career he insisted on the importance of hygiene, fresh air, regular baths, frequent change of clothing and bed linen, healthy and plentiful nutrition, a balanced alcohol intake – and, despite his reputation for quarrelsomeness, human kindness.[35]

In 1825 Barry's position as Colonial Medical Inspector at the Cape fell victim to the Colonial Secretary, Sir Richard Plasket's decision to replace the post with a Supreme Medical Committee after taking offence at what he considered the Inspector's obstructionism, intemperance and insubordination in highlighting severe failures in the system.[36] A decade on, at St. Helena, incensed at the 'disgusting circumstance' to which local women patients, many of them prostitutes suffering from venereal and other diseases, were subjected, Barry called a halt to the 'greatest irregularities' arising from the use of male hospital attendants and 'immediately hired a respectable woman of color as Matron'.[37] Ten years earlier, in 1827, he had published a medical treatise on the herbal treatment of syphilis and gonorrhea.[38] In Corfu, his rehabilitation regime for wounded soldiers from the Crimea led to a substantial fall in the death rate at Scutari.[39] In his last posting, in Canada, he lobbied for separate accommodation for married soldiers to spare army wives the violation of privacy to which they were otherwise exposed in communal living and sleeping quarters.[40] If Barry was dedicated to humanitarian and medical reform, he also showed considerable concern for some of the causes (such as the ill-treatment of women, particularly prostitutes) that the rising generation of Victorian feminists, led by figures like Josephine Butler, were to take up at the end of the decade that saw his death.[41]

Uncompromising in his effort to uphold professional and humanitarian standards, whatever the personal fallout, undiplomatic in his impulsiveness, provocative to the point of impertinence, Barry faced demotion and relocation, one court-martial and another formal arrest that, but for the intervention of Lord Raglan, might have seen him court-martialed for a second time.[42] Though 'capable of generous feeling, and of gratitude to those who were kind to him', as a medical colleague wrote after his death, his 'irritable and impatient temper brought him into constant collision with authority'; when 'anything touched his importance, his anger knew no bounds; there was no authority or station which he (secure in his own importance) would not set at defiance.'[43] Ultimately, the annoyance he had caused to the establishment deprived him of public accolades and a dignified retreat from his career. For all his pioneering achievements and his lasting impact on medical practice, the formal recognition he craved was withheld, leading later commentators to conjecture about Florence Nightingale's potential role in blocking special honours.[44] Barry's 1859 appeal against his forcible retirement on the grounds of his health ends with the statement that he was 'loath to close a career which impartially may be deemed to have been a useful and faithful one without some special mark of her Majesty's gracious favour', an assertion that in an earlier draft had been worded more strongly as an entitlement: 'he has proved himself more than ordinarily zealous and useful during a long career in Her Majesty's Service ... [and] trusts that he has sufficiently shown that he has a claim to some consideration not to say indulgence, from the authorities under whom he is placed.'[45] No such distinction was bestowed.

A groundbreaking medical reformer, Barry created a stir – for good or for bad – also with his eccentric personality. Julie Wheelwright suggests that his 'swagger' may have served to 'mask fears of detection'.[46] Playing *va banque* in the style of Edgar Allan Poe's 'Purloined Letter' – flaunting his difference as a mark of individuality in order to avert suspicion – must have been exhilarating even if it was a risky game with high stakes. Diminutive in stature, with delicate small hands, and dandyish, even flamboyant in appearance and behaviour, Barry had, as Count Emmanuel de Las Cases noted in 1817, 'the form, the manners and the voice of a woman'.[47] The British naval officer and later admiral William Henry Dillon, who had required Barry's professional services in September 1816, recalled in his *Narrative of My Professional Adventures* of 1856 that '[m]any surmises were in circulation relating to him; from the awkwardness of his gait and the shape of his person it was the prevailing opinion that he was a female'.[48] Holmes rightly questions the extent to which Dillon, who was suffering from a 'violent inflammation in both eyes' at the time, could have been in a position to observe Barry at such close quarters; but his words, published eight years before Barry's death, suggest that, at least in the early stages of his career, Barry's ambiguous gender prompted speculation.[49]

As an accomplished raconteur, with a 'style of conversation ... greatly superior to that one usually heard at a mess-table', Barry was often invited to social functions.[50] The Earl of Albemarle, who visited the Cape in 1818, was bemused when, on being told that Barry was 'the most skillful of physicians, and the most wayward of men', he 'beheld a beardless lad ... with an unmistakable Scotch type of countenance – reddish hair, high cheek bones. There was a certain effeminacy in his manner, which he seemed to be always striving to overcome.'[51] (See Fig. 2.1). Albemarle's reminiscences, published in 1876, carry echoes of the myth that had developed. These include hearsay about Barry's noble lineage as the 'legitimate grand-daughter of a Scotch Earl' (presumably Lord Buchan)[52] who took up her disguise 'from attachment to an army surgeon

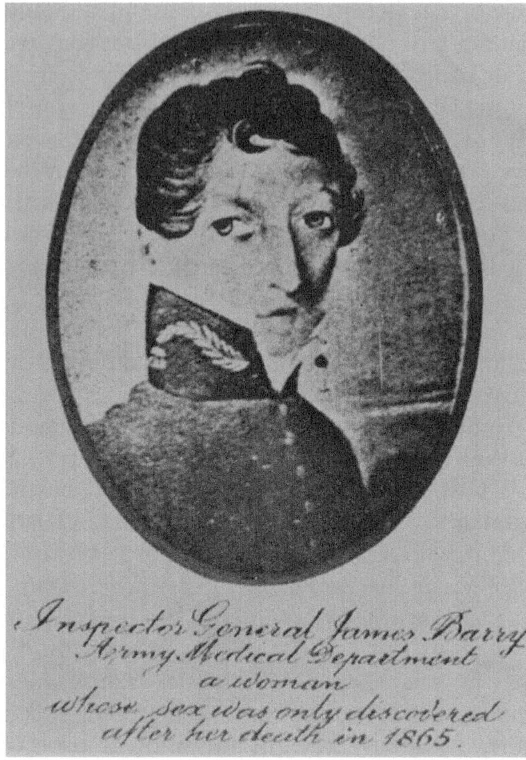
Inspector General James Barry
Army Medical Department
a woman
whose sex was only discovered
after her death in 1865.

Fig. 2.1 James Barry; portrait (L002265), reproduced courtesy of the Museum of Military Medicine

who has not been many years dead' (intriguingly, the Irish-born Barry is here assigned 'unmistakable' Scottish origins inherited from her reputed Scottish father).[53] But Albemarle's account resonates with de Las Cases's 1823 description of the 'absolute phenomenon' Barry represented at the Cape.[54]

Witty at society gatherings, charming and flirtatious with the ladies,[55] but with a reputation for being excessively short-tempered whenever he encountered instances of abuse or when his professional judgment was called into question, Barry was frequently the object of gossip.[56] The most injurious scandal arose in 1824 over the nature of his relations with his employer, Charles Somerset, resulting in an anonymous placard being displayed in Cape Town's most public thoroughfare, the Heerengracht, accusing Somerset and Barry of buggery.[57] Coinciding as it did with a

Commission of Inquiry into Somerset's governorship of the Cape following complaints about his autocratic regime, overly lavish lifestyle and clampdown on freedom of speech, the 'placard affair' with its allegation of sodomy was calculated to demolish the governor's moral credibility. While Barry was not the primary object of vilification, inevitably his reputation and morality too were marred, with references to 'Dr. Barry's wife' pointing to his sexual inversion as well as to Somerset's patrician depravity.[58] The threat of degeneracy having infected the bloodline of the Cape administration was exacerbated when a petition brought to the British Parliament in 1825 asserted that Somerset had 'committed an unspeakable atrocity with his reputed son', combining the imputation of homosexuality with incest.[59] Though Somerset was cleared of charges of corruption, the libel was a contributory factor in his departure as Governor of the Cape in 1826.

Barry's notoriety became legendary after his death when the woman who had laid out his body insisted that not only was it that of a 'perfect female', but that 'there were marks of her having had a child when very young.'[60] This claim was never corroborated for, despite contemporaneous (and later) statements to the contrary, no autopsy was carried out on the body, which had already been buried.[61] In the absence of a body, what came to be scrutinized in twentieth-century biography was the brief correspondence between Staff-Surgeon McKinnon, who, having known Barry for over a decade, had recorded his male sex on his death certificate without a physical examination and the Registrar General who sought clarification on the case.[62] Intriguingly, this leaves us with a professional exchange between men about sensational revelations about a male colleague disclosed by a nameless female servant whose voice assumes as much of a spectral presence in the tale as does that colleague's female body. Not having been paid for her labour by Barry's landlady, the layer-out sought to reclaim her expenses from the attendant doctor and, when this failed, presumably sold her story to the press.

When news of the late Inspector General's 'secret' first broke in the Dublin-based *Saunders's News-Letter* on 14 August 1865, the charwoman's discovery was referenced to 'two nurses' (the layer-out and, as Michael du Preez and Jeremy Dronfield have brought to light, the younger maid employed in the house, Sophia Bishop, who was almost certainly not party to the discovery). Barry's death is here relocated to a more exotic earlier setting (Corfu rather than metropolitan London).[63] Following a condensed version in the *Manchester Guardian* on 21 August, a longer piece, in the *Medical Times and Gazette* on 26 August (reproduced by the *Timaru Herald* on 25 November and, in French translation, by the *Revue Étrangère*), included the original with corrections and a commentary that undercut Barry's professional achievements by essentializing him, not only as a mere woman, but as that archetype of female inconsequence, an elderly spinster with a fondness for pets.[64]

'[T]he indubitable fact', lent prominence in *Saunders's News-Letter*, that 'a woman was for forty years an officer in the British service, had fought one duel, and had sought many more, had pursued a legitimate Medical education, had received a regular diploma, and had acquired almost a celebrity for skill as a Surgical operator', in other words, that Barry had proven that women could excel in 'male' professions and even the most masculine of rituals (duels), was now vehemently cast in doubt: 'As to the "firmness," "skill in operating," "decision of character" etc … there may be a question; but about the querulousness, irritability, and quarrelsomeness, there can be none.'[65] This reads like damage limitation; as an organ of the male medical establishment, the *Medical Times and Gazette* had a stake in protecting the reputation of the profession, hence the insinuation that Barry, under present conditions, would not pass muster; when the deceased had been admitted half a century earlier, 'the Professional qualifications required for the service were not of the highest order'.[66] Ironically, the discourse of professional standards that Barry had been so determined to uphold and improve was misappropriated to discredit him.

The initial newspaper reporting was followed by letters from contemporaries who had been acquainted with Barry and vouched with equal force of conviction for either of his genders. Barry's odd appearance, high-pitched voice, strange habits, dandyish outfits, shortness of temper, love of animals, weddings and christenings were all cited as markers of his femininity.[67] Closer colleagues were more concerned with highlighting Barry's credentials as an individual; whatever his body ('male, female or hermaphrodite'), McKinnon affirmed that Barry had been 'a pleasant and agreeable man … [who] behaved himself like a gentleman.'[68] (By implication, the cultural spectacle that was being created over his body was lacking in the very attributes that distinguished gentlemanly codes of conduct.) McKinnon's focus on Barry's personal qualities proved the exception among medical and military colleagues.

More official responses by senior army officers engaged in complicated mental acrobatics to assert that, while Barry had been singularly dysfunctional in masculinity, he had still been an anatomical man. Thus Edward Bradford, Deputy-Inspector-General of Hospitals, who recorded first meeting Barry in Jamaica in 1832, presented a medical case history that sought to contextualize Barry's feminine traits through both birth defects and family anomalies. Key aspects of Bradford's narrative influenced subsequent biofictional accounts such as 'A Mystery Still' (1867). '[B]orn prematurely' to parents who had the misfortune to die both at the same time, Barry had been adopted by 'persons of high rank' whose patronage he enjoyed throughout his career. In 'appearance and manners ... most singular', with 'the voice ... of an aged woman', he took great pains to catch the public eye with his ostentatious behavior and showy attire (an absurdly overlong sword and spurs). Extravagance in self-presentation was accompanied by other eccentricities like a diet of 'milk and fruit'. Driven by a 'singular craving for authority and power', Barry did not baulk at physical combat (the reference here is to the duel Barry fought with Somerset's Aide-de-Camp, [Abraham] Josias Cloete, about one of Somerset's female visitors).[69] This, however, as Bradford implied, was testament to Barry's impetuous and shrewish temper (i.e. effeminacy) rather than to more manly qualities since, 'when suddenly called on for a duty he disliked, he went to bed, and wept like a child till the danger was passed' (femininity is here equated with infantilism).[70]

And yet, all of these peculiarities notwithstanding, and though Barry had been 'quite destitute of all the characters of manhood', speculation about his sex was 'too absurd', for, as Bradford concluded, 'There can be no doubt among those who knew him that his real physical condition was that of a male in whom sexual development had been arrested about the sixth month of foetal life': an astonishing claim, given that Barry's origins (least of all the history of his birth) were not known for another 120 years.[71] Bradford's unconvincing deduction was correctly dismissed by the French medical press as a tactical move to deflect attention away from the army. René Arnold writing in the *Revue Étrangère* suggested that Barry was much more likely to have been a hermaphrodite, 'one of these beings resembling the fabled son of Hermes and Aphrodite, participating in both sexes without belonging to either'.[72] Indeed, by placing emphasis on prenatal irregularities, Bradford hinted at Barry's intersexual condition: embryogeny of the time (and also today) ascribed various anomalies in the development of the genitals, including hermaphroditism, to 'arrest undergone' *in utero*.[73]

In his endeavour to shield the military from public ridicule, Bradford co-opted Galenic ideas of 'genital homologies' that Thomas Laqueur has conceptualized as underpinning the 'one-sex model': the notion that, as Katharine Park and Robert Nye explain, 'male and female genitalia developed out of the same anatomical structure'.[74] Whereas women and men constituted radically different entities in the two-sex model, in the one-sex paradigm, Laqueur argues, 'pairs of ordered contrarieties played off a single flesh ... Fatherhood/motherhood, male/female, man/woman ... masculine/feminine ...were read into a body that did not itself mark these distinctions clearly.'[75] Michel Foucault notes that this facilitated the recognition of intersexuality, a diagnosis less easily accommodated by the 'reductive oversimplification' of the nineteenth-century two-sex model that sought to delimit bodily ambiguity with the qualifier 'pseudo'-hermaphroditism.[76] While Foucault's and Laqueur's argument of an historical shift in the eighteenth century from ancient one-sex model to modern two-sex model has been contested,[77] it is worth noting that in Herculine Barbin's near-contemporaneous case medical opinion concurred in masculinizing the subject's intersex condition.[78] This may offer a context for Bradford's contradictory logic: with the one-sex model intersexuality could be interpreted as incomplete male development.[79] The professional urgency to protect the military establishment made it imperative to uphold the principle that Barry had incontestably been a man, however defective the nature of his sexual organs; to acknowledge that a woman could have infiltrated the army undetected was too embarrassing to countenance.

Until the discovery of Barry's birth identity as Margaret Bulkley, this line of reasoning continued to be invoked to support the argument of Barry's male sex. Thus in 1970 South African scholar Percival Kirby took umbrage at biographer Isobel Rae's references to Barry as a woman and instead diagnosed Klinefelter's syndrome (a genetic condition of boys being born with two X chromosomes, now seen as part of the wider intersex spectrum) to maintain that Barry was 'definitely a male, though one who was unfortunately feminine in external appearance'.[80] Kirby's feminine-looking man resonates with Bradford's Victorian-Galenic man with imperfectly developed genitals. Like Kirby a century later, Bradford sought to contain popular interest in women's challenge to dominant social structures with a story about a dysfunctional but nevertheless indisputably male body.

As Holmes points out, the marked reticence with which the flurry of sensational newspaper reports about Barry was addressed by the authorities and the peculiar silence of the London press signals how much was at stake for the military and medical establishments.[81] The doors of the former remained resolutely closed to women doctors until the First World War,[82] while the latter had only just begun to accommodate women among its ranks. If Barry's retirement in 1859 had coincided with the first officially accredited female physician, British-born but US-trained Elizabeth Blackwell, being entered on the British Medical Register, it was only the year after Barry's death, 1866, that Blackwell was joined by a second, now UK-educated, woman, Elizabeth Garrett.[83] As a graduate of Edinburgh University in 1812 who took up his first post in 1813 and whose career extended over forty-six years, Barry had prefigured women's entry into the medical profession by half a century. What was even more extraordinary was the idea that a woman could have attained such senior positions as Staff-Surgeon, Colonial Medical Inspector and Principal Medical Officer, ultimately to be entrusted with the highest-ranking medical appointment in the military, Inspector General of Hospitals.

If Barry was a woman, how had she succeeded in passing as a man? Geertje Mak notes that, before the advent of late-nineteenth-century sexology, sex was assigned in three ways: by 'inscription in the social community', through 'representation of the body', and by the 'representation of the self'.[84] Given the exclusion of women from British higher education and the professions until the latter part of the nineteenth century, a medical officer's sex was inscribed as male both by his community (university teachers, the British military, colleagues, patients, the law that denied women access to the medical profession) and through self-presentation. Though Barry's ambiguous body (Mak's second category of inscription) encouraged rumours about his sex, only two such accounts were published during his life-time.[85] Frequent regimental relocations brought changes in community that offered opportunities for reinscription through renewed self-representation when the public perception of Barry's body had entered a crisis point, as after the libel affair in the Cape.[86] How are such processes of inscription reflected in biographical, biofictional and biodramatic approaches to Barry? What motivation and agency is Barry granted? How do neo-Victorian biographilic renditions relate to the Victorian response? Is Barry depicted as female, male, intersexual, transgender? These are among the questions to be examined in the next two sections, which consider the posthumous cultural construction of Barry from the later-Victorian to the contemporary period. In the first instance, what are the key textual strategies and 'writing games' of Barry life-writing?

Writing Games with Doctor James: Sexual/Textual Hybridities

In reflection of Barry's gender hybridity, a pronounced feature of Barry biographilia is textual hybridity, manifested in what in the introductory chapter was noted as the blurring of genre boundaries, as when biographies embed fictional passages or biofictions profess to historical veracity.[87] The latter is illustrated in George Edwin Marvell's *Cape Times* story 'The Mystery of the Kapok Doctor' (1904), which purports to be the transcript of a memoir authored by Barry himself. Intended for publication after his death, the papers 'passed into the possession of a relative of the writer's', only promptly and 'most unfortunately' to have been 'stolen or destroyed' when, in an unguarded moment, he left the room.[88] Marvell's is a tired example of the trope. A more notable case of a self-declared 'fiction founded on fact' is Olga Racster and Jessica Grove's *The Journal of Dr. James Barry* (1932).[89] The Preface introduces the novel both as a 'document' and as an 'almost unbelievable romance', implying that Barry's achievement of passing as a man without unsexing herself by losing her inherently female sensibility is matched by the authors' equivalent aptitude in creating 'feminine' romance from 'masculine' research.[90] Barry's incorporation of one sex into another is mimicked on the formal level by the framing device of the Preface's authorial contextualization and the Appendix's biographical-historical verification which enclose the 'buried' tale that Barry 'might herself have written'.[91] The emphasis on historical accuracy is undercut by markers of anxiety about 'the *degree* of authenticity which the story *claims*' (emphases added) and 'the danger *which lies in turning scanty fact into fiction*' (emphases in original).[92]

The awkward linguistic about-turns with which the textual frame seeks to validate the authorial project mirror on the extradiegetic level the intradiegetic protagonist's fears about the credibility of her act. Just as Barry is troubled by the thought of 'shameful failure' in her impersonation of masculinity, so Racster and Grove apprehend criticism of their authorial performance, in particular their assimilation of history into fiction, while at the same time expressing discomfort with too formulaic an approach to genre: 'No matter how much history itself may lie, an unreliable manuscript is considered reliable if provided with footnotes. But how tiresome the story becomes when encumbered with references!'[93] The critique of normative and purist genre (and gender) conceptualizations (no genre – nor gender – is unadulterated if 'history itself may lie') is promptly followed by a display of the authors' proficiency in meeting conventional standards of professional practice (such as the citation of sources).[94] By implication, their 'unreliable', even deceitful (lie-laden) feminine fiction attains the authority of (masculine) history.

If Racster and Grove's novel illustrates the complex manoeuvres involved in the biofictional claim to authenticity, it also evidences the second inflection of hybridity often found in Barry biographilia, and that is the double, sometimes triple titling strategy of individual works, as if Barry's 'chameleon figure' with his multiple identities could only be represented adequately by multiple editions.[95] Thus *The Journal of Dr. James Barry* was accompanied by a near-identical edition (issued by a second London publisher), *Dr. James Barry: Her Secret Story*.[96] A more recent example is Patricia Duncker's novel *James Miranda Barry*, published in 1999 by Serpent's Tail (reissued in 2011 by Bloomsbury), whose 2002 US edition (by Harper Perennial) appeared as *The Doctor*: an intriguingly bland choice of title, so pointedly devoid of the hint of transgender in Barry's middle name, but which appears conceived as contextual information relevant to the original edition for which it furnishes a subtitle: *James Miranda Barry: The Doctor*. The Harper Perennial cover illustration with its oddly apparelled antagonists engaged in a sabre and sword fight raises questions about the titular hero and what his medical role might entail; the pictorial allusion to duelling and play-acting, though fully intelligible only after consumption of the novel, offers a further commentary on the hero's mysterious identity (see Fig. 4.3 in Chapter 4).

The paratextual hybridity of Rachel Holmes's biography is even more striking. Published in 2002 by both Penguin and Random House, *Scanty Particulars* draws ironic attention to the speculative nature of all historical enquiry into the subject of Barry. (The title's erotically suggestive connotations, to contemporary readers, belies its origin; it is derived from an 1895 second-hand account of Barry's student years in a letter to the *Lancet* and in its Victorian usage was meant to convey the paucity of biographical information on the doctor.)[97] The variation in subtitle and other paratextual elements such as cover illustrations indicate that different aspects of the Barry myth are pitched at different international target audiences. For while the UK edition of *Scanty Particulars* and its subtitle promote mystery and a Victorian surgeon's 'remarkable' life, US readers are promised a more spicy outlook of 'scandal' and the revelation of an 'astonishing secret' by 'Queen Victoria's most eminent military doctor'.[98] The allusion to a prurient secret by a high-ranking army officer, placed in the implicit context of Victoria's reputed prudery, hints at sexual transgression; as does, in more subtle ways, the cover illustration (Fig. 2.2). Here Barry is featured as a Victorian gentleman turning his back on (or returning from?) an encounter with another gent, whose hat is doffed in acknowledgement and whose face, and identity, like Barry's, are hidden from view.

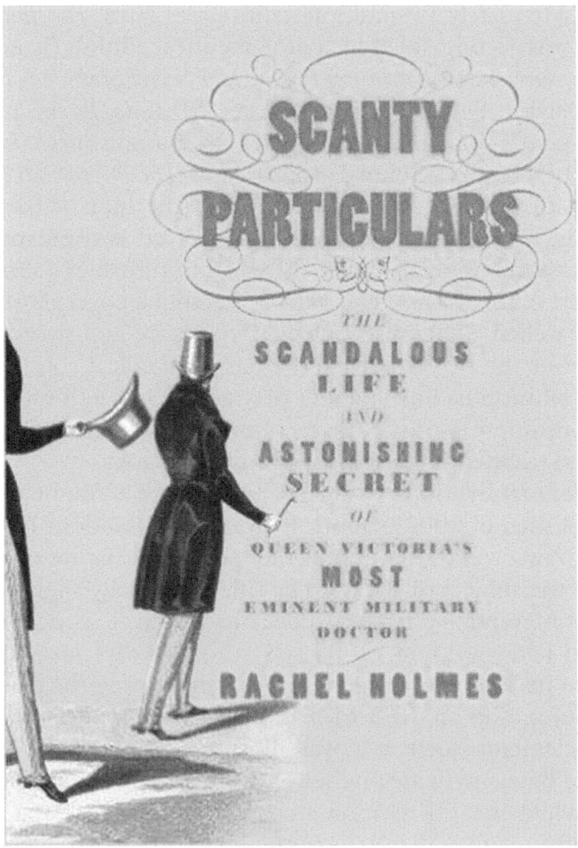

Fig. 2.2 Cover of the US edition of Rachel Holmes's biography *Scanty Particulars* (Random House, 2002), courtesy of Penguin Random House LLC Permissions Department

The Penguin edition offers an even more prototypical inflection of the Barry myth with its striking adaptation of a photograph of the ageing Barry flanked by his black servant and white dog Psyche – the two companions so prominent in biographilia from 'A Mystery Still' onwards. These two quasi-alter egos represent the Other in racial and species terms to Barry's gendered Other (Figs. 2.3 and 2.4). By association with the contemporaneous Anglo-Irish poet Mary Tighe's much-admired rendering of the classical myth, *Psyche, or The Legend of Love* (1811), Barry's

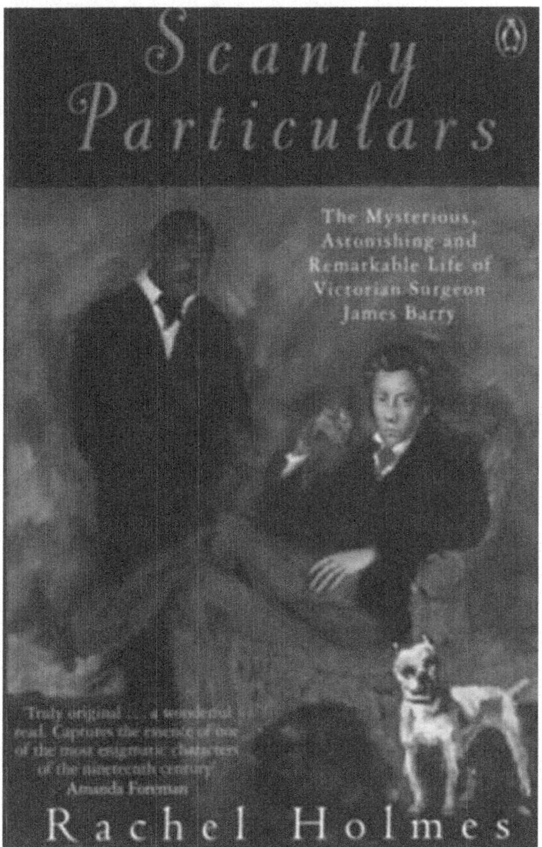

Fig. 2.3 SCANTY PARTICULARS: THE MYSTERIOUS, ASTONISHING AND REMARKABLE LIFE OF VICTORIAN SURGEON JAMES BARRY by Rachel Holmes (2003). Copyright © Penguin Books, 2003

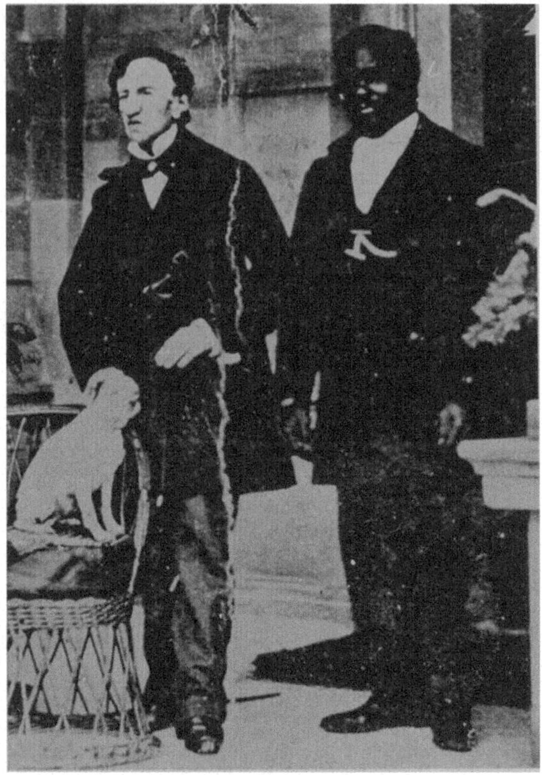

Fig. 2.4 James Barry; portrait (L0022267), with servant and dog, reproduced courtesy of the Museum of Military Medicine

choice of a name for his poodle, Psyche, simultaneously hints at a secret love affair and at 'English' Barry's Irish origins.[99]

Significantly, the re-imagined Barry's gaze (Fig. 2.3) poses a direct (metatextual) challenge to the reader's scrutiny. Whereas the historical Barry of the original photograph (Fig. 2.4) bears a distinctly cross and forbidding facial expression and looks sideways, away from the lens, the reconstructed Barry engages with the reader and is additionally, through the closer positioning of the two characters to each other and the other man's attentive focus, placed in an affective relationship to another person. This Barry is not the detached, sullen figure he appears in the photograph and that he is so often represented to be in biographilia.

The titular and visual juxtaposition of the two editions of Holmes's biography is both mirrored in and inverted by their content. The Random

House volume is shorter, with material cut from the Preface and the chapters. But though in content more diluted, this edition has a references section, whereas the Penguin edition lacks formal authentication of source materials other than through a select bibliography.

The third incarnation of the text, published by Tempus (The History Press) in 2007, reproduces the US edition with a new title that blends together the key referents of the preceding versions while also drawing on the trope of secrecy established by two earlier biofictions: *The Secret Life of Dr. James Barry: Victorian England's Most Eminent Surgeon*.[100] The titular alteration from 'Queen Victoria's Most Eminent Military Doctor' (Random House) to 'Victorian England's Most Eminent Surgeon' (Tempus/History Press) performs a curious historical and geopolitical shift from the broader compass of the British empire (and army) to high-Victorian England (and domestic surgery). The cover illustration (Fig. 2.5) reproduces a partial aspect of a portrait of the middle-aged Barry.

As with the US edition of *Scanty Particulars*, we are denied full sight of the face.[101] This is not so much a play on the ultimate 'unknowability' of the subject, as, rather, an implicit promise of disclosure. For however much the historical Barry may have wished to escape scrutiny, his cut-off eyes suggest that he is caught in the gaze of the afterworld, powerless to challenge our appropriative desire (or, as in the UK edition's cover, to engage with us in an exchange of looks). Once the reader opens the book, it is implied, the cover will be lifted on Barry's 'Secret Life'. This presents us with a very different version of the Barry depicted in the original portrait (Fig. 2.6).

With its full-frontal face and expansive body movement, the original features a self-assured man of authority, in full possession of his destiny (and with a distinctly masculine posture that demands leg room). By contrast, the Tempus cover emphasizes concealment and withdrawal (with invisible legs that readers may even expect to be crossed in a feminine parallel to the right arm's shielding impulse). Denied the power of the gaze, this Barry appears to have neither vision nor confidence. The left arm no longer marks out the extensive physical space (and social and professional pre-eminence) that Barry claims for himself but instead turns into a protective gesture, implying a desire to cover the body and keep others at bay.

Holmes's editions thus mimic aspects of Barry's gender performance in both visual and textual forms. In invocation of the idea of a 'third' sex, we are presented with three different versions of the biography, symbolizing

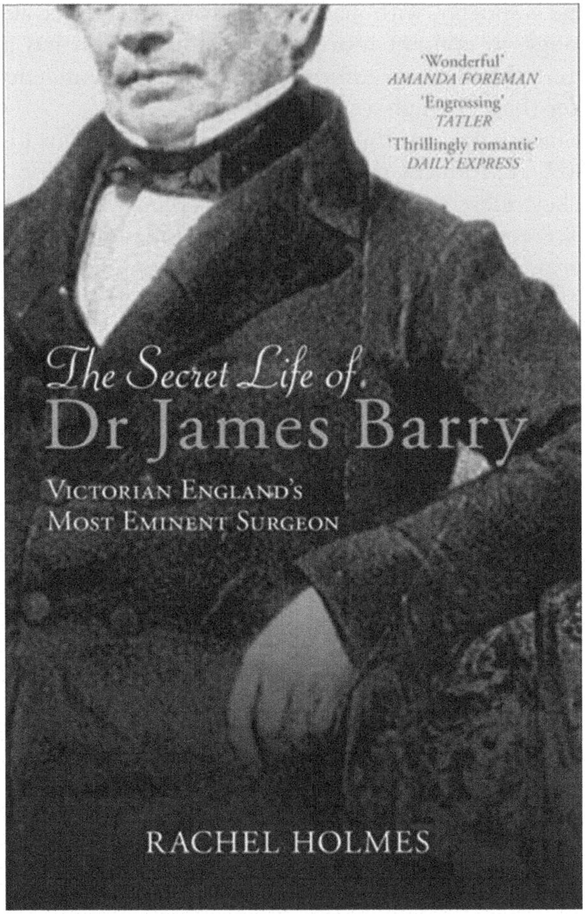

Fig. 2.5 Cover of Rachel Holmes's biography *The Secret Life of Dr James Barry* (Tempus / The History Press, 2007), reproduced courtesy of The History Press

three potential sex/gender positions embraced by Barry. There is first the misdirection of forbidden sexuality set up by the paratext (the covers and titles' allusion to sexual secrets), an impression consolidated by the first half of the biography, which withholds crucial knowledge of Barry's female birth identity: the uninitiated reader is thus encouraged to place the presumed affair with Somerset and ensuing libel case within a homosexual

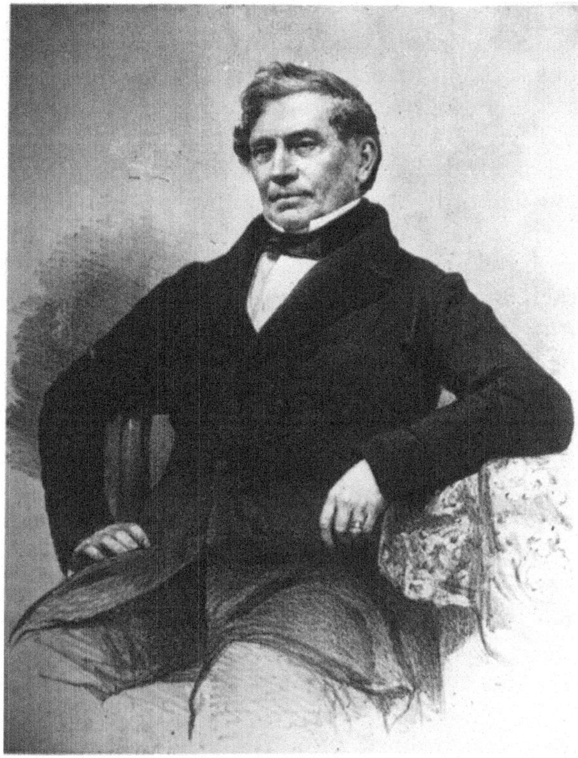

Fig. 2.6 Portrait of James Barry, founder of Barry Brothers and Nephew and member of the Legislative Assembly at the Cape, reproduced courtesy of Western Cape Archives and Records Service, Cape Town, South Africa (reference number M774)

context. It is only with Barry's death that Holmes discloses the matter of his disputed sex. Was Barry, then, a biological woman whose male impersonation became internalized over time, engendering a trans identity? Ultimately, Holmes's overriding argument is that of intersexuality,[102] a case that is developed in great depth by the final chapters, with the effect of making readers review Barry's life story and the earlier chapters from an entirely different angle. In this way the textual ending returns us to the beginning, prompting us to reread Barry's biography and this time picking up on the clues that were always already there.

Holmes's work is not the only instance of the biographilic game with textual diversity as a marker of sex/gender instability. Other texts pinpoint the interplay of binaries – the effeminate man, the female warrior – in Barry's subject constitution. The most notable example of such textual/ sexual doubling is *A Modern Sphinx* (1881), the first novelistic response to Barry, by Ebenezer Rogers, an army officer whose claim to first-hand knowledge of Barry rested on his story of their having shared a cabin on board a ship bound for Barbados in 1857, when 'in harsh and peevish voice', Barry would order the (then twenty-two-year-old) 'youngster' to 'clear out' whenever he wanted to dress.[103] Rogers's laborious adventure-cum-sensation novel appears the prototype of what Henry James had in mind when he compared Victorian three-deckers to 'large loose baggy monsters, with their queer elements of the accidental and the arbitrary'.[104] Applied to the publishing history of Rogers's text, James's famous dictum highlights a gender hybridity that unwittingly retraces Barry's. The association of scatterbrained excess with femininity (floppy fleshliness) queers the male author whose disturbed textual body politic evidently required the guiding hand of a female virtuoso to restore order. It was none other than Mary Elizabeth Braddon who edited Rogers's unwieldy three volumes down to a more readable single volume, issued as *Madeline's Mystery* in 1882.[105] As in the case of Holmes's biography, Rogers's novel saw a third version in 1896 when the original 1881 text was reissued in a three-in-one-volume de-luxe edition of *A Modern Sphinx* with seven illustrations and an introduction that drew on Rogers's 1895 correspondence in the *Lancet*.[106]

The male-to-female-to-male authorial interactions that shape Rogers's three incarnations of his novel exemplify a third characteristic of biographilic hybridization: intertextual cross-fertilization. Thus biographies may draw on earlier biofiction for historical authentication and these fictional sections then transmigrate, as documentary records, to later novels, drama or critical literature. The origin of much of this cross-textual interpenetration that has given sustenance to the Barry myth, and which also informs Rogers's text, is a story that was published two years after Barry's death in Dickens's journal *All the Year Round*, 'A Mystery Still'.[107] Unsigned, the story has not been formally credited to Dickens's authorship but is often referenced to Dickens in Barry biographilia. Parts of the text indeed have a Dickensian texture that makes it tempting to speculate that Dickens might have edited and revised the story in some way, perhaps by exerting editorial control as Braddon did of Rogers's novel; or even that he might have had a hand in the composition of some passages.[108] The first of the biofictions, 'A Mystery Still' is a witty piece that masquerades as a witness account in invocation of the flurry of newspaper reports published in the wake of Barry's death two years earlier. Barry's enigmatic character is explored through a narrative of contradictions that casts him simultaneously as a freak and medical pioneer, swashbuckling trickster and love-torn heroine. This tale set the pattern for almost all subsequent Barry biographilia. What, then, are the key tropes of the Barry mythos, as reflected in what I term the 'Barry archive'?

The Barry Archive: Victorian to Neo-Victorian Life-Writing and the Construction of the Barry Mythos

My concept of an archive is indebted to Halberstam's notion of a clearly demarcated textual corpus as 'a productive narrative, a set of representations, a history, a memorial, and a time capsule' that helps to shed light on sociocultural formations.[109] Comprising biography, biofiction and biodrama from 1865 to 2016, the 'Barry archive' is such a 'collective cultural product' that allows insight into the narrative construction (and also circumvention) of this historical transgender figure over the last 150 years. With at least one feature film confirmed as being in preparation, the archive is a growing cultural resource.[110] The purpose of this chapter section is to identify shared narrative traits across biographilic forms that sustain the idea of an 'archive' while also taking note of differences in the representational strategies of texts across time and genre. In order to elucidate the formation, development and modes of articulation of the Barry *mythos*, the textual corpus is discussed in chronological order and by genre.

In the direct aftermath of Barry's death, it was inevitable that the earliest texts to construct important facets of the Barry myth were biographically-inflected obituaries, press notices and individual responses. With the first biography not published until the mid-twentieth century, it is in biofiction – 'A Mystery Still' and Rogers's *A Modern Sphinx* (and variants) – that the Barry mythos found its first significant expression. Victorian biofiction highlights the perplexing oddities of Barry's character (a travestied form of early sexological readings of his queerness) only to heteronormalize his transgression in a backstory of lost love. This sexual/textual strategy of attenuating the threat of gender crossing by reinventing the female man as a romantic heroine is a marked feature also of early twentieth-century biographilia. This is exemplified by the first stage version (a text that preceded their later novel by over a decade), Olga Racster and Jessica Grove's *Dr. James Barry: A romantic play founded on South African history* (1919, produced at the St. James's Theatre, London). Infused with melodrama, the (in the words of the Lord Chamberlain's Office) 'longwinded and improbable' plot presents Barry as a fugitive wife who takes up medicine and a posting abroad to escape domestic violence at the hands of her dissolute aristocratic spouse, only to be tripped up by her entrapped femininity when she falls in love with a fellow officer.[111]

Near-synchronic in publication date, the first twentieth-century novel, Réné Juta's *Cape Currey* (1920), also weaves a tale of love and loss, concluding with the sensational disclosure of a secret over and above Barry's female sex. Here the 'unnatural' imposition of masculinity on the female body and mind has punitive repercussions on Barry's son, the product of a romantic entanglement in girlhood (Barry Junior is revealed to be a beautiful but fatally diseased young man).[112] In contradistinction to this text, which is narrated from the perspective of Somerset's daughter Georgina, Racster and Grove's *Journal of Dr. James Barry* (1932), a novel based on their earlier biodrama, for the first time projects Barry as a focalizer; the first-person narrative of a fictional memoir encourages readers to sympathize with the protagonist's dilemma. The novel illustrates Max Saunders's concept of 'pseudo-autobiography', a sub-category of autobiografiction that mimics autobiography, not to parody it but to authenticate itself: the equivalent in textual performance to Barry's male impersonation.[113]

Much narrative space in the novel is given to the heroine's learning process in enacting masculinity; if masculinity is but an act, not an essence, this also reveals femininity as a strategic rather than 'inherent' gender identity. Most of the women characters are shown to go to considerable lengths to deploy their seductive charms to turn men's heads for their own empowerment: the emphasis on their performative talent and the artificial nature of femininity strengthens the argument for dissociating gender from sex. The belief in anatomy being destiny is particularly strongly challenged in the figure of Barry's friend Sophie, a young woman who unsuccessfully seeks to gain access to medical training and in the course of the narrative turns into a proficient nurse with exemplary courage and skill. While her motivation for a medical career is her 'feminine' drive to alleviate human suffering, she is depicted as resembling Barry in uniting within herself both 'feminine' and 'masculine' traits: 'born to be a physician', she 'is the man in woman's clothes' to Barry's 'woman in man's clothes.'[114] Sophie's case substantiates the idea that gender performance can be a productive means of bridging the gap between private and public personae, and between psychological 'essence' and bodily appearance.

That in the new century Barry's life was revisited by authors based in South Africa (Marvell, Racster and Grove)[115] may derive from the fact that his first, and longest, posting had been at the Cape (1816–1827), where a descendant of the child he had delivered by Caesarian section became the first Prime Minister of the South African state.[116] It is a singular irony that a humanitarian reformer like Barry, who secured the freedom of at least one slave, should have become the godfather of a family dynasty that was to take a leading role in the Apartheid regime; even more so that the first play to celebrate Barry's achievements should have adopted a pro-slavery stance: in a digression to the main plot of Racster and Grove's biodrama, Somerset makes the astonishing claim that 'no portion of the community is better off or happier than the domestic slave' and sets forth his 'enlightened' vision for a benign form of paternalistic slavery in South Africa.[117]

Importantly for this particular inflection of the Barry myth, the early twentieth century was a time of intense concern about gender relations unsettled by the Great War. As shell-shocked men returned from the front to find themselves displaced at work, women were urged to rediscover their femininity and indulge in romance: a desire bound to founder in the aftermath of the war and its casualties. The story of a woman like Racster and Grove's Barry who, by shouldering 'male' responsibilities, was able to attain a position of public authority while missing out on love and human companionship would have held considerable symbolic significance in this period.

If early twentieth-century biofiction and biodrama blend aspects of Victorian sensation with post and interwar sentiment and inject a South African nationalist perspective into the Victorian adventure plot, mid to later-twentieth and early twenty-first-century biographies blur genre boundaries by adopting the narrative strategies of fiction in their portrayal of Barry's (hi)story. The legacy of Victorian biofiction, in particular 'A Mystery Still', is conspicuous here, in that (as is explored in more detail in Chapter 3) key aspects of this tale are co-opted as quasi-documentary source. This fictionalizing impulse is also in evidence in the use of long promotional subtitles that mimic the textual paradigms of the eighteenth and nineteenth-century novel and add sensationalist undertones. At the same time the appeal to readers' appetite for the spectacular combined with ground-breaking archival research that uncovered Barry's origins. Thus Isobel Rae's *The Strange Story of Dr. James Barry: Army Surgeon, Inspector General of Hospitals, discovered on death to be a woman* (1958) drew on papers held by the War Office, including Barry's career summary, 'The humble memorial of Dr. James Barry', revised as 'Memorandum of the Services of Dr. James Barry' (1859).[118] Rae established Barry's family connection to the history painter and his group of influential friends. In *The Perfect Gentleman: The remarkable life of Dr. James Miranda Barry, the woman who served as an officer in the British Army from 1813 to 1859* (1977) June Rose traced Barry's identity further, not to the niece (as in Rae) but to one of the daughters of the painter's sister. On the basis of handwriting samples, Rachel Holmes's *Scanty Particulars* (2002) followed art historian William Pressly's lead in confirming Barry's identity as the elder of the two daughters. The most recent biography, by the urologist and Barry historian Michael du Preez and the novelist Jeremy Dronfield, *Dr. James Barry: A Woman Ahead of Her Time* (2016), sheds light on the afterlives of the Bulkleys, especially Mary-Anne's later trajectory,[119] and, drawing on census information, establishes the existence of two female servants in Barry's final lodging house: the layer-out who broke the story and the younger, then still unmarried and childless Sophia Bishop, a housemaid employed by Barry's landlady: a crucial discovery since all previous work misidentifies the charwoman as Sophia Bishop.[120]

In contradistinction to the two twentieth-century biographies which, written at the dawn, then in the sway of second-wave feminism, construct Barry as a biological and psychological woman determined to make her way in a man's world and therefore passing herself off as male, the early twenty-first-century work by Holmes advances a case for reading Barry through the physical condition of intersexuality.[121] In support of her premise, Holmes draws extensively on Barry's M.D. thesis on the female hernia, a medical complaint that can be mistaken for descending testicles in intersex individuals.[122] None of these biographies is what Garber calls a 'normalization' narrative, intended to 'recuperat[e] social and sexual norms' in transvestite performance, the way early twentieth-century fiction and drama do.[123] Yet in their juxtaposition of cross-dressing woman and intersex subject, the texts invoke the parameters of the Victorian social progress or physical malfunction narratives and in the process, as LGTBQ+ writer Hamish Copley points out, risk erasing the possibility of transgender readings of James Barry.[124]

This is illustrated in du Preez and Dronfield's biography, which goes to great lengths to impute an irrepressible femininity to Barry, contending that 'James' was no more than a male persona, a mere 'disguise ... obscuring without ever fully concealing the girl beneath': once a girl, it appears, forever a girl, even when the person in question is a septuagenarian male.[125] 'Margaret' is here conjured up as the 'authentic' identity, an 'irremovable stowaway' hiding in the seams of 'James's' breeches, always threatening to erupt from behind the mask: this, the authors argue, is the reason for Barry's eccentricity and lifelong 'struggle to master' masculinity: 'Margaret never could succeed in imitating the male persona entirely – it was ... not in her'.[126] Even though she might clad herself in the outer apparel of manhood, 'the shadow that the candle threw on the wall was as sinuously feminine as ever.'[127] (Judging by Barry's portraits, his figure, though certainly petite, was anything but of the womanly kind).

Such emphasis on Barry's 'feminine' anatomy and disregard of his evident ease as a man of authority (see Fig. 2.6) sits oddly with the biography's simultaneous tribute to his exceptional record as a military surgeon. Not only was his performance of professional masculinity convincing enough for him to be entrusted with high office, again and again, but after five decades of living as a man it is implausible that he could have retained a strong female sense of self discarded at the age of twenty. As in Victorian depictions of Barry, the 'truth' of the *body* is cast as a non-negotiable *mental* condition closely tied to gender normativity, irrespective of the impact of transformative experience on identity, so that even after a lifetime as James, 'Margaret' would still have hankered after 'bringing her dresses out of storage'.[128] Incapable of crushing her biologically inherent urge for a culturally codified expression of femininity (manifested in the desire for an arbitrarily gendered dress style), Margaret was forced to conceal and repress her 'real' self. In an ironic counter move, the authors contain Barry's breaching of sex/gender boundaries within an endnote that only the inquisitive reader is likely to locate, referencing the potential of transgender only to foreclose it:

> This consistent failure to shed her femininity is one of the strands of evidence against the idea that Margaret/James had a transgender personality. She may have been bigender, but we have no evidence for this; she lived one part of her life exclusively as female, and the other (with limited success) as male. By modern definitions, it is not altogether certain that she counts even as a transvestite, since the decision to live as a man was apparently motivated more by ambition than identity.[129]

Given the extent of contemporary cultural and political interest in transgender identities, it is startling that this most recent twenty-first-century text reverts to the cyclical logic of Victorian gender essentialism. It was only by suppressing her 'natural' feminine instincts that Barry was capable of achieving the groundbreaking work that singles her out as a pioneer of medicine (du Preez and Dronfield even suggest that if the Army Medical Department had put Barry in charge of Scutari, the Crimean War would have taken a different course); and yet by prioritizing professional over affective life choices, Barry inevitably failed as a woman, just as she equally failed the test of masculinity in that her feminine desire for sumptuous clothes and her female body characteristics always shone through.[130] That Barry could have started off as a gender impersonator determined to study for a profession and make her way in the world and, in the course of years, have turned into a crosser defining himself through his new identity is obviated by a biologically determinist approach that appears to refute the possibility of (historical) transgender identity altogether.

Du Preez and Dronfield's biography illustrates the legacy of Victorian gender normativity in contemporary life-writing. This legacy also surfaces in work that seeks to contest what might be called the 'repressive hypothesis' of the Barry mythos by endowing the cross-dresser with a modern insouciance about sex. An example is Jean Binnie's bioplay *Colours*, produced by the Abbey Theatre, Dublin and Leeds (now West Yorkshire) Playhouse in October 1988.[131] With her unfailingly female sense of self, strong heterosexual orientation and powerful libido, 'Jane' Barry could be taken for a postfeminist send-up of Barry tropes. Indeed, in an interview Binnie noted that she wanted her play to appeal to teenage girls. That this involves (consensual) under-age sex without strings with a number of men who are between two to three times the protagonist's senior in years may have a different resonance thirty years on, in a time of intensifying concern about the prevalence of child and teenage sexual grooming.[132]

In the play, after indulging in joyful sex with each of her three mentors (David Erskine; General Miranda; and Arthur Wellesley, not yet of Waterloo fame),[133] the fourteen-year-old responds with great equanimity to her pregnancy, succeeds with supreme confidence in commandeering the support of all the co-fathers and, leaving her child in the care of her mother, throws herself into her medical studies. Her military career offers her easy access to the company of men; frustration arises, however, from having to contain her desire in the presence of so many enticing athletic bodies. The invocation of an embodied and highly sexed Barry inverts gender stereotypes, as when, referring to tasty male bums as mouthwatering plums, she compares the temptation they exert to that of chocolates that one knows must not be touched.[134] After her youthful peccadillos, however, she only allows herself one further affair, with Somerset, in which she duly takes the lead; and promptly conceives again (this child, however, is miscarried).

Ultimately, for all of her display of sexual agency, Jane's autonomy is heavily compromised by her emotional and psychological overdependence on her father, the painter James Barry, whose illness sparks her wish to take up medicine, whose sexual lawlessness she emulates, and who even in death guides her every step (the painter's ghost takes material shape and interferes in the events). With his insistent demand for a description of the 'colours' (sensual impressions) of her experiences, Barry Senior partakes of her life, indeed lives on through her. Jane never escapes her father's influence, nor does she wish to. It is no accident that her lovers are all father figures (and, with the exception of Somerset, the men he picked out for her) and that she launches into her affairs in the aftermath of his death. Her entire life's course and every impulse are shaped by identifying herself in and through her relation to men. Her later rape by a corrupt army commander whom she sets out to 'seduce' to her vision of reform by, of all things, disguising herself as a woman stands as a reflection of this Barry's entrapment within male-dominated scripts.

Such a script also decrees maternal instincts, a notion that comes under considerable strain in a plot that depicts Jane's relations with her baby daughter as merely instrumental (as a means to secure her mentors' material support of her career aspirations) and yet has her drop everything decades later, despite the lack of any contact over the years, when news reaches her of Marion's illness. There is little credibility in Jane suddenly being overcome by the love of her child; nor would Marion at this stage even be a child. More convincingly, Jane's conflicted relationship with her own mother ('Aunt' Isabel, the painter's sister) and that mother's profound resentment of her male-identified daughter offer a probing, if brief, foray into the psychodrama of woman-to-woman relations. Here, too, a woman's transgressive sexual desire (in Isabel's case, incest) ultimately strips her of agency, thus underwriting the trope of chastisement (the woman who dares must get punished, one way or another).

While contemporary Barry biographilia can thus have the effect of reinforcing gender essentialism, other work explores gender variant and queered narratives. Inflections of transgender discourse in late-twentieth-century and more recent biographilia often develop from within plots that, initially at least, cast Barry as a cross-dressing woman with an (albeit conflicted) female gender identity and heterosexual orientation. The biographilic Barry's desire is usually directed at one of two men: Somerset or Cloete, or both, in succession or simultaneously, in an Eros/Agape divide. Somerset is the off-stage lover in Frederic Mohr's (David McKail's) 'solo' play *Barry: Personal Statements* (1984).[135] The play was first produced on the stage in the US and the UK in 1983/1984 and revived for the stage in 2008.[136] Mohr's biodrama engages with second-wave feminist concerns in portraying Barry as a dedicated medical reformer inspired by a Scottish Highlands wise woman and herbalist.[137] Barred from higher education and the medical profession on account of her sex, Barry is persuaded by her mentors to resort to stratagem, but her passion for her vocation does not preclude a love affair with Somerset. The first of the two monologues, set in 1819, presents the expectant mother who has gone into hiding to give birth to her child, the second, forty years later, the pre-eminent Deputy Inspector-General preparing for a duel. Whereas the young Barry participated in such a ritual because she felt rejected in her sense of womanhood (due to Somerset's attention to a sexual rival), the ageing general is instead precipitated into action in order to defend his masculinity. The cause of the duel is a junior officer's taunt: 'The young fool … must be taught his lesson. "Old-womanish", indeed. I'll give him "Old-womanish!"'[138]

Having successfully passed as a man for all of his adult life and career, Barry is shown to have shifted in identity, from a woman grounded in her pregnant body to a high-ranking professional man offended by aspersions of femininity. Barry's inner sense of masculinity, however, is fragile: hence his duel, and his dismissal of medical women like Florence Nightingale for lacking 'manly' qualities: 'She is not a gentleman!' Ironically, Nightingale's rank as a lady and the advantage she took of her social influence to achieve her ends compounds her unsuitability. The tenor of Barry's objection to Nightingale – that she is not and never will be a 'gentleman' – signals his intermediacy of both class and gender. Barry may have a female body, but he defines himself by the mental, behavioural and moral attributes of manhood.[139] In the process of reaffirming the patriarchal axiom of male superiority, femininity is downgraded as professionally and ethically unsound. Barry therefore cannot conceive of himself other than as a man.

This queering of Barry's identity is a notable feature of contemporary biodrama. Sebastian Barry's one-act *Whistling Psyche* (2004) also draws on the juxtaposition of Barry and Nightingale to focus on the characters' self-reflections in the form of soliloquies that gradually develop into a disjointed dialogue. Set in a Victorian railway station, in an eerily quiet, Beckettian waiting room symbolic of the limbo between life and death (as well as of Barry's liminal gender), the play explores the similarities in their life choices, reformist vision, and personal sacrifices.[140] As in Mohr's text, Barry seethes with professional and gender-inflected resentment at Nightingale's public celebration as a medical pioneer when she 'did no more than I had been doing for thirty years, and that without changing out of her skirts'.[141] Nightingale's strategic deployment of womanliness contrasts with Barry's neutralization of hers. For just as the titular Psyche, Barry's poodle (a key trope in the Barry mythology) remains intangible despite being invoked throughout by Barry's whistles, so too Barry's femininity and female body have dematerialized not only in her professional but also her sexual life. Her sole experience of intimate bodily exchange, her affair with Somerset, was initiated as a gay encounter and conducted in the darkness and silence of the night, in 'a realm of story and dreams'.[142] Transgender is here encoded through the queering of a 'straight' libidinality.

That queer sexuality is not of necessity subversive in itself is further problematized in Kit Brennan's two-act, larger-cast *Tiger's Heart* (1996), winner of the 1994 Canadian National Playwriting Competition, which depicts Somerset's (homo)sexual aggression as an abuse of power that parallels his corrupt governance practices.[143] Titled after *Henry VI*, Part III (Act 5, Scene 7: 'O tiger's heart, wrapped in a woman's hide'), the play investigates Barry's self-liberation from the patriarchal sexual politics that cost both her biological sister and her sister's namesake (one of Barry's patients) their lives. Withdrawing from Somerset, Barry projects her personal-political insurgence into a cross-racial heterosexual relationship with her African servant Dantzen (Dantzen or Danzer, the name of Barry's servant at the Cape and in Mauritius), but tragically disregards the fatal danger in which she places her black lover.[144]

Both *Whistling Psyche* and *Tiger's Heart* establish analogies between Barry's hybrid gender position and the breaching of other category boundaries such as race and ethnicity. As Roy Foster notes with reference to *Whistling Psyche*, Barry's 'own confusion of gender and destiny ... mirrors the uncertainty of Ireland's position in the Victorian empire – part colonized, part colonizing, neither the one thing nor the other'.[145] Barry's Irishness predisposes her/him to challenge dominant hegemonies and identify with the 'plight of all the unfortunates around me': slum populations, slaves, prostitutes, prisoners, lepers, lunatics.[146] The only member of the colonial elite who 'attempts a correct pronunciation' of non-Anglophone names and appears to understand the native Bantu language, the Barry of *Tiger's Heart* is pitted against the men who wield racial and sexual power (Somerset is pointedly played by the same actor as the slave trader and his aide-de-camp Cloete is doubled up with the Hunter figure who kills Dantzen).[147]

Barry is also juxtaposed to the women who in their disempowerment, shared across differences of class and ethnicity, act as inverted mirror versions of what she escaped by renouncing her femininity: her Irish sister Maggie, the victim of sexual assault and murder; the identically named English wife of an East India Company clerk who, after her husband's desertion having turned to prostitution, languishes and then dies in prison of the combined effects of battery, syphilis and leprosy; Lady Mary, the imperial wife and mother who almost perishes in childbirth.[148] As in *Whistling Psyche* and in Mohr's play, Barry's freedom and agency are premised on her identification as a man and specifically a gentleman.[149] Crucially, however, they are additionally dependent on emotional and sexual detachment. The moment Barry acts on her desire, she becomes vulnerable (to Somerset's manipulations; to pregnancy); the moment she falls in love and enters a relationship, she makes others vulnerable (Dantzen is murdered because of her transgression). Loneliness and aloofness are thus the price Barry has to pay for the empowerment gained from crossing gender boundaries.

If biodrama pinpoints solitude as a key determinant of Barry's life, contemporary biofictions develop scenarios that involve Barry in passionate and sometimes long-term relationships (heterosexual, lesbian and queer), projecting a modern erotic self-awareness and self-confidence into the body of the nineteenth-century cross-dresser or transgender individual. This is the case in Patricia Duncker's postmodernist renditions in short story and novel formats which play with Barry's shifting sex/gender positions, as a lesbian who finds recognition and friendship in a community of indigenous women ('James Miranda Barry', 1989) and as a gender-variant character (*James Miranda Barry*, 1999) who, after a lifetime as a man, desires to come out as a woman in his retirement but is prevented from doing so by his female partner, who is anxious to avert charges of lesbianism.[150] From childhood, Barry moves seamlessly between gender categories, simultaneously perplexing and fascinating her/his environment; as an adult s/he epitomizes the idea of an intermediate, 'third' sex/gender whose erotic allure feeds the straight and gay fantasies of women and men in equal measure.

The indeterminacy of Barry's gender is, in Duncker's novel, reflected in a body that resists easy classification. When the girl that is later to become Barry's lover seeks to establish whether her friend is 'really a girl', or rather the boy she is dressed up to be, and checks for tell-tale physical signs, 'she looked at me, puzzled and amazed ... Then she burst out laughing, withdrew her hand and kissed me. "Well, you're a sort of a girl, I suppose. But definitely not like me."'[151] Queered by the suggestion of intersexuality, Barry's transgender identity serves to confound contemporary reader expectations about gender, sex and sexuality. The nineteenth-century protagonist is here cast futuristically in the twenty-first-century category of the transcender: a 'girl *and* a boy, a girl *in* a boy, a boy who is a girl, a girl who is a boy dressed as a girl, a girl who has to be a boy to be a girl'.[152]

A different version of the (post)millennial resonance of Barry's gender variance is presented in Anne and Ivan Kronenfeld's counterfactual novel *The Secret Life of Dr. James Miranda Barry* (2000). Adventure and sensation tale, romp and neo-historical chick lit in one, the text dramatizes the problems faced by career-minded women who want to have it all. Its unambiguously female protagonist boasts an extraordinary capacity for survival under the most challenging of conditions (the aptly-named Pandora starts her narrative trajectory as a seven-year-old Parisian street girl orphaned by the French Revolution who lives rough and fends for herself, undaunted by the threat of violence and with a partiality for philosophical ruminations far beyond her years). Guided by her adoptive father Miranda, she dons trousers and a male identity in order to practice the profession of her choice. After years of battling her passion for Miranda's son Leander and his wish for a conventionally domesticated wife, she eventually capitulates to her sexual and reproductive desires – 'I do so want a baby'[153] – but following the infant's death resumes her career to stem a cholera epidemic in Paris before joining the regiment of her by now suitably reconstructed, egalitarian-minded Major husband as staff-surgeon. The grand finale sees the couple preparing to attend the graduation ceremony of the first (but, unbeknown to all bar the main protagonists, in reality second) British woman doctor, Elizabeth Garrett.

The conflict between personal ('female') and professional ('male') fulfilment is explored in two further biofictions, Florida Ann Town's novel for the Young Adult market, *With a Silent Companion* (1999), and Sylvie Ouellette's French-language *Le Secret du docteur Barry* (2012). Part novel

(Margaret Bulkley's girlhood and transformation into James) and part biography (Barry's medical career), *With a Silent Companion* offers an apt illustration of the tensions involved in straddling gender and genre categories: with each genre acting as a disruptive 'silent companion' to the other, the text fails to perform convincingly either as fiction or as biography.[154] Its novelistic aspect identifies the roots of Margaret's gender imposture in the child's frustration with the limitations of girlhood and her desire for adventure which, fired by her awareness of social injustice, provide fertile ground for Buchan and Miranda's experiment.

Margaret's Irishness, a catalyst of her determination to challenge the status quo, serves as a test case for learning to negotiate the interplay of essence (her inner sense of identity) and performance. For just as Margaret picks up an English accent by listening to how Londoners speak, and in the process comes to pass as English, so too does she train herself to master the act of masculinity by observation and mimicry. However, her new life comes at the cost of any personal intimacy: as the student recognizes, 'Friendships were too dangerous … And romance would be impossible'.[155] This message is brought home with a vengeance during the scandal prompted by the sodomy libel, which, though fabricated, leads to Barry's resigned conclusion that she 'could never allow herself to become closely involved with another person', however innocent their relations might be.[156] Her mental resistance to the idea of any physical attraction to Somerset betrays her self-repression (and possibly the author's reluctance to engage young readers in explorations of desire), compounding the implausibility of a never entirely fleshed-out character.[157] Barry's subsequent self-caricature by adopting an exaggerated display of masculinity to conceal her lack of an inner life parallels the author's attenuation of her heroine into a wooden figure purged of any interiority or life-like emotion.

Self-restraint is also the keynote of the mature Barry in Ouellette's novel. Initially, however, Barry abandons herself to an affair with Somerset, the intense sexual passion of which is fuelled by their shared excitement about her gender duality. In contradistinction to Somerset's more explicitly gay libidinality in *Whistling Psyche* and *Tiger's Heart*, Ouellette's governor is impelled by sexual fetishism focused on Barry's clothed and unclothed body. He loves undressing the boy to reveal the girl underneath, whom he then arrays – re-genders – in female underwear, corset and scarlet dress, to start the process all over again: 'Was it, then, that duality that excited him so much? Was it the idea to join himself to a being who, in the eyes of the world at least, seemed to be a man?'[158] The text plays with Eve Kosofsky Sedgewick's conceptualization of the triangulation of desire by turning the gender bender's body into a fantasy of both gay and straight gratification, positioning Barry as her own rival to the shifting tastes of her lover-commander.[159] It also explores twenty-first-century interest in crossed sexual appetites: problematically, of the barely teenage Margaret for the middle-aged Miranda, Somerset's for the bisexual and transgender fantasies that can be enacted with Barry's androgynous flesh, and a male official's and female officer's wife's craving for Barry's male body. In the midst of all these sexual obsessions, one character, Barry's duelist Cloete, having accidentally discovered her sex when tending to her wound, offers admiration, respect, and love. While reciprocating his feelings, Barry, however, is too frightened of the consequences for her identity, too firmly tied to her career and hence her masculinity, to indulge what to her, too, is a profound attachment. Ultimately, the very success of her gender imposture turns into a trap since her performance, as in Judith Butler's model, has become essentialized, imprinted on her flesh: 'son personage lui collait à la peau'.[160]

The publication over recent years of a number of both English and foreign-language biofictions that seek to capture a popular readership of different age groups and the development of a biopic, *Dr. James Barry* (co-produced by Rachel Weisz, who is also in the lead role, and with the screenplay, written by Nick Yarborough, drawing on Rachel Holmes's biography), indicates the broad contemporary appeal of the James Barry story.[161] In its inflection in popular culture, the story of the cross-dressing woman is typically embedded in a heterosexual romance plot. This is reflected in the earlier development of a (now probably stalled) feature film, *Heaven and Earth* (directed by Marleen Gorliss and with Natascha McElhone in the lead role). The title plays on the story's Cape location ('Hemel en Aarde') while simultaneously raising expectations of a passionate love story (plot outlines indicate that Somerset sacrifices his career to protect Barry).[162] Romantic love galvanized by a 'discernable sexual' pull is also invoked in du Preez and Dronfield's 2016 biography; though 'what manner of love it was, from either side, would be impossible to identify with certainty': a coded reference to the queer desire that scandalized contemporaries of the 'placard affair' and that is explored more explicitly in twenty-first-century biofiction and biodrama.[163] The epistemological crossings involved in the collaboration of a scientist (du Preez) and a creative writer (Dronfield) point to the genre experimentation that is a constitutive feature of Barry biography.

As indicated at the start of this chapter, 'Doctor James' has also inspired contemporary music culture with Gilmore & Roberts's lyric in the style of an Irish folk ballad. Referring to Barry's 'tales of success' as 'a mystery', Gilmore calls on 'Doctor James' to 'Tell me your secret' so as to recuperate her/him as 'a well-known figure in our history' – a statement the ambiguity of which mirrors Barry's, for does 'our history' refer to the British or (given Barry's Cork origins) the Irish nation, the history of women and feminism, the history of transgender, or all of these in conjunction?[164] The multiple readings that the figure of Barry invites are in tension with the gender-binarity of the discourses used to explore that figure's story. This is exemplified nowhere more prominently than in the problem of pronouns, the 'pronomial dysphoria' that Marjorie Garber identifies as a 'constant pitfall in discussions of the transsexual phenomenon.'[165]

Pronomial (Mis)Appropriations: 'I Must Still Use the "Masculine"'/'I Must Retain the Feminine Gender'[166]

How to refer to an individual's intermediate gender position in a linguistic system that operates through the principle of binarity? The power of gendering, like that of naming, works both ways: gender codification and naming are deeply imbricated with social, racial and imperial classification models; but, as Halberstam reminds us, 'claiming a name [gender] or refusing to and thus remaining unnameable' (of no fixed gender) confers agency on the subject.[167] And yet to respond to Barry's idiosyncratic and iconoclastic self-performances from a contemporary perspective by resisting the normative principle of gendering would disregard the historical conditions of Barry's life and career.[168] Equally problematic is the impulse to essentialize Barry as female on the grounds of the layer-out's testimony of the 'facts' of the body she examined.[169] Nonetheless, for four of his five twentieth and twenty-first-century biographers (Rae, Rose, du Preez and Dronfield) Barry's birth identity and presumed body constitute the 'truth' of his identity: a woman in disguise yet always a woman, Barry is constructed as a gender impersonator not a transgender person. This is also reflected in critical works of second-wave feminism such as Elizabeth Longford's: 'An eminent surgeon in the fighting forces who went through normal life as a man, but whom nobody in fact considered normal … James Barry may possibly have been "intersex" but is far more likely to have been a woman'.[170]

Conversely, should we, like Rachel Holmes, embrace Barry's self-identification as a male, even if we speculate, as Holmes does, about his potential intersexuality or consider (in David Getsy's terms) his 'transgender capacity', believing his identity to have been located in the in-between, what Garber calls the 'third term'? In such cases, does the use of the male pronoun delimit the 'space of possibility' for the disruption of all categories that Garber envisages?[171] Similarly, if we conceptualize Barry through Halberstam's paradigm of 'female masculinity' as constituting not androgyny but 'total ambiguity', do we lose the fluidity of this ambiguity by the constraint of restricting ourselves to one or the other pronoun? And what pronoun do we prioritize for a female man? '[W]hen a woman is mistaken consistently for a man', Halberstam argues, 'it is safe to say that what marks her gender presentation is not androgyny but masculinity'; intriguingly, however, this masculinity is marked by the female pronoun ('a woman ... her').[172] Do we reference gender or sex? Halberstam draws on Butler's point that '[w]hen the constructed status of gender is theorized as radically independent of sex, gender itself becomes a free-floating artifice, with the consequence that *man* and *masculine* might just as easily signify a female body as a male one, and *woman* and *feminine* a male body as easily as a female one'.[173] Yet the dilemma of the pronoun remains in place. Similarly, in her study of historical cases of intersexuality, Geertje Mak proposes to adopt an 'almost random' use of male and female pronouns, but this leads either to tortuous sentences or to an inadvertent reconsolidation of normative gender/sex discourses.[174]

Contemporary non-binary use of the singular 'they' or neologisms like 'per/per/pers/pers', 'e/ey/em/eir', 'sie/sir/hir/hirs', 've/ver/vis/vers' and 'zie/zim/zir/zirs' are more suited to twenty-first-century ambigender, agender, intergender, pangender, third gender, genderqueer and genderfluid subjectivities; it is questionable whether such terms can do justice to Barry's likely sense of self after fifty-six years of living as a man (from 1809 to 1865).[175] One option might be to replace pronouns with Barry's initials, JMB, but this strategy too falls short ('when Barry took up JMB's first appointment'). Were it not for the complexity of such a venture, the virtuoso omission of all gender signifiers by the Oulipian French writer Anne Garrétta might offer itself as a model; as Emma Ramadan (Garrétta's translator) notes, not only do we never discover the gender of the first-person narrator of *Sphinx* (1986), nor that of the narrator's lover A***, but 'at no point does it [their gender] matter to the story'.[176] This, of course, is the crux of the matter, for in Barry's case gender – and the tension between gender identity and gender representation – does matter because that is precisely what is under investigation in the cultural remediation of the figure. My approach in this book is informed by contemporary LGTBQ+ policy of following the preference of the individual in question; in Halberstam's words, to 'adapt to a pronoun system based on gender and not on sex, based on comfort rather than biology'.[177] This study therefore employs the male pronoun as a marker of Barry's choice of a masculine identity, except for contexts and texts where Barry is treated as a female; I use both pronouns where a text or passage deliberately projects Barry as occupying Rogers Brubaker's 'trans of between' ('either/or') or 'trans of beyond' ('both/and') positions.[178]

The complexities of referencing Barry were apparent from the start. Staff Surgeon McKinnon's response to the Registrar General was carefully worded to avoid the use of pronouns.[179] By contrast, the newspaper correspondent who broke the story, in *Saunders's News-Letter*, interrupted the narrative about the discovery of Barry's female sex with a parenthetical explanation for the choice of male pronoun: '(for I must still use the "masculine")'.[180] The opposite was the case when, thirty years later, a reader correspondence developed in the *Lancet*, and Ebenezer Rogers, the author of *A Modern Sphinx*, quoted from the letter of a general who had known Barry when serving in the West Indies and who, after initially stumbling over the pronouns ('I knew him, or her, in Jamaica … I do not think he, or she, wore a ring'), came to the conclusion that in speaking of his former colleague he 'must retain [or, rather, assert] the feminine gender'.[181] In either case the use of the imperative 'must' reaffirmed the rule of law that Barry had so spectacularly breached. Another contemporary instance of pronomial confusion originates from the dean of McGill Medical School, Dr. G. W. Campbell's recollection that if, when he attended the Inspector General in 1859 in the early stages of his own career, he 'had not stood in awe' of Barry's formidable rank and achievements, 'I would have examined him – that is her – far more thoroughly. Because I did not, and because his – confound it, her – bed-room was always in almost total darkness … this, ah, crucial point, escaped me.'[182]

Even more remarkable is the mixture of gender references in a letter Florence Nightingale addressed probably to her sister Parthenope, Lady Verney, shortly after Barry's death in 1865, in which she gave a vivid account of their clash ten years earlier. Barry, then stationed in Corfu, had turned up in Scutari on his way to the Crimea without official orders, with the express intention, as he jokingly remarked in a letter to Dr. James Henderson (the surgeon who stood in for him as a locum during his absence), to 'lionis[e] or rather vagabondis[e]'.[183] More likely he wished to inspect the hospital facilities and management, secretly hoping that he might find grounds for complaint to corroborate his private sense of grievance on having been denied service at the front.[184] Whatever caused his ill temper on the day their paths crossed, Barry evidently could not resist the opportunity to harangue Nightingale in the presence of a military audience. As Nightingale recalled in anger,

> I never had such a blackguard rating in all my life – I who have had more than any woman – from this Barry sitting on (her) horse, while I was crossing the Hospital Square, with only my cap on, in the sun. (He) kept me standing in the midst of quite a crowd of soldiers, commissariat servants, camp followers etc etc, every one of whom behaved like a gentleman, during the scolding I received, while (she) behaved like a brute.
>
> After (she) was dead, I was told (he) was a woman. …
>
> I should say (she) was the most hardened creature I ever met.[185]

The letter records Nightingale's unabated outrage at her treatment, but it also offers intriguing insight into her mental (trans)gendering of Barry into what Sam Ward (the brother of Julia Ward Howe) some twenty years earlier had called 'a kind of moral hermaphrodite' with reference to George Sand.[186] Nightingale starts and ends with her knowledge that Barry was (believed to have been) a woman. In the recollection of the scene, Barry is pictured as the man who so rudely confronted her, but one whose claim to 'proper' masculinity was in doubt even then given his discourteous behaviour, so much at odds with the conduct of the other males present, gentlemen every one of them. Small wonder, then, if 'he' was really 'a woman'. Barry was thus doubly guilty of violating gender norms, both as a woman who masqueraded as a man and as a man who didn't know how to treat a woman like a 'gentleman'. (As noted previously, in Mohr's *Barry*, Nightingale's words are markedly turned against her: here it is Nightingale who, from Barry's perspective, fails to meet the mark in gentlemanly codes).

The high-handed nature of Barry's put-down of Nightingale has been read as female rivalry (the resentment by a woman who has played by male rules of another woman's deployment of femininity to sidestep them) and in *Whistling Psyche* is presented as anger at seeing a younger, professionally less qualified rival honoured for her own long-standing achievements.[187] But there is also a strong sense of Barry's male-identified dismay at finding a woman meddling with what should remain a man's business. It was Barry, after all, who could boast of an extraordinarily high survival rate for wounded Crimean soldiers, and yet whose desire to be posted to the

Crimea was frustrated because Nightingale had got there first (how much the official put-down of his formal request continued to rankle with Barry is suggested in his later listing the Crimea as one of his official postings).[188] Nightingale's oddly modern-sounding collocation of interchangeable gender pronouns testifies to the complexities of Barry's gender identity.

If biodrama visualizes Barry's play with shifting roles and identities, this fluidity is more difficult to reconcile with the biographical project of telling the life story of a single individual (other than in fictional mock biography such as Virginia Woolf's *Orlando*). For all their focus on the slipperiness of gender, Barry biographies predominantly adopt a single pronoun. Thus in their reading of Barry as a woman who impersonated a man to escape poverty and lead an independent life, Isobel Rae and June Rose use the female pronoun throughout. Even when biographers problematize their pronoun choice, the 'real' James Barry still tends to be cast as a woman. This is prominently manifested in du Preez and Dronfield's work, whose subtitle leaves no room for uncertainty about Barry's sex ('A Woman Ahead of Her Time') (Fig. 2.7).

While, with its blanked-out face,[189] the cover engages with Barry's unstable identity, the 'Authors' Note' explains that the use of pronouns

> var[ies] according to situation, depending on whether s/he is appearing in the persona of the male 'James Barry' or that of her original female identity; between these extremes, Barry is referred to as either 'he' or 'she' depending on whether the viewpoint is 'his' outer persona or 'her' inner self.[190]

This results in rather stilted prose, as when the authors reflect on what Barry's course of action would have been if on entering the British Army he had had to undergo a physical examination: 'if such an examination had been required in 1813 – would James have tried to game the system … Or might Margaret have sent her alter ego on a different course, perhaps trying to establish him as a social practitioner in the world of her mentors …?'[191] The imposition of 'outer' and 'inner' identities creates the impression that Barry suffered a quasi-schizophrenic split, hence perhaps his irrational outbursts of temper and general intractability:

> A gulf had grown between James and the Margaret Bulkley who had first put on this disguise … It was Margaret who possessed all [the new knowledge, experience and skills], and … yet outwardly she had no existence. This struggle with identity was difficult, and must inevitably exact a price; a price in emotional stress that would grow with the passage of years.[192]

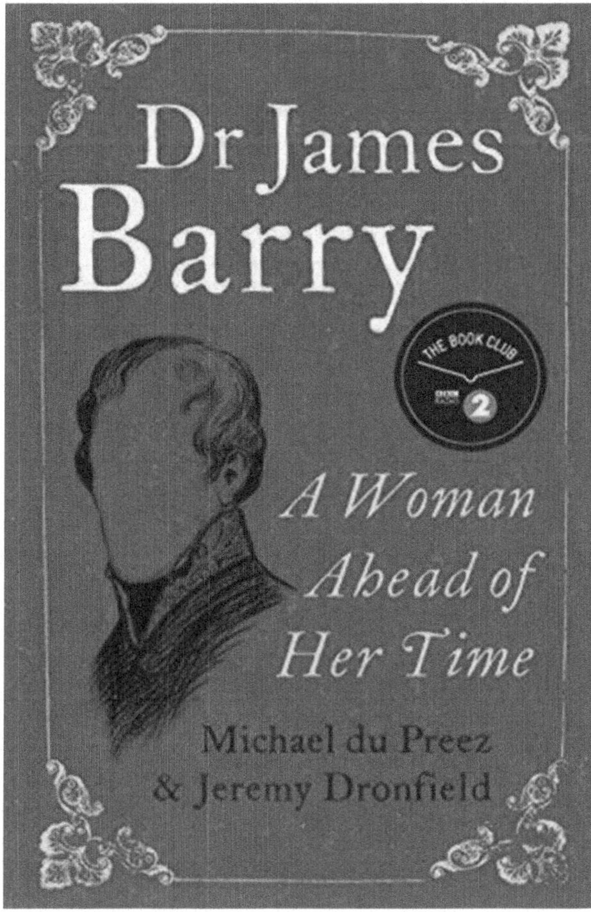

Fig. 2.7 Cover of Michael du Preez and Jeremy Dronfield's biography *Dr James Barry*, first published in the UK by Oneworld Publications, 2016, reproduced courtesy of the publisher

In the representational emphasis on a divided sense of self, the potential of transgender is passed over and Barry is pathologized.

In contrast, Rachel Holmes, who places Barry in an intersexual context, adopts the male identity he espoused. Significantly, in contradistinction to the other biographies, her (sub)title does not reveal the sex of the 'Victorian Surgeon James Barry'. The text opens programmatically with an epigraph by transgender activist and writer Leslie Feinberg: 'There are no pronouns in the English Language as complex as I am.'[193] This should alert the reader to the pronominal games-playing of the ensuing text, but Holmes's circumvention of pronouns in the prefatory section is so skilful that their absence may not be registered at first reading. The Preface magisterially sidesteps pronomial identifiers altogether, thus offering, in the linguistic medium, an illustration of Barry's resisting gender performance. Holmes's different conceptualization of Barry entails a different telling of the story, one that breaks with the convention she identifies as consisting in selecting 'the end as the beginning', Barry's death and the revelation of his female body (which constitutes the opening of Rae, Rose, du Preez and Dronfield's biographies).[194] Instead, as Chapter 4 explores in more detail, Holmes starts with the making of Dr. James Barry: his medical studies, the 'birth' of his identity.

The four pronoun choices of Barry's immediate contemporaries – 'she' of the female body, 'he' of the male career, pronoun avoidance to pay tribute to the moral attributes of the gentleman, the 'she/he' hermaphrodite or split self – find an echo in biographilic representations of Barry. Stage drama offers ample opportunity for embodying Barry's gender instability in the juxtaposition of female actor and male persona. This is made explicit in Brennan's *Tiger's Heart* in the stage direction that 'The actor playing BARRY needs to find the male side of the character, for BARRY's disguise is authentic, having by now lived the lie for ten years': 'living the lie' here slips into an expression of 'authenticity'.[195] Barry's body/mind duality is mirrored in the doubling up of the other characters, with the same actor playing two or more roles, each being identified by a mask.[196] Barry's masquerade is thus both singular (by virtue of his being the only character to be paired with an actor rather than another character) *and* representative (all identities are masks, all roles authentic disguise).

Biodrama thus lends itself with particular force to a metadramatic visualization of the tension between performance and identity. Both Racster and Grove's and Mohr's plays introduce the audience to a manifestly female character (an aristocratic wife, an expectant mother) who then turns herself into or reveals herself to be passing as a 'man'. Mohr's heavily pregnant 'woman of twenty' starts her monologue with a reference to her imminent confinement ('my time is near') before outing herself: 'Yes I do have a pretty little head, but I cannot toss it in disdain at love-sick young men, because I am one too. … Except that I am not really a man … But I live as one … and doubtless will do until … I take off the mask. If I ever do ... or can.'[197] Part Two depicts a sexagenarian Inspector General telling mess-table anecdotes about soldiers having involuntary erections in the presence of a fancied commander. The difference in gender performance between the two 'Personal Statements' signals the change in gender identity Barry has undergone in the intervening years. The juxtaposition of the two characters – one in white, the other in black, one young, the other old, one a woman, the other a man – is so persuasive that spectators may only gradually realize in the course of the second part that they are, in fact, one and the same person.[198] Similarly, Racster and Grove's Prologue, which ends with Lady Barrymore's decision to leave her abusive husband, is followed by a first act set in the Cape, depicting a boisterous and flirtatious dandy who prides himself on his sex appeal ('You see, I'm attractive! There is no doubt about that') before referring to his 'woman's instinct in man's clothes': it is only at this point that the veil is lifted for the audience, who now recognize Barry as the fugitive Lady Barrymore.[199]

Unlike the third-person mode that is constitutive of biography, biofiction permits a wider range of perspectives. In texts written in the third person in which he is not the main protagonist, such as Ebenezer Rogers's *A Modern Sphinx* and Renée Juta's *Cape Currey*, Barry appears as enigmatic to the reader as he is to the main focalizer (Lord Charles's daughter Georgina in *Cape Currey* and a range of Rogers's cast of characters in *A Modern Sphinx*). In keeping with Patricia Duncker's point about the popularity, in neo-Victorian fiction, of fragmented or unreliable first-person narration, a more prominent choice is what Marie-Luise Kohlke terms 'autobiofiction', fictional autobiographies that encourage closer reader identification with the protagonist (examples are Racster and Grove's *Journal* and Duncker's story 'James Miranda Barry').[200] The use of the first person opens up a space for readers to probe different identities and to reimagine Barry as female or transgender, with a heterosexual or lesbian orientation.

By contrast, third-person fictions with the titular promise to unveil Barry's secret, such as the Kronenfelds' *Secret Life*, cast Barry unambiguously as female. In further illustration of this principle, Ouellette's *Le Secret* frames Barry's femininity with an introductory chapter that reveals only gradually what the male adolescent's secret consists in (at which point the male pronoun of the opening shifts into the female – 'elle' – for the remainder of the text) and an Epilogue set after Barry's death and discovery of his female body in which Cloete and Dantzen, the two men who have loved Barry, talk about him in the male pronoun in order to honour his lifelong male identity in the face of the revelation of his body's secret.[201] The kinship that is here established between the two men, with its hint of what Elizabeth Freeman has called 'queer belonging', points to the potential of a queer community *à trois* that might have been forged in Barry's lifetime, but that the heteronormative narrative frame and pronomial structure always proscribed.[202]

The most playful and complex treatment is provided by Duncker's two versions of 'James Miranda Barry' that act like refracting mirrors of each other (from 'I/she' to 'she/he/I'). While the short story interrupts the first-person thoughts of its (initially ungendered) narrator with the memory of a critical moment in childhood that marked the turning point from female to male identity, the novel alternates between chapters (parts) voiced in the first and third person. The first, third and final two chapters record the first-person impressions of the child (who is referred to by others in both genders), the experiences of the graduate doctor and then senior military physician, and the thoughts and emotions of the retired, private individual. The second and fourth chapters, about Barry's studies in Edinburgh and his posting in Corfu, adopt a third-person perspective and the male pronoun. The shift in narrative voice effects a tangible break with Barry's childhood and evokes his sense of disorientation in adapting to his new identity: 'I feel like two people. One of them is true and one is a charade. I don't know which one is real. And mostly I feel that neither one really exists.'[203] As Eveline Kilian notes, Barry's split self is also dramatized in a mirror scene at the start of part three, in which the apprentice doctor stares at his reflection in the sea at Portsmouth Harbour:

> I catch sight of myself in a long, ruffled sheet of sea water and I am fearfully humiliated. There stands a small, peculiar figure, dressed in a scarlet jacket and grey trousers, with a full-length overcoat tailing across his narrow shoulders. The coat is too long and the figure looks grotesque, a puppet dressed in a carnival costume.[204]

Arguably, however, self-alienation is here no longer rooted in gender confusion but, rather, in Barry's professional sense of failure and guilt: he has just lost a patient. A decade on, when he takes up his position in Corfu, by now in full enjoyment of a formidable medical reputation, he is entirely comfortable with his identity; here third-person narration and free indirect speech serve to reflect on the allure he exerts on others, men and women alike, who muse about 'What was so hypnotic, strange and intense about this man, which began to appear like a deliberate tactic to beguile and seduce?'[205] Fluctuations in narrative perspective can thus connote self-estrangement but also a gender hybridity that is experienced as empowering.

Duncker's and Ouellette's shifting pronouns and points of view, the use of masks and doubling in Brennan's dramaturgy, the juxtaposition of two characters who act as versions of each other in Sebastian Barry and Mohr's plays, the framing devices presented in biographers' choice of titles and cover images, the authorial commentary that in Racster and Grove enwombs the first-person narrative of the fictional diary: the structural composition and paratextual strategies of biographilic works frequently offer a metatextual illustration of the cover acts of Barry's gender performance. The textual frames visualize and re-enact Barry's bodily camouflage: a camouflage accomplished with the help of vestments – a version of Garber's 'foundation garments' that facilitate the transvestite act.[206] For in order to reconstitute himself as male, every day afresh, by donning the sartorial accoutrements of masculinity, Barry must first wrap up and neutralize the female body. It is not only Barry's outer garments – the cocked hat, the stiff collar, the padded shoulders, the overlong sword, the high-heeled shoes – that form a key component of the Barry myth; Barry's inner garments, too – his towels – constitute a biographilic trope, signalling his agency and self-empowerment while at the same time referencing the vulnerability of his masquerade.[207] In Racster and Grove's *Journal*, the fugitive Lady Barrymore, now a medical student, gains in masculine self-confidence after wrapping herself in several layers of towels: 'I am enormously pleased with myself. … Bolt upright and hard-muscled – apparently – I am estimated to be more of a man … someone who even rouses envy, and a little disturbance among young women. … I am rapidly becoming one of the best fencers among the University students.'[208]

Here the stiff towels constitute a quasi-bodily prop for 'hard-muscled' masculinity. But Barry's towels can also denote the danger of exposure through a literal uncovering of the body, a stripping away of the protective cover; this is most conspicuous in the duel and bedroom plots that are discussed in more detail in the next chapter. The towel trope was first introduced in 'A Mystery Still': 'Six towels were among the invariable items of his toilet, and though Black John never assisted at it personally, he was aware that his master wrapped these cloths about him; whether he did so for warmth, or to conceal any personal defects in his emaciated form, was a mystery.'[209] The unwrapping of this mystery, an unwrapping that is prototypically concerned with uncovering the secrets of the body, is the driving force of the Barry myth.

CHAPTER 3

Myths and Afterlives: Foundation Stories and Body Plots

[E]njoying a reputation for considerable skill in his Profession, … [h]e was clever and agreeable, save for the drawback of a most quarrelsome temper, and an inordinate addiction to argument … He was excessively plain, of feeble proportions, and laboured under the imperfection of a ludicrously squeaking voice … He … died about a month ago, and … was discovered to be a woman! … This is all that is yet known of this extraordinary story. The motives that occasioned, and the time when was commenced this singular deception, are both shrouded in mystery. … There is no doubt whatever about the fact, but I doubt whether even Miss Braddon herself would have ventured to make use of it in fiction.

Saunders's News-Letter (14 August 1865)[1]

[B]iofiction … thrives on an inherent sense of simultaneously seductive and transgressive violation grounded in a composite and reciprocal self-Othering. The Othering of the historical subject in the process of fictional life-writing simultaneously Others the writing/reading self.

Marie-Luise Kohlke, 'Neo-Victorian Biofiction' (2013)[2]

Biographies, like lives, are made up of contested objects – relics, testimonies, versions, correspondences, the unverifiable. What does biography do with the facts that can't be fixed, the things that go missing, the body parts that have been turned into legends and myths? … Some body parts, literally, get into the telling of the stories, in the form of legends, rumours or contested

A. Heilmann, *Neo-/Victorian Biographilia and James Miranda Barry*, https://doi.org/10.1007/978-3-319-71386-1_3

> possessions. Body parts are conducive to myth-making ... There is a tremendous fascination with the bodily relics of famous people ... These 'body-part' stories play into the subject's posthumous reputation ...
>
> Hermione Lee, *Body Parts* (2008)[3]

> [Q]ueer genders profoundly disturb the order of relations between the authentic and the inauthentic, the original and the mimic, the real and the constructed ... [T]here are no true accounts of 'passing lives' but only fictions, and the whole story turns on the production of counterfeit realities that are so convincing that they replace and subsume the real.
>
> Judith Halberstam, *In a Queer Time and Place* (2005)[4]

Barry's story has all the characteristics of sensation fiction: there is the distinguished military surgeon of exceptional talent whose physical oddities prompted comment which, fuelled by his fiery disposition, resulted in frequent altercations, and whose sex, when revealed after death, engendered mystery tales around his origins and motivation. The 'production of counterfeit realities', which is the fictionalizing impetus that Halberstam identifies as instrumental to the re-presentation of trans lives, was in evidence from the first newspaper report on James Barry. In examining the Victorian foundation myth and its neo-Victorian remediation, this chapter places particular emphasis on biofiction in order to probe the contention that sensation is the archetypal medium of biographilic engagement with Barry. Given that 'Miss Braddon herself' did in fact make a contribution to the cultural history of the Barry legend, what inflections does the 'seductive and transgressive violation' that Marie-Luise Kohlke pinpoints as a defining trait of biofiction take in the composition and evolution of this particular story? What (metatextual) processes of Othering and dissociation might ensue from intradiegetic acts of voyeuristic appropriation? And if, as Hermione Lee argues, life-writing relies on the myth-making attributes of its protagonists' 'body parts', what, in textual terms, are the 'bodily relics', the plots, of the Barry mythology? What 'new stories emerge', Kathryn Hughes asks in *Victorians Undone*, when the material reality of the Victorian body and its various constituents are considered 'at the moment they created crises in individual lives'? How might the stories of such crises feed readers' appetites for 'breath, movement, touch', for sensation in its most essential sense? (Hughes' book might in itself serve as an illustration of the sensations and bodily reactions called up by such 'embodied history'.)[5] In seeking to address these questions, the chapter investigates the central 'body narratives' that have shaped the Barry mythos.

It begins with the Victorian foundation stories, extending Kohlke's model of biofictional strands to the broader category of life-writing to conceptualize Barry archetypes across the range of biographilic forms.

Narrative Archetypes of Barry Biographilia: Celebration, Appropriation and Sensation

In her incisive typology of neo-Victorian biofiction, Kohlke defines three specific modes: 'celebrity biofiction', 'biofiction of marginalised subjects' and 'appropriated biofiction'.[6] Celebrity biofiction 'speculates about the inner lives, secret desires, traumas, and illicit pursuits of high-profile public figures, …highlights tensions and discrepancies between public and private personas, with transgressive desires providing a frequent focal or fissure point.'[7] Because it seeks to pry into the secrets of the 'great', 'celebratory or commemorative' elements are often accompanied by 'irreverent or prurient' impulses.[8] As noted in the introductory chapter, it is precisely the scopophilic drive of such narrative strategies that sustains their allure. While, as Kohlke argues, celebrity biofiction may at times overlap with aspects of the second type, in the main this latter strand, 'biofiction of marginalised subjects', is impelled by a 'revisionary and political' impetus that 'seeks to restore voice to the historically voiceless … [and] commemorates not just the marginalised subjects, but the injustice of their historical disregard and silencing.'[9] 'Appropriated biofiction', the third sub-genre, by contrast, parasitically feeds on historical subjects for entirely self-serving purposes. No longer concerned with the play with authenticity and simulation, it turns its subject matter into what Helen Davies has conceptualized as a 'ventriloquist's puppet' by attributing 'elements of real lives to someone else entirely or us[ing] these lives as springboards to launch into blatantly counterfactual fabrications'.[10] That A.S. Byatt's *Possession* is included in this category is surely overstating the case, but Kohlke – as much as Byatt – raises important questions about the ethics of appropriating factual lives for voyeuristic and fetishistic consumption.

Informed by a desire to ground their representation of Barry in historical, political, psychological or sexological-physiological contexts and as such invested with the (feminist, intersex or trans-inflected) project of recovering forgotten lives, biographical, biodramatic and postmodernist explorations tend to fall into the first two sub-genres, while most biofictions across the time period (Victorian, early and later twentieth century and present-day) are more closely aligned with Kohlke's 'appropriated' stance. An intermediate case that might be called 'mock or parody biofiction' is presented in 'A Mystery Still' of 1867.[11] A short story masquerading as a documentary newspaper report, the tale's claim to presenting a witness account was taken at face value from the start. In the course of a reader correspondence in the *Lancet* in 1895, one of Barry's former senior fellow-officers recalled it as being 'pretty nearly correct', and Ebenezer Rogers, the author of the first full-length novel, which heavily draws on the tale in its reinvention of Barry as Dr. Fitzjames, praised the piece as an 'inspired article' that for a time was the 'talk of the town'.[12] With its multiple genre crossings, the story cuts across Max Saunders's biografictional sub-categories of 'mock-biography' and 'pseudo-biography'. Saunders distinguishes between mock-biografictions that 'adop[t] a pseudo-biographical strategy to parody or satirize' biography and pseudo-biografictions that 'borro[w] biographical form to lend verisimilitude', seeking to 'provide convincing impressions of authentic life-writing'; both forms serve humorous or parodic purposes.[13] Parody is key to 'A Mystery Still': its witty memorialization became the foundation text of the Barry myth.

Building on earlier newspaper reports and letters by Barry's contemporaries published in the wake of his death and on pictorial representations such as a cartoon (which Rachel Holmes attributes to Edward Lear)[14] of an elderly Barry in Corfu and the photograph of Barry in his retirement (Figs. 3.1 and 2.4), 'A Mystery Still' established in readers' minds a vivid impression of the 'queer' little doctor, '[f]rail in body, unique in appearance, and eccentric in manner' who 'ensured respect by his capacity', 'kept a black servant, a serviceable pony, and a small dog called Psyche' and was known for his 'kindness for the poor'.[15] Even if Barry was caricatured as a 'tame imp', the story painted a kinder picture than the anonymous cartoonist.[16]

That the cartoon's satiric depiction focuses on Barry's military dress while dispensing with the companions (the black servant, the pony) that are the staple of the myth from 'A Mystery Still' onward may indicate how powerful a challenge Barry's appropriation of a 'male' uniform and its accessories (the horsehair whip, pointedly flaccid) was felt to be.[17] As Marjorie Garber has noted with reference to Dr. Mary Walker, the US dress reformer who acted as assistant surgeon of the Union Army from 1864, even when nineteenth-century women made no attempt to pass as men, the 'spectacle of women in men's clothes, or at least in men's

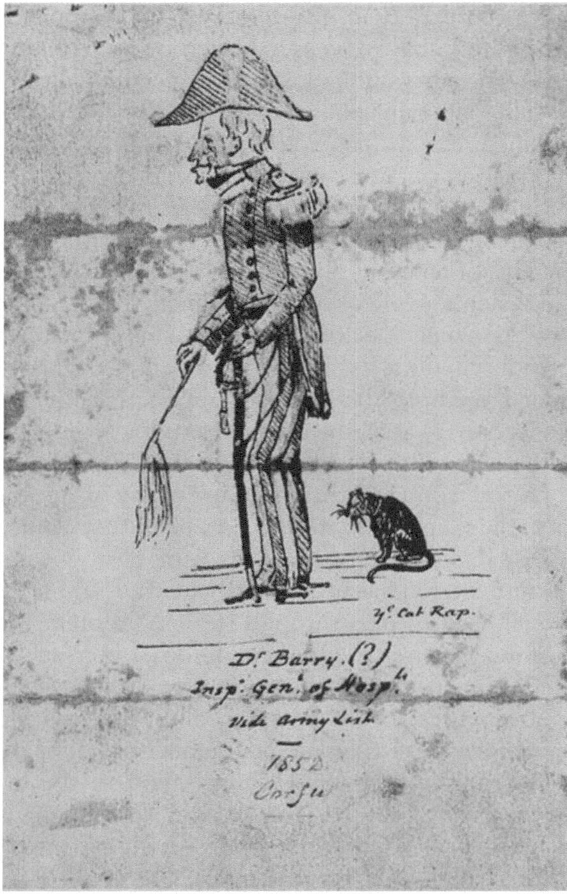

Fig. 3.1 James Barry; portrait, cartoon (L0022269), reproduced courtesy of the Museum of Military Medicine

uniforms' was still considered offensive because it suggested that masculinity and masculine authority in themselves were merely sartorial, accoutrements that could be slipped on, not biological attributes intrinsic to the male body. Walker's self-presentation 'in full masculine apparel, from striped trousers and frock coat to high silk hat', attracted similarly parodic treatment to Barry's.[18]

The resonance and contested nature of images of women in male garments associated with public office is indicated by the publication date of 'A Mystery Still'. The story about a woman's exceptional career in a prototypically masculine domain coincided with parliamentary debates about extending the franchise to women householders on the same terms as men under the Second Reform Act. 'A Mystery Still' preceded by two days John Stuart Mill's speech, on 20 May 1867, urging the House of Commons to amend the bill by replacing 'man' with 'person'.[19] Mill argued that the idea of retaining an artificial 'separation between women's occupations and men's – of forbidding women to take interest in the things which interest men – belong[ed] to a gone-by state of society'.[20] Even more aptly, he cited the example of Elizabeth Garrett who, 'from an honourable desire to employ her activity in alleviating human suffering', had 'knocked successively at all the doors through which, by law, access is obtained into the medical profession' and, with all resolutely shut in her face, found a 'narrow entrance' through the Society of Apothecaries; but 'so objectionable did it appear to that learned body that women should be the medical attendants even of women, that the narrow wicket through which Miss Garrett entered has been closed after her, and no second Miss Garrett will be allowed to pass through it.'[21] 'A Mystery Still' makes a related point: in the absence of legal recognition, subterfuge was the only way for a gifted woman to make her way into the profession, thereby 'effect[ing] ... great cures' for the benefit of all.[22] Placed in the context of Mill's political endeavour to implement equality of opportunity for women, the story makes an implicit contribution to the debate about women's rights by paying tribute to one woman's outstanding capabilities and achievements. This is one of the reasons why it ends with the revelation of Barry's unambiguously female gender.

Primarily, of course, 'A Mystery Still' is about the sheer 'audace', the extraordinary nerve, daring and resourcefulness of the personality in question and about the turns and twists in the plot.[23] As such, it is a story about story-telling, a metafictional tale that reflects on the making of the myth. In the very process of constructing the mythos, the author called satiric attention to the exaggerations and contradictions the Barry story had already started to engender: '[d]espite his shuffling gait, he might have been no more than thirty, although he had been an M.D. nearly twenty-four years!'[24] (It is tempting to identify a Dickensian wit in the turn of this phrase: the temptation in itself, of course, serves as an illustration of the counterfeiting game with 'authentic' and imagined, 'real' and fabricated representations; fittingly, therefore, the satirical exaggeration of Barry's tender age was taken at face value and reproduced as biographical information in later newspaper reports.)[25] In similarly ironic manner, Barry's identity as a gentleman is referenced only to be quantified in relation to his slight build (size and physique here implicitly standing in for sex): 'a gentleman every inch of him: though this is not literally saying very much for him, seeing he was but a little man.'[26] The parodic hyperbole of the text was subsequently misconstrued as factual information; thus Olga Racster and Jessica Grove's play *Dr. James Barry* (1919), Reginald Hargreaves's 1930 Barry chapter in *Women-at-Arms*, June Rose's biography of 1977, *The Perfect Gentleman*, and, more recently, Florida Ann Town's biographically-inflected novel *With a Silent Companion* (1999) echo 'A Mystery Still's' invocation of Barry's odd inconsistencies as a vegetarian who 'abhorred apples and potatoes' as 'filthy roots'.[27]

Perhaps influenced by the earlier first-hand account by Edward Bradford, Deputy-Inspector-General of Hospitals, who in 1865 had issued the only semi-official response to the discovery of Barry's sex, 'A Mystery Still' embellishes the story of Barry's patronage.[28] When calling on readers to take note of the enigma of Barry's origins and identity ('who he was, or what he was, never ceased to be a question of debate'), the text alludes to his high-born friends, ever ready to shield him from the repercussions of his 'irritable temper' and iconoclastic attitude to authority figures, and hints at a blood connection with nobility: 'His influence had been at work for him before he landed. He was released from arrest'.[29] This point would find an echo in biodramas by Racster and Grove in the early and Jean Binnie in the later twentieth century.[30] Rachel Holmes surmises that the Somersets and Beauforts played a significant if covert role in Barry's fortunes, such as when Barry was set free without charge on his forcible return to Britain in 1838: 'Here as elsewhere, when a Somerset appears in Barry's story, official records disappear'.[31]

The text's rhetoric of insinuation left its imprint on late-nineteenth-century accounts by Ebenezer Rogers (Dr Fitzjames is the niece of an earl) and Mark Twain ('she was a daughter of a great English house, and that was why her Cape wilderness brought no punishment') and also influenced turn-of-the-century sexologists (Havelock Ellis, in an echo of the Earl of Albemarle's comments of 1876, refers to Barry as 'the granddaughter of a Scottish laird').[32] In the popular imagination the tale was further embroidered in the early twentieth century. George Edwin Marvell's formulaic sensation story 'The Mystery of the Kapok Doctor', published in 1904 in the Christmas annual of the *Cape Times*, re-invented Barry as Joan Augusta Fitzroy, thus associating her with the Somersets (Lord Charles's brother, Fitzroy Somerset, later Lord Raglan, was a powerful ally for the historical Barry) while at the same time affording her royal origins by turning her into the Prince Regent's illegitimate progeny.[33] This is the implied context for Racster and Grove's melodramatic play of 1919 and later novel *The Journal of Dr. James Barry* of 1932, where a profound mystery hangs over Lady Barrymore's high-born origins that Lord Charles is 'not free to tell'.[34] By contrast, the cocky Assistant Staff-Surgeon of Colonel N.J.C. Rutherford's 'Dr James Barry' (1939) is only too well-aware of his lofty provenance and in his aggressive pursuit of advancement uses every opportunity to boast of 'the blood of princes [that] flows in his veins'.[35]

The story of Barry's parentage sparked by 'A Mystery Still' also inspired implausible conjecture in later twentieth-century biography: June Rose speculates about an illicit affair between Lord Charles Somerset's grandmother, the Bluestocking Frances Boscawen (1719–1805) and the Sea Captain John Barry, James Barry Senior's father, having produced Mary Anne, James Barry Junior's mother, born 'long after [John Barry's] wife had passed childbearing', thus turning the younger James Barry into a niece of Charles Somerset.[36] Rose's biographical suppositions influenced Frederic Mohr's *Barry: Personal Statements* (1984), which adopts the story of Barry's illegitimate roots as the grand-daughter of Mrs. Boscawen.[37] The prevalence of the trope suggests that illegitimacy stands in for gender transgression in the Barry mythology; the measure in which Barry's crossing is perceived as deviant is reflected in the sensationalist pitch of the narrative. Illegitimacy is combined with incest in Binnie's *Colours* (1988/89), which makes Barry the product of a sibling relationship (between her 'Aunt' Isabel and James Barry the painter); inspired by the bohemian irregularity of her family circumstances, the protagonist goes on to conceive two children from altogether four fathers (her first-born, a daughter, is the love-child of her three co-mentors).[38]

Most recently, Michael du Preez and Jeremy Dronfield have sought to identify biographical sources for Barry's reputed child, born (as the layer-out claimed) in Barry's teenage years.[39] This child, they propose, was passed off as Margaret's 'sister' (the existence of a second Bulkley daughter is documented), named Juliana after her great-grandmother (Juliana Barry; a young, unmarried dressmaker called Juliana Bulkley was traced by the biographers as being resident in Cork in 1826).[40] The narrative amplification of this sub-plot to the Barry story offers an ironic comment on Ina Schabert's and more recently Michael Lackey's differentiation between biography's focus on 'accurate representation' and biofiction's foregrounding of 'imaginative creation': the 'imaginative reasoning of a writer of fictional biography', Schabert argues, 'tends to be much bolder than that of the biographer'.[41] Barry biographilia exemplifies consistently that such generic demarcations cannot be upheld. For as du Preez and Dronfield contend, Juliana Bulkley was the product of rape, by Margaret's uncle, Mary Anne's delinquent brother Redmond Barry. Redmond found refuge with the Bulkleys in 1802 but committed some offence so loathsome that he was 'run ... out of town on a rail' by them a year later. The collapse of the Bulkley family shortly after is attributed primarily to this catastrophe, which changed Margaret's life forever. Small wonder, perhaps, if she assumed a male persona, given that a 'normal' development (love, marriage, and a family) had been wrecked for her.[42]

Given the biographilic impetus for sensation, Barry cuts a singularly sad figure as a gender transgressor. It is striking that, reminiscent of Thackeray's ironic narrative method in *Vanity Fair*, the Barry puppet of 'A Mystery Still' is granted a happier trajectory than is the case elsewhere since he is, for the greatest part of the story, cast as the agent of his destiny.[43] Ultimately the text constructs the persona of a swaggering daredevil who 'defied the rules of the [military] service with impunity', as when, faced with disciplinary action at having deserted his post and returned to Britain without leave of absence, he 'coolly' claimed that he 'ha[d] come home to have [his] hair cut.'[44] There is a hint of Austen's Frank Churchill here that intimates concealed business of some kind.[45] The factual Barry, while posted as Staff-Surgeon in Mauritius, did return to Britain without official leave in 1829 on hearing of Lord Charles's serious illness, and attended Somerset until his death in 1831.[46] The parodic fictionalization of the incident in the anecdote of the haircut is echoed throughout Barry life-writing, from Ebenezer Rogers's *A Modern Sphinx* (1881), Racster and Grove's play, Rutherford's 'Dr. James Barry' (1939) and novel versions of the early twentieth century through Elizabeth Longford's historical account in *Eminent Victorian Women* (1981) to Anne and Ivan Kronenfeld's biofiction *The Secret Life of Dr. James Miranda Barry* (2000), the *Oxford Dictionary of National Biography* entry of 2004 and du Preez and Dronfield's 2016 biography.[47] The trope is so well-established that it has spawned its own twists; in Binnie's *Colours* it is Joseph, 'Jane' Barry's faithful black servant, who comes up with the story, to the great amusement of the authorities, thereby securing his master's acquittal in the court-martial.[48]

Like the myth itself, and like Barry biographilia more generally, 'A Mystery Still' is marked by conceptual and generic instability. The story starts with a psychologically insightful point about Barry 'afford[ing] a good illustration of the triumph of mind over matter'[49] and continues by dramatizing his highly idiosyncratic character, raising probing questions about his background. This is followed by a movingly realistic sense of the urgency with which Barry, struck down by serious illness, appealed to a friend to ensure his body would be buried in his clothes, without a physical examination (an anecdote co-opted from Edward Bradford's account).[50] Yet the piece ends on a note of sentimental fabrication that is at variance with the previous rhetoric of mockery which undercut the clichés that were in circulation about Barry: 'his reasons for leaving England were very sad: a broken-off engagement with a young and beautiful creature'.[51] Intriguingly, this reference to a romantic entanglement is followed by an allusion to Barry's hidden female body swathed in layers of towels.[52] Does this suggest, then, that the love affair was actually of a same-sex nature, or does the 'young and beautiful creature' reference a man (in analogy to 'Dr Barry's wife' in the placard affair)?[53] In a similar manner, the story's reference to the doctor's insistence on 'periodical blood-lettings either by leeches or lancet' stands in odd contrast to the real-life Barry's medical practice: one of his first reforms was to do away with leeches and bleeding.[54] After the deathbed revelation of Barry's sex, the text closes on a dramatic finale that invokes the conventions of the fable:

> A nobleman's valet came for the [dog]; settled accounts with Black John, even to giving him the return passage-money to the island whence he came; and no one has since appeared claiming any relationship with the eccentric being, who was even more mysterious in death than in life.[55]

The sentimental desire for narrative closure provided by this fairytale ending haunts Barry biography of the twentieth century: the scene is related as a contemporary witness account in Hargreaves's *Women-at-Arms* and as hearsay in Isobel Rae's *The Strange Story of Dr. James Barry*, where it is complemented by a companion tale about a mysterious black box Barry had deposited with the McCrindles, friends in Kingston, Jamaica, and which, according to their son (writing to the *Glasgow Herald* in 1949, 84 years after the event) was collected in equally enigmatic fashion: 'a body servant, a black soldier, called at my parents' house … and told them that a footman in livery called at the hotel and took away the black box'.[56] McCrindle's family anecdote having become Rae's addition to 'A Mystery Still's' fable is further embellished in Rose's *Perfect Gentleman*: here it is not one but 'two footmen in gorgeous livery' who 'called at the lodgings … and removed all her belongings – including her poodle … her diamond ring and the mysterious black box. Her Negro servant apparently went back to Jamaica, his passage paid by an unknown benefactor.'[57] Rachel Holmes, while discussing the gifts Barry made to the McCrindles, is the only biographer to dispense with the romance of the footman and the black box.[58]

In contrast, du Preez and Dronfield's *Dr. James Barry* adds yet more flourish to the mythodrama by speculating that the black box may have contained intimate letters from Lord Charles that the Somersets would have wanted to secure. The biography concludes by supplementing the retrieved box, its secret forever guarded, with another container that yields the sensational: Barry's Ghost of Femininity Past. When Barry's battered travelling trunk, having been passed on after his death to his agents' manager, coincidentally called Mr. Barrie, was opened, it revealed 'a collage of fashion plates clipped from ladies' magazines – a parade of gowns, crinolines, bonnets, hats and coiffures pasted to the musty leather: a catalogue of loss and longing.'[59] Surely a biographer's extravaganza if ever there was one: the spectacular discovery of evidential material that corroborates conjectures of Barry's lifelong desire to recover his lost femininity throws into relief the urgency of the biographilic impulse that seeks to return the crosser to the counterfeit of conventional gender normativity.[60]

As the nineteenth century came to a close, the sentimental turn in 'A Mystery Still' that would see a revival in later twentieth-century and contemporary renditions was refracted into different narrative directions. Mark Twain, who enjoyed crossing gender boundaries in his own fiction, offered readers a North-American inflection of the tale when he had Barry, after disgracing herself with her aristocratic family in the old world, 'cho[o]se to change her name and her sex and take a new start in the [new] world.'[61] In American frontier style the newly masculinized Barry becomes a 'duel[list] of a desperate sort' who 'killed his man'.[62] As John Leigh notes, Twain was divided between satirizing what he regarded as 'sham-duels' (duels not intended to result in the death of either of the combatants) and admiring 'real' duels, fought unto death; the latter exerted a 'singular fascination' on his imagination.[63] That his Barry does not recoil from risking his own and taking another man's life enhances his virility while paradoxically adding to his moral credentials. To counterbalance these aggressive tendencies and ease the transition of his narrative from the 'wild young fellow' with 'plenty of pretty girls … none of [whom] could get hold of his heart' to the 'daughter of a great English house', Twain references, as the apex of Barry's 'mastership of his profession', the Caesarian section he conducted, 'sav[ing] both mother and child'. Textually, the birth of the child also delivers up the woman in the male impersonator: 'It was then discovered that he was *a woman*.'[64]

Barry's feminization was not solely the work of male writers, however; late-century feminists, too, were at pains to normalize women who passed as men while co-opting their cross-dressing acts for the political struggle for equal rights. The transgender potential hinted at fleetingly in the 'queer' Doctor James of 'A Mystery Still' and in Twain's dandy-duelist is played out in the crossed desires that girls performing boys could arouse in their hapless male friends, but in the women themselves it is neutralized in their protest against their social, educational and professional dispossession. This is illustrated in Sarah Grand's bestselling New Woman novel of 1893, *The Heavenly Twins*. In Grand's text one of the titular twins, the tomboyish Angelica, thwarted in her artistic and intellectual ambitions, assumes the guise of her twin brother Theodore, nicknamed Diavolo. When her identity is revealed to the stunned musician she has befriended, and as the recognition dawns on him that he has been falling in love with the boy that never was, she denies that she ever had any romantic interest in him; instead, what prompted her to take up her disguise was the need to set herself free, physically, mentally, and artistically. '[H]aving once assumed the character', she tells him,

> it came naturally: and the freedom from restraint, I mean the restraint of our tight uncomfortable clothing, was delicious. I tell you I was a genuine boy. I moved like boy, I felt like a boy; I was my own brother in very truth. Mentally and morally, I was exactly what you thought me[.][65]

It is boyhood, rather than manhood, that liberates the girl. Neither a girl denied the right to self-determination nor an adult man burdened with responsibilities, the boy is the embodiment of transgender fluidity *par excellence*. Here the counterfeit, because it is self-fashioned, is a reflection of the creative agency and imaginative capacity of the artist: as Angelica points out, her boyhood self (like all selves) is essentially a performance, the 'exercise of the actor's faculty', and as such also comparable to the act of 'creat[ing] a character as an author does in a book'.[66] If becoming a boy is coterminous with coming into full possession of one's faculties, crucially, it is also equated with the freedom to assume a professional or artistic role of one's choice (a middle-class wife, Angelica is prevented from pursuing her interest in public musical performance which, dressed as a boy, she is able partially to realize). To vindicate herself for the deception she practised on her friend, she invokes two role models: the writer and artist George Sand and the 'Inspector General of the Army Medical Department', Dr. James Barry.[67] In order to attain a position of authority in a world governed by men, Grand implies, a woman had to embrace a male persona even if, as in the case of Barry, this might entail an impersonation so permanent that the mask eventually grew into the flesh. Yet this had nothing to do with any kind of transgressive sexual disposition; rather, it was entirely bound up with the quest for artistic self-realization and the struggle for sex and gender equality.

In contradistinction to Grand, fellow New Woman writer Ménie Muriel Dowie asserted that 'there [was] no longer any need for [women] to put on the garb of men in order to live, to work, to achieve, to breathe the outer air'.[68] Yet her edition of women warriors' memoirs, published in the same year as Grand's novel, indicates the strong symbolic meaning she too attached to historical instances of female cross-dressing. Like Grand, she emphasized modern women's sexual self-sufficiency and focus on their professional self-development, establishing an explicit juxtaposition between the earlier women's 'coarse grimy sensuality' and love of 'being ever at masquerade' that drove their swashbuckling pursuit of adventure and the much more serious-minded, morally upright and educated New Woman who, impelled by a 'fine purpose', wished to make a contribution to the world as a 'social regenerator'.[69] In castigating women warriors for their dependence on men, Dowie downplayed their use of romantic expediency narratives to justify their assumption of male personas. As Grand's reference to James Barry indicates, this was a much more congenial example of male impersonation.

The Amazon in men's attire remained an important part of feminist iconography and took on key significance for the suffragettes in the early twentieth century. Though Cicely Hamilton's *Pageant of Great Women* (1909) omitted Barry from its line-up of women warriors (Christian Davies, Hannah Snell, Mary Anne Talbot), probably because no female name could be attached to the personality (today Barry does make an appearance in suffrage history),[70] it was precisely the lack of accounting for an exceptional woman that is likely to have fired up the distinguished actress Sibyl Thorndike's enthusiasm for taking on the lead role in Racster and Grove's play.[71] In response to the traditional narrative that sought to stabilize Barry's gender crossing by motivating it with reference to a romantic entanglement (the 'follow your man' trope that earlier women cross-dressers had invoked in their memoirs), early twentieth-century feminists like Racster and Grove constructed Barry as a woman compelled by an unhappy marriage to sacrifice her wish for a conventional life to the advancement of an independent career.[72]

The endeavour to clear Barry of any imputation of selfishness by locating the origin of her move into medical studies and a public life in adverse domestic circumstances sometimes led to Barry serving as a tool to denigrate feminism as sex-starved neurosis. In Hargreaves's 1930 account, Barry constitutes 'an almost perfect example of the penalties to which Nature condemns the individual who seeks to impose a deliberate condition of frustration upon the urge towards a perfectly normal expression of that individual's sexual life'.[73] Invoking the longstanding cliché of an early disappointment in love, Hargreaves came to the (in the absence of any evidence) startling conclusion that '[w]ith the temperament of an odalisque, [Barry] forced herself to the restraint of an anchorite, with what consequences to nervous fibre and energy her frequent outbreaks into unreasonable querulousness bear abundant, if pathetic witness'.[74] Hargreaves' portrait of Barry as a cantankerous misanthrope whose unhappiness derives from sexual repression has some resonances with George Moore's early twentieth-century novella 'Albert Nobbs' (1918/1927) about a cross-dressing head waiter in a Dublin hotel. Ever fascinated by the strange turns that frustrated desire could take, and with a particularly keen interest in repression and sexual pathology, Moore was much more supportive of women's rights than Hargreaves, but he too saw sexual self-denial, in women and men, as the root of all evil.

Moore's eponymous hero/ine Albert takes up her disguise partly because of unrequited love but, more crucially, to escape sexual harassment and poverty. As a male waiter Albert can make multiple times the starvation wage he earned as a woman and even set aside a store for bad times. Henceforth all emotional life is replaced with income generation. Both money and feelings are stashed away until a chance encounter with a transman, the happily married house painter Hubert Page, leads Albert to realize the extent of his desolate state. Lonely and cut off from life, condemned to 'live without man or without woman, thinking like a man and feeling like a woman', Albert is 'neither man nor woman, just a perhapser'.[75] The story ends badly when Albert's failure to secure a wife culminates in death. His posthumous exposure as an imposter has repercussions also on Hubert who, by now a widower, finds himself propelled into a return to femininity and heteronormative marriage.

If commentators like Hargreaves co-opted early twentieth-century sexual science and its recognition of female desire in order to pathologize feminism, and experimental writers like Moore approached gender migration primarily through a psycho-sexual lens, sexologists, like fin-de-siècle feminists, dissociated cross-dressing from sexual desire. Whereas feminists focused on female transvestism as a means to an end (professional and economic self-realization; a life of one's own), sexologists directed attention to crossing as an end in itself: transgender identity. Magnus Hirschfeld, in his study on *Transvestites* (1910), defined the yearning to inhabit the outer garments and inner self of the opposite sex as an 'independent complex ... which cannot be ordered according to recognized models' such as fetishism or auto-eroticism, emphasizing that it 'must be considered separately' from sexual orientation.[76] His anecdotal synopsis of 'Miss Anne Barry's' life refers to Barry's 'sharp tongue', conflict with the authorities, and duel but offers no interpretation of the case.[77] Havelock Ellis's similarly brief discussion, though almost entirely derivative of earlier sources such as 'A Mystery Still' and the Earl of Albemarle's memoirs, concludes that '[t]here is no indication of any sexual tendency in her history, whether heterosexual or homosexual, and we may believe that, as is fairly common in this psychic anomaly, the sexual impulse was not strong, and, therefore, easy to divert and sublimate in this transformation.'[78] To sexologists, cross-gender performance was in itself a libidinal drive. In Ellis's words,

> A man who 'plays a part' during the greater part of his active life and continues to play it long after the active phase of his life is over, plays it, moreover, with such ability and success that no one suspects the 'masquerade,' is, we may be sure, fulfilling a deep demand of his own nature.[79]

Barry's story is embedded in *Eonism* (1928, vol. VII of Ellis's *Psychology of Sex*) and preceded by a much more detailed account of the gender-fluid Charles-Geneviève, the Chevalier D'Éon de Beaumont (1728–1810). The Chevalier inspired Ellis's conceptualization of what he had previously called 'sexo-aesthetic inversion', a term he ultimately found as 'unsatisfactory' as Hirschfeld's 'transvestism': the latter was 'altogether inadequate, since a longing to wear the garments of the other sex is only one of the traits exhibited, and in some cases it is scarcely or not at all found', while the former 'may wrongly suggest that we are here concerned with homosexuality, though that is usually not present'.[80] Rather, 'Eonism' defined a psychological condition 'in which the subject more or less identifies himself or herself with the opposite sex, not merely in dress, but in general tastes, in ways of acting, and in emotional disposition.'[81]

In sex/gender inversion of Barry, the Chevalier was 'commonly regarded as a woman', but after death found to be an anatomical male. The parallels to Barry are striking: 'He was of nervous disposition but restless and adventurous, courageous and full of energy, even quarrelsome and irascible. He became one of the best swordsmen of his time … Though sometimes lacking in judgment, he was of high intelligence and sagacity … He appears to have had no known sexual relationships either with women or men, notwithstanding various romantic legends which circulated concerning him'.[82] For all these similarities, D'Éon was in fact, in modern terms, a 'transcender' to Barry's passer.[83] In contradistinction to Barry, D'Éon throve on the performance of gender fluidity. Since D'Éon presented her/himself alternately in both sexes and refused to identify either as the 'true' identity, to the point of prompting bets and court suits being placed on the question, s/he proved considerably more unnerving to contemporaries, so much so that her/his sex was officially declared female in Britain, prompting Louis XVI to follow suit; on returning to France, D'Éon was forced by royal edict to live as a woman. While this differentiates D'Éon's from Barry's experience, in both cases 'exile, or repatriation – geographical displacement' was, Garber notes, 'directly linked to gender "determination," the erasure of ambiguity.'[84]

As the examples discussed indicate, Barry life-writing addresses this ambiguity in different ways: by inventing an elaborate story of origins as in Marvell's 'The Mystery of the Kapok Doctor', or by imaginatively filling out what is known of Barry's life in order to bring the inner person to life. In this respect, 'A Mystery Still' and Barry biographies can be placed in the context of the two approaches Kohlke defines within the celebrity strand of biofictional writing, 'tunnelling' and 'infilling'. Tunnelling, she argues, '"fleshes out" a life with alternative competing versions and counter-identities', whereas infilling consists in 'writing someone a missing interior life … Put differently, one asks of its subjects: who were they *really*? The other asks: who *were* they?'[85] Given the impenetrability, for early biographers like Rae and Rose, of who Barry was, his black box and footmen may be intended to meet the demands of recovering a family and emotional ties for Barry, to bestow on him the 'happy ending', albeit posthumously, that he is deemed to have deserved so as to obviate the punitive message inherent in a life spent on medical and humanitarian reform that terminated in lonely and insanitary death followed by sensational public exposure. The desire for elaboration and the desire for alternative scripts go hand in hand and are therefore incorporated simultaneously in many of the texts: hence the consistent shifts in narrative modes in 'A Mystery Still'. In the case of the most recent biography, on the other hand, the amplified story of 'Margaret's' inner life constructs a Freudian figure of mourning and self-estrangement that more closely resembles George Moore's sad and withdrawn 'outcast from both sexes' than the successful professional who still had a private life with friends and a substitute family. As in Moore's 'Albert Nobbs' novella, this other Barry finds that 'the clothes she wore smothered the woman in her; she no longer thought and felt as she used to when she wore petticoats, and she didn't think and feel like a man though she wore trousers. What was she? Nothing, neither man nor woman, so small wonder she was lonely.'[86] The crosser's sense of feeling cut off from others is a frequent lament in Barry biographilia; Albert's sentiments find an eacho in Binnie's *Colours*.[87]

Not all reinventions of Barry are necessarily of the empathetic kind; the early fictions in particular construct a heavily clichéd character. Kohlke's third type of fictional life-writing, 'appropriated biofiction', and her differentiation between 'glossed' and 'divergent or alternative' biofiction of the 'appropriating' kind offers a useful further paradigm. 'Glossed' biofiction draws on 'made-up characters and plots, which are nonetheless extensively modelled on famous historical subjects, their lives, writings and/or art'. The primary objective of 'glossed' biofiction, Kohlke contends, is not to shed greater or new light on historical subjects but to '"raid" individual histories for raw materials, distilling a quasi "essence" of past personalities and providing a short-hand stereotypical gloss on memorable/scandalous aspects of their lives and times'.[88] The factual individual in this way becomes a type. Examples of such flat character presentation can be found in early twentieth-century Barry biographilia, Racster and Grove's play (the subsequent novel with its first-person narrator presents a more individualized figure) and Réné Juta's *Cape Currey* (1920). While in these texts the characters are nominally based on Barry, Lord Charles, his daughter Georgina, and Cloete, the plots are only loosely related to historical events. Thus *Cape Currey* places the 'placard affair' and the commission of inquiry into Somerset's conduct in the context of a tale about crossed desire, fiery Amazons, bar fights, and exotic adventure in an atmospheric South African landscape setting, and Racster and Grove draw on Barry's humanitarian concern for the treatment of prisoners and lepers and dismissal of unqualified apothecaries to add corruption, arms dealing and a roué's designs on Barry's providentially recovered step-sister Lavinia.

In 'appropriated' biographilia Barry is flattened to a stereotype, as illustrated in Marvell's 'The Mystery of the Kapok Doctor' (the titular kapok refers to the material with which the coat was padded to give the wearer the appearance of a more masculine build). In a story-line heavily over-invested in cliché, the infant that is to become Barry is snatched from the bosom of her loving and cruelly betrayed mother one winter's night in the wake of Christmas (the mother duly dies of a broken heart). Abducted by a muffled man with a gold signet ring (the ring, like the box, are signifiers of Barry's superior pedigree), the child is taken to a secret location where she is carefully educated for the next decade and a half until at sixteen her parentage is revealed to her by persons unknown, after which, in a confrontation with her father, the Prince Regent, she declares that, in memory of her mother's tragic fate, she will 'abjure womanhood' and 'appear henceforward before the world as a man' so as to 'win a name for [her]self no matter where, no matter how'.[89] Her royal patronage protects her on her journeys. In the Cape the allure she exerts on women causes her to become embroiled in a number of sword-fought duels; Cloete is here recast as Lieutenant Mannering. Somerset does not know her secret but acts as her patron in the hope of royal favours; they fall out when Barry champions the freedom of the South African press. This Barry only briefly comes to the semblance of life in his dalliance with Aletta, a young Boer woman who is also the object of Mannering's desire (and who after the duel becomes Mannering's wife).

Marvell's Barry throws herself into a life of adventure and thrives on her assumption of a male identity: 'I forgot my womanhood. I became more truly a man than a woman.'[90] And yet the materiality of the body always threatens to rupture the masquerade, however accomplished; an elderly lady patient comments on Barry's gentle hand and feminine powers of empathy and to a military colleague he 'look[s] more like a woman than a man.'[91] Appropriated biographilia essentializes the body, whose inexorable laws always end by disciplining the spirit of the impersonator. This is also manifested in Racster and Grove's protagonist, a reluctantly cross-dressing damsel in distress whose show of masculine prowess in battling a fraudster culminates in a hysterical weeping fit behind closed doors:

> ... (Sobs louder and is evidently hysterical)
> (A knocking is heard at the door)
> SOMERSET: Lord madam! Pull yourself together. This is awful. Think of the rascal thoughts these men will have if they find you like this.
> (Barry sobs without ceasing while the knocks continues [*sic*]. Finally LORD CHARLES HENRY SOMERSET picks BARRY up in his arms and distractedly carries her off left. ENTER CAPT. KEPPEL centre. He looks round in surprise and gives a suggestive whistle).[92]

Barry's *impromptu* sword fight with an embezzler after he made lewd remarks about a female friend, Lavinia (who in her capacity – unbeknown to others – as Barry's step-sister acts as an alter ego and a reminder of herself as a woman) thus serves to throw into relief the fragility of Barry's performance of masculinity. Having wounded (penetrated) her adversary, Barry collapses into feminine hysteria as her 'real self' reclaims possession of her body. Femininity is equated to infantilism, and she is carried offstage by Somerset, her protector, who knows her 'true' identity as Lady Barrymore. That the scene is witnessed, and misinterpreted, by an outsider (Captain Keppel, the future Lord Albemarle) offers an implicit gloss on the factual sodomy libel, which consequently appears grossly misconstrued.

Similarly, in Juta's *Cape Currey*, Barry's male façade crumbles in the course of two duels, though the primary reason for the demise of her manhood under the onslaught of her 'overstrained nerves' is the exposure of her most guarded secret.[93] Since the third-person narrative offers readers little insight into Barry's thoughts and we are increasingly distanced from the character the more Georgina comes into focus, Barry assumes an ever more wooden appearance; the pull 'he' exerts on the much more animated and individualized Georgina seems implausible. In the final part of the novel Barry is altogether drained of life as, in brusque succession, she is cast into extravagant Gothic and sensation scenarios. The text perpetuates the myth of the woman who sacrificed everything for the man she loved, whom she followed 'all over the world', only to be settled with an ailing son whose physical condition reflects the father's moral corruption – a lurid adaptation of Mary Shelley's Frankensteinian script of the monstrous progeny that is born from gender misappropriation.[94]

The real-life Barry's humanitarian concern for the welfare of lepers is here co-opted for sensational overkill. Barry's 'real' secret is not so much her female sex (which Georgina detects much earlier after Barry is wounded in a duel) as the existence of a beautiful but leprous son, looked after by mute servants and confined to a remote house by the hills, where he is discovered by Georgina's Amazonian friend Aletta.[95] As the woman and the youth are about to embrace, he is shot dead by a servant to prevent infection. The bandages that conceal the son's diseased flesh invoke the cloths that hide Barry's female body, signalling an equally 'diseased' condition. Unsurprisingly, Barry is desperate to 'lay down his … burden, all the play acting over, all the strain, … working the whole of the life'.[96] After a second duel, when Cloete accidentally uncovers her sex and is sworn to secrecy, Barry is so world-weary and defeated that, like Lady Barrymore in Racster and Grove's play, she too has to be carried off.[97] The most enduring impression the reader retains of *Cape Currey* is that of the fainting Barry, the secret of whose body has been divested of its male cover – an image indicative of a text that disintegrates into what can be called 'sensation biofiction'.

Sensation is a recurrent mode of Barry life-writing. The first bionovel on Barry, Ebenezer Rogers's *A Modern Sphinx* (1881), falls into this category, though sensation fiction 'proper' had well passed its prime by the 1880s. The titular invocation of the sphinx serves to appeal to readerly tastes for the exotic; colonial adventures take up considerable space in the narrative. Half lion, half woman; seductive, inscrutable and threatening all at once: the sphinx also stands for the mix of sentiments – fascination tinged with fear, desire with dread – prompted by the gender crosser.[98] An example of sensation biofiction, *A Modern Sphinx* can be placed into Kohlke's model of 'divergent or alternative biofiction', that is biofiction that takes the process of fabulation further than the 'glossed' variety, prompting questions about the ethics of '[r]epurposing real lives for … sensational effects'. Biofiction of such inflection, Kohlke argues, constitutes 'a vampiric and cannibalistic enterprise … the stealing of a voice, life, and identity rather than a body'; this is the grave-robbing enterprise depicted in James's *The Aspern Papers*.[99] The moral justification for such appropriation, Rogers implied in public correspondence, derived from his personal knowledge of the subject. As a young officer, he had met Barry on board a ship and claimed that, since they had served together in the West Indies, he 'had particular opportunities of observing her habits'; in letters to the *Lancet* in 1895 and the introduction to the (third) 1896 edition of his novel he cited other senior officers who had known Barry in support of his portrait.[100] But in constructing his narrative version of Barry he drew exclusively on existing tropes.

The publication history of Rogers's novel offers insight into the way in which Barry was made over into marketable produce in order to sell something other than his own story. Featured as the crabby Principal Medical Officer Dr. Fitzjames, Barry, up until the final volume, is a side kick to an elaborate sensation plot about the mysterious origin and attempted seduction of a mixed-race girl, interwoven with a complicated narrative of colonial corruption and lost and reclaimed inheritances. Despite Rogers's conviction that 'the mere fact that Dr Barry's career is touched on ought to ensure readers', the novel did not take off. Though it was 'extensively advertised at the time of publication', he had to concede in January 1882 that it had 'failed to produce interest.' A 'cheap edition', he was sure, 'would sell well; as this is not, however, the opinion of Mr Maxwell [the publisher]', he mournfully commented, 'my work is doomed to die.'[101] Evidently, however, he was able to change Maxwell's mind, and to persuade Mary Braddon (Maxwell's long-standing partner and since 1874 his wife) to lend a helping hand into the bargain, for the novel was reissued later that year as *Madeline's Mystery,* having been edited down into one volume by Braddon. If, fifteen years earlier, *Saunders's News-Letter* had proclaimed the material too much to handle even for the Queen of Sensation herself, now a triumphant Rogers was elated to announce that 'Miss Braddon has, in fact, *dared*!'[102]

For all of Rogers's excitement, however, Braddon did not make that much of an intervention. Her amendments mainly concern a tightening of the plot narrative and, intriguingly, a toning down of some of the more suggestive and challenging aspects of the story.[103] Thus the erotic allure of mixed-race women is contained, the Creole heroine is racially purified in name, and an allusive bed-share scene in which the exposure of the doctor's secret is prevented by his dog attacking a fellow-officer who attempts to 'slip quietly under the mosquito-net' next to his master is dropped from *Madeline's Mystery,* thus purging the original narrative of its play with the homosocial implications of the passage.[104] Braddon, it appears, exercised editorial control not to amplify but to restrain potentially subversive subject matter.[105]

Even Braddon's brand was not enough to make a success of the novel. When public interest in Barry resurfaced fourteen years later in a reader correspondence in the *Lancet,* Rogers seized his moment and, after drawing attention to the earlier incarnations of his book and Braddon's contribution, had the remainder of his original sets bound into a one-volume illustrated 'de luxe' edition (1896) which he then advertised to the *Lancet* correspondents, taking care this time to make the connection between Fitzjames and Barry explicit: 'You are aware that my novel, "A Modern Sphinx" (Dr. James Barry or Fitzjames) ... has been republished in one volume, with seven illustrations ... application for which should be addressed to me'.[106] The inclusion of portraits of Barry here serves the 'trailer' function that Julia Thomas has identified as a constituent part of Victorian illustration.[107] To make sure readers could not possibly overlook the context, the frontispiece (Fig. 3.2) reproduces a Barry prototype that provides a visual reinforcement of the textual representation of Fitzjames as a 'caricature of a man'.[108] In their shared emphasis on the comic clash

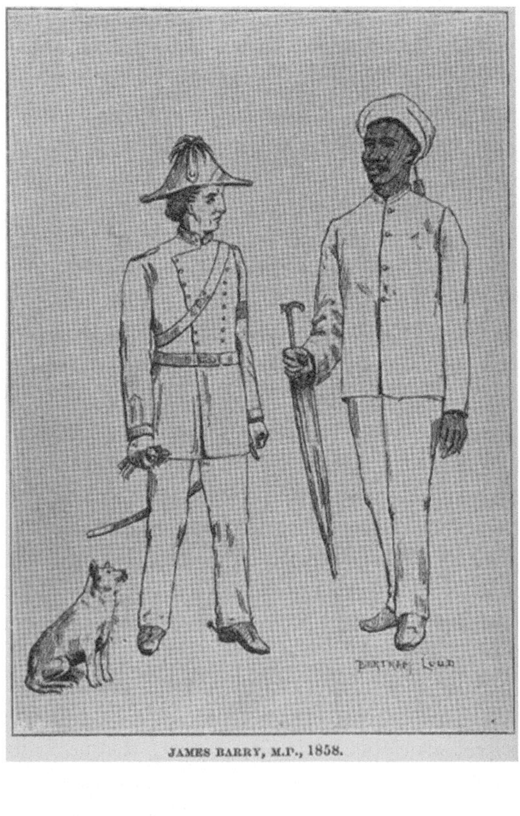

Fig. 3.2 © The Library Board: C.194.a.672 Frontispiece: 'James Barry, M.D., 1858' [also referenced as 'James Barry (with servant and dog) by Bertram Loud'], Ebenezer Rogers, *A Modern Sphinx* (De luxe edition, 1896), reproduced courtesy of the British Library

between the doctor's diminutive size and his excessive display of military regalia, text and image mimic earlier representations in 'A Mystery Still' and the Corfu caricature (Fig. 3.1):

> [T]here, ... feeling his way very gingerly along the fresh-washed decks, was Dr. Fitzjames in full uniform, with cocked-hat shrouding his shrivelled features and a tunic that seemed to bury his small frame out of sight, while a big sword rattled in its brass scabbard in consonance with big brass spurs affixed to his two-inch heels, and in his hand he carried a huge umbrella, overshadowing the *tout ensemble*...[109]

In adaptation of 'A Mystery Still', Fitzjames's uncertain sex is displaced into a play with the gender associations of umbrella and sword that foregrounds the former (femininity), while the latter dangles behind his legs. The illustration adds the other two staple ingredients of the myth, the black servant and the poodle (here recast as a terrier).

The positioning of doctor, servant and poodle replicates the extant photograph of the historical Barry (see Fig. 2.4); the caption explicitly references Barry rather than his novelistic alter ego Fitzjames. In his third attempt at pitching himself as an author, Rogers was at pains to authenticate his work with visual references to documentary material. His remediation of the Barry trope in its turn came to inspire later work. The cover of Isobel Rae's *Strange Story* is manifestly indebted to Rogers's frontispiece and almost assumes the semblance of a follow-on still with its opened umbrella and Barry's more expansive body language (Fig. 3.3). As a source text, *A Modern Sphinx* is thereby accorded a measure of the 'authenticity' that Rogers so aspired to, while the first biography, by inference, takes on aspects of a fiction sequel.

A second illustration in *A Modern Sphinx* (Fig. 3.4) is adapted from a cameo portrait of Barry. This Barry is featured with elongated eyebrows and lips shaped into a diffident (sphinx-like?) smile, lending him a more feminine facial impression than the original miniature on which the image is modelled (Fig. 3.5). As Rogers duly noted, the portrait highlighted 'the unmistakeable [*sic*] female characteristics of Barry's features.'[110]

With the link between Fitzjames and Barry firmly established, the text employs the full battery of Barry clichés: 'Bombastic in speech and repellent in manner', Dr. Fitzjames is a teetotaller and vegetarian who in order to have access to fresh milk at all times insists on travelling with his goat.[111]

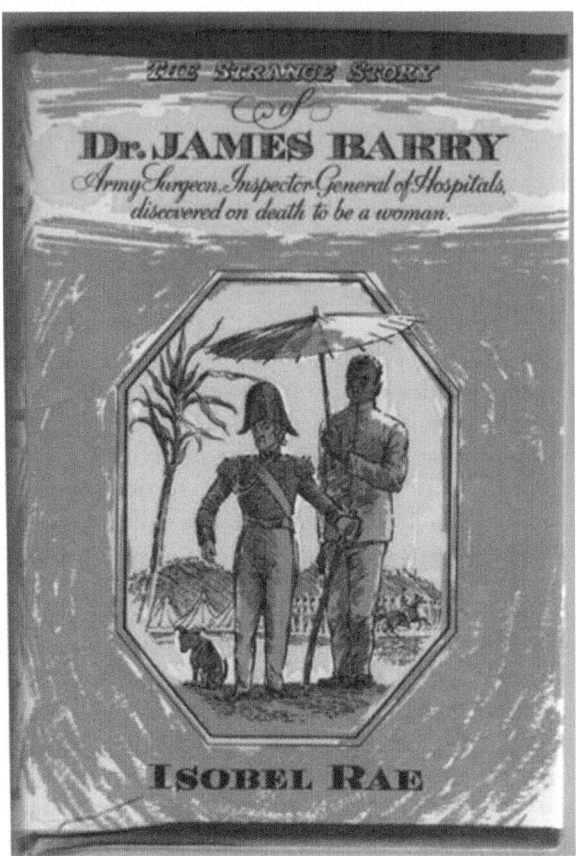

Fig. 3.3 Cover of the first biography, Isobel Rae's *The Strange Story of Dr. James Barry* (Longman's, Green and Co, 1958)[112]

But for all his oddities he is singularly popular with the ladies and sought after for his 'social attainments'.[113] While respected for his superior medical knowledge and the nurturing care he bestows on ailing patients, he is resented for his pomposity and the patronage he enjoys in high places, a privilege that has secured him fast-track promotion over others. His attachment to outdated codes of behaviour makes him into 'one of these fossils that have survived the duelling age'; after being injured in one such ritualistic exchange, he sequestered himself and would not permit

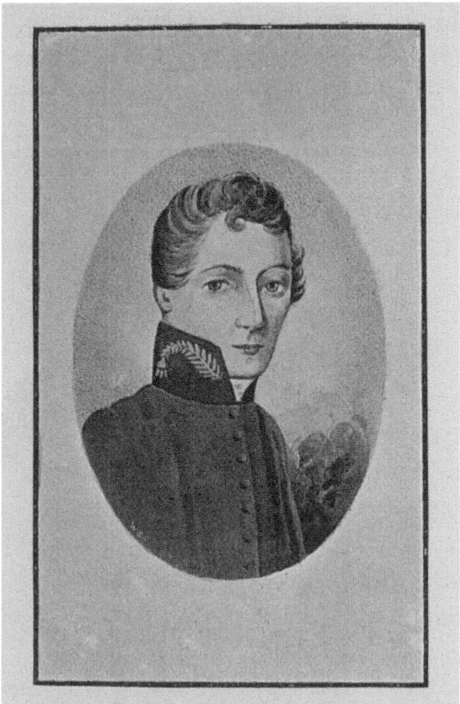

Fig. 3.4 © The Library Board: C.194.a.672: 'James Barry, M.D., 1834' [also referenced as 'Jms. Barry, from Netley Hospital Mess'], illustration 3 in Ebenezer Rogers, *A Modern Sphinx* (De luxe edition, 1896), I, p. 185, reproduced courtesy of the British Library

examination of his wound.[114] This display of bravery was, however, followed by apparent cowardice when he subsequently refused to take up another challenge even though his reputation was at stake (in the novel it is this refusal to honour the rites of manly conduct that leads to his arrest and forcible return to Britain). As one of the characters exclaims, 'What a curious mixture of frivolity, arrogance, cleverness, exclusiveness, and sociability went to make up that man's character'.[115]

Even more than in *Cape Currey*, Barry/Fitzjames is marginalized in the text and only assigned a more significant role in the last volume, when he becomes a key agent in the resolution of the dis/inheritance story. The plot is heavily co-opted from Victorian sensation fiction and melodrama, crossed with what Elaine Showalter has called 'King Romance', the imperial adventure story.[116] Set in the tropical environment of British Guiana

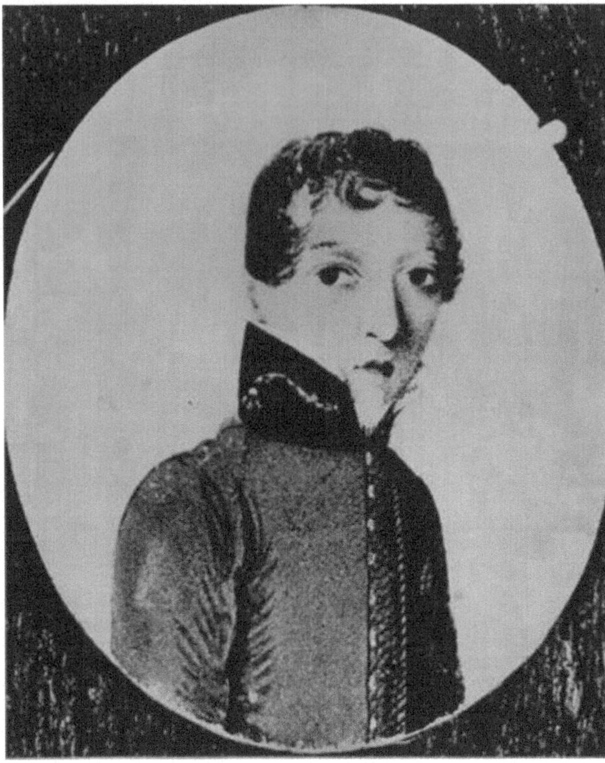

Fig. 3.5 James Barry; portrait, youth (L0022263), reproduced courtesy of the Museum of Military Medicine

(close to the Windward and Leeward Islands where the factual Barry had postings, and in direct proximity to Miranda's Venezuela), the different plotlines are interspersed with dramatic episodes: hunting in exotic locations, a picnic that turns into a deadly battle between a jaguar and an ant-bear (a scene that bears some resemblance to Rider Haggard's later description of the lioness and crocodile fight in *She*), indigenous live-burial rites, canoe outings that end tragically under waterfalls. The text is also awash with the tropes of sensation fiction: several characters have either been entrapped in fake marriages or, if legally married, have the documentary evidence of their legitimate claims destroyed by arson attacks (in adaptation of the destruction of birth records in Wilkie Collins's

The Woman in White). Though the villains of the novel are all male, female duplicity and corruption play their part in the treacherous plots of the men. One of the colonial wives has a fatal 'taste for strong narcotics' combined with adultery, and the woman whose husband she is plotting to steal is a mistress of feminine artifice thanks to 'the skill of a Parisian *artiste*'; her dramatic transformations and use of stage props (make-up, wig, gauzy fabrics) are reminiscent of Braddon's Lucy Audley and Louisa May Alcott's Jean Muir, while at the same time hinting at Fitzjames's own masquerade.[117]

The central plot is organized around Creoline Barrett, daughter of the mixed-race Creole beauty Evangeline, who, heavily pregnant, was abandoned by her English husband (whose father, having fallen out with his titled relatives in Britain, misappropriated a country estate on Guiana by means of fraud and a fake marriage). After Evangeline's death the infant is adopted as their own by a childless rector couple, the Barretts, and is told her history on her seventeenth birthday. A beautiful and guileless girl, she is courted by, and falls in love with, the unscrupulous Major Catherwood, who plots to marry her to get hold of her money and then to abandon her. Revealed to be none other than Creoline's biological father, Catherwood meets his grisly end in the aftermath of a train crash when he travels back to Britain to accede, as the heir apparent, to the Seskinore earldom his father had lost. A rival claimant is Catherwood's cousin and adversary, Mortimer Whitlington, the detective figure in the text. Initially introduced as a morally suspect character (a correspondent in a divorce case with a 'sinister countenance ... soft sensual eyes ... [and a] compressed mouth with lines of cunning and selfishness'),[118] Whitlington proves to be an upright English gentleman. This is categorically not the case for the lawyer Mr. Grey who, having risen to the office of Administrator-General by fraud, embezzlement, arson and murder, gets his just deserts in a sensational trial that ends with his death sentence. Before his friends can save him from execution with an indigenous drug that temporarily induces a near-death state, he falls victim to his love-crazed cousin's murder-suicide. His widow instantly sets out to lure the next powerful man into her web. False clues, multiple identities, dark family secrets (including fear of hereditary madness), fraudulent marriages, lost and recovered patrimonies, adultery, bigamy and incestuous desire, arson, murder, poison, opium addiction and fatal train crashes, even an amputation – Rogers's novel creaks under the heavy weight of its sensation machinery.

As if that were not sufficient, in his introduction to the 1896 edition Rogers lays claim to a near-prophetic vision. His invention came true, he asserts, when, the very week after the novel's publication, the then Administrator-General of Guiana was 'suspended from office, in consequence of an alleged deficiency of 20,000£ in his accounts'. Given that the 'amount, method, and history of the real and fictitious embezzlement are *strangely similar*', Rogers could not help but wonder if 'the wretched man … [had] read my serial novel, and copied the crime? Did the Governor and Executive Council also imitate the loose conduct of their prototypes in my story?'[119] By inference, if Rogers was capable of anticipating colonial affairs with such shrewdness, his representation of Barry had to be reliable. Rogers went one step further by implying that not only did his work provide truthful insights into Barry's character, but that it was in fact a homage to the doctor: 'James Barry ought to be regarded as the wonder of the 19th century, and to be worshipped and pillared and be *Madame Tussaud* [*sic*] in consequence.'[120] And yet, where were the official markers of distinction? Why, despite her 'abnormal back door influence', did Barry not receive the honours she deserved on retirement:

> quite … unduly, she was most strangely overlooked in the distribution of honours at the close of campaigns, or on Her Majesty's birthdays; … *why* were James Barry's war services, if any, ignored? *Why*, if she deserved the distinction, by long, faithful and courageous service and conduct, why was she not dubbed a K.C.B.? *Why*, we cry in despair and astonishment, *why* was this female Aesculapius, who served in every part of the Empire… *and in the Crimea*, *why* was she not given a simple C.B.[?][121]

Having established his credentials as the champion of the disinherited (an extradiegetic extension of one of the plotlines), Rogers permits himself to speculate about the inner life of Barry ('what a life of repressed emotions must hers have been?') before arriving at the most suitable choice of genre for doing his subject justice: 'what a subject for melodramatic treatment Miss Barry's character would be!'[122] Barry's melodramatic 'life of repressed emotions' comes to light in the penultimate chapter, 'Home at last', in a letter read out after Fitzjames's death by Mrs. Elrington, an officer's wife (herself a cast-off heiress) who became his confidante after she tended to him during an illness. Fitzjames's 'full confession as to my extraordinary career' echoes the performative memoirs of swashbuckling cross-dressers such as Hannah Snell's 'full and true account' of her 'Surprising Life and

Adventures' (1750) or Mary Anne Talbot's equally hyperbolically titled 'extraordinary Adventures' (1809).[123] The reader now learns that Fitzjames, alias Jessie Pownall, is the missing niece of the Earl of Seskinore (a version of Somerset/Fitzroy), who made her his sole heir after she entrusted him with her secret: that, having been disowned by her relatives for contracting a romantic marriage to a physician, and without other means to support herself, she decided after his tragic death to 'unsex' herself by assuming his position (an astonishing feat, accomplished without the benefit of prior study). Significantly, the plan to impersonate her deceased husband ripened during the latter stages of pregnancy – an impulse that, Fitzjames admits in the convention established by *Lady Audley's Secret*, 'may have been fostered and stimulated by puerperal mania, although it must be admitted that there was much method in every plan I conceived'.[124]

In its depiction of the after-story, the posthumous revelation of Fitzjames's secret, the text calls itself into question in a rare gesture of self-mockery (if self-mockery it is). This parodic element also underpins the rumour mill to which Fitzjames's death gives rise: 'It's a gent that's been murdered by his niggar servant, I hear … and when his wife arrived this morning … and heard the news, she dropped down dead too'.[125] There is even a hint of embryonic metatextuality when, in an echo of the *Saunders's News-Letter* correspondent, Fitzjames's solicitor is plagued by pronomial confusion, as if to signal the way in which after Barry's death the public truth of the body overwrote the inner truth of the self: 'if ever I cared for a human being I did for him, her, I mean. … He, I mean she, went even beyond me in her expressed contempt of women in general.'[126] Ultimately, the novel ends with the conclusion that 'none of [us] appear able to fix his personality'; as one of Rogers's characters exclaims, in intertextual cross-reference to the first of the Barry biofictions, 'Fitzjames will remain a mystery still'.[127]

If anything, *A Modern Sphinx* testifies to the mythmaking qualities of the Barry story as one that could be attached almost indiscriminately to any plotline to inject narrative frisson. Keen to promote circulation of his rambling three-decker, Rogers sought further to validate and raise interest in his depiction of Barry by publishing an account, allegedly told to him by a colleague, of how his sex was discovered by a party of officers in Trinidad when they tended to the feverish Barry: 'on throwing back the sheets from off the unconscious "Doctor" it was seen that she was a woman – and upon recovery of her senses she made those present swear that her secret would not be disclosed until after her death.'[128] This is, again, the stuff of sensation fiction. Stripping the body of the male impersonator of its illicit trappings (professional qualification – 'Doctor' – here being aligned with purloined male anatomy) means to restore the order fractured by the gender bender. However doubtful the biofictional credentials of Rogers's novel, his titular sphinx is, nonetheless, an apt metaphor of the hybrid, forever indeterminate body that defies the endeavour to heteronormalize the transgressive subject. The sphinx remains defined by indefinability.

Intriguingly, this indefinability is reflected in the very title selected for the text – for who is the 'modern sphinx'? Since Fitzjames is not revealed to be a woman until the end and since the heroine, Creoline Barrett, is a straightforward not inscrutable character, the title is yet another false clue. Braddon's revised edition, *Madeline's Mystery*, more appropriately highlights the (renamed) protagonist and the mystery that attaches not to her personality but to her parentage and racial identity. That Creoline/Madeline is of mixed race (as a Quadroon, her mother had one black grandparent, and her father turns out to have a similar background) adds an important dimension to the novel's engagement with Barry in pointing to the parallels between race and gender passing. Creoline's alabaster complexion and 'faultless countenance' invoke a fluidity of the raced body that by inference can be applied to the gendered body, too.[129]

The novel also problematizes the notion of miscegenation, for Creoline is one of many mixed-race daughters. White male colonials are shown to be in the habit of taking indigenous mistresses or inveigling them into fake marriages; the fact that none of the mixed-race mothers survives offers an implicit commentary on their exploitation and hints at the legacy of slavery. The children of these unions (in the novel always female), if the offspring of wealthy fathers, may be coveted for their 'darksome voluptuous bust[s]' and may even have been educated in English finishing schools (albeit to little intellectual effect); but they are as incapable of breaking through the 'barrier of colour' as are their materially less fortunate sisters.[130] Differences in racial purity are correlated with sharp class distinctions; half-sisters who share the same father stand in the relation of mistress and maid, again recalling slavery (the murder victim, Angeline, is her white half-sister's maid, and she is killed by the man her sister loves to the point of self-destruction).

Unsurprisingly, the novel is marked by racial cliché: 'most coloured Creoles' are 'vain, saucy, obstinate, and capricious, [i]ndolent in domestic matters', with 'showy' but 'questionable' accomplishments, their ideas firmly 'centred on dress and the frivolities of fashion' and tireless in their pursuit of pleasure; yet they possess 'a certain languid coquettishness' and a sensual allure that 'captivated imperceptibly'.[131] But the mystery and murder plots undercut some of these stereotypes. Fearless and vocal in standing up for her rights, Angelina is also clever (with the exception of Whitlington, she is the only character to have pieced together the story of Grey's crimes), while Creoline illustrates that it is nurture rather than nature (or 'race') that shapes individual development. When she learns about her mixed-race origins and the story of her adoption, not only does she spearhead the establishment of a foundling hospital, she also begins to conceive of herself as a 'friend' of the indigenous population and, indeed, as one of them: 'for am I not in reality of the same class – the same race?'[132]

The ending of the novel sees Creoline and her children comfortably ensconced in the uppermost reaches of English society, as the wife of Colonel Seagrave and close friend of the Earl of Seskinore and Lady Cheetham (Fitzjames's daughter, who has had her heirloom restored to her). With the murder of Angeline and the geographical displacement of Creoline, their potential to contest racial hegemonies on Guiana has been lost, but the latter's social elevation in England carries racial hybridity into the heart of Empire. In this respect Braddon's renaming (taming) of Creoline into a more Europeanized, Caucasian Madeline diminishes the challenge of an otherwise explicitly creolized heroine.[133] Creoline and Fitzjames are not closely connected in the plot; yet the fact that Creoline ends by moving in the circles that would have been Fitzjames's had she lived to reveal her identity effectively racializes the Barry story. For all its weaknesses, this establishes a link of sorts between Rogers's Victorian sensation novel and Kit Brennan's postmodernist play *Tiger's Heart* (1996), discussed in the next chapter. Here the tentative analogy implied in *A Modern Sphinx* between racial and gendered hybridity is developed into an explicit exploration of gender and race crossing as acts of resistance to the dominant order: 'Our histories on our bodies, all the world can read; but a body's just the border of a place they will never possess.'[134] It is precisely this struggle over the possession of Barry's body, and that body's resistance to appropriation, that was key to the Barry story from its very inception.

Body Mnemonics: Barry In and Out of the Looking Glass

If this chapter began by tracing the foundation narratives that have given shape and form to the Barry myth, its second part examines the 'body mnemonics' of that myth: the constructed memory traces of Barry's subject constitution, the imagined journey of 'becoming James' through pivotal scenes of transformation, crisis and exposure. The journey motif in Barry biographilia coheres with the conventions of contemporary transgender narrative. As Rogers Brubaker notes,

> journeys of self-discovery, self-transformation, and self-realization, stories of transgender migration have a satisfying narrative form. They begin with a divided self, in a condition of pain, suffering and alienation; they pass through crises or critical turning points on the way; and they culminate in the overcoming of alienation and the affirmation of the true self.[135]

This narrative trajectory, however, finds altered expression in Barry biographilia, not least because the historical subject's story is bounded by death and exposure. In contradistinction to contemporary 'body narratives', the last stage of the journey, in Jay Prosser's words 'corporeal and social transformation/conversion; and finally the arrival "home"', often in the sense of reassignment surgery, is necessarily figured differently in life-writing that focuses on pre-twentieth-century subjects.[136] Thus in neo-Victorian Barry biographilia transformation and transition are not the end point but, after an introductory, contextualizing phase, typically constitute the start of the protagonist's story of crossing. Transformation here is of a sartorial and social, not corporeal nature, and consists in costume change and a move from domestic to public spaces. The ensuing narrative focuses on the processes and practices of performing in the new gender identity while negotiating the ever-present risk of discovery in both professional and private contexts. The triple pattern Prosser identifies for transsexual autobiography – 'departure, transition, and the home of reassignment'[137] – in Barry narrative is represented by three moments of transition that are dramatized in episodes that feature three different experiences of conflicted and shifting gender identity: departure through self-refashioning in the looking glass; trial by duel; dénouement in the bedroom. This dénouement can take three different forms: exposure (the deathbed revelation), comic circumvention, or queer subversion.

As the point of departure, the mirror scene is inherent to transgender narrative. Prosser notes that it represents

> a convention of transsexual autobiography … A trope of transsexual representation, the split of the mirror captures the definitive splitting of the transsexual subject, freezes it, frames it schematically in narrative. The difference between gender and sex is conveyed in the difference between body image (projected self) and the image of the body (reflected self). … Looking into the mirror is [also] a figure for the autobiographical act: autobiography is ostensibly anyway the literary act of self-reflection, the textual product of the 'I' reflecting on itself.[138]

In neo-Victorian Barry life-writing, however, the mirror scene is presented from another angle through a different ontology. Where transgender autobiography is about evidencing an *a priori* identity that is firmly grounded in the protagonist's childhood experience of having been 'born into the wrong body'[139] and the purpose of the narrative is, initially, to convince the clinician and, in a second stage, the general reader of the authenticity and conclusiveness of this identity while offering support through role model function to the transgender community, Barry biographilia, by contrast, explores a separate scenario. Here, the protagonist is not so much propelled by a sense of 'wrong embodiment'[140] as by a desire for self-development. Transgender is rarely a point of departure but more of a gradual process in which a performative act over time becomes internalized. Therefore the vestments of the 'new' identity, when tentatively, playfully slipped on in front of the mirror, may initially prompt a feeling of alienation rather than home-coming. Predominantly (though not exclusively: Duncker and Holmes afford counter-examples), the point of the mirror scene in Barry life-writing is not to offer proof of transgendered authenticity before the event but to fashion an identificatory model for the non-transgender reader to 'understand' and sympathize with Barry's journey. Placed in Barry's subject position in front of the mirror, and looking at Barry the woman looking at the newly born man emerging from the glass, the reader is encouraged to become personally invested in the protagonist's successful performance.

Like the mirror scene, the duel and bedroom plots focus on the contested body and its liminal state between femininity and masculinity. All rely on a reader to give these moments meaning. Passing narratives therefore, as Monique Rooney argues, represent the passer as a figure who paradoxically embodies fragmentation and doubleness at one and the same time: a split self in transition, in-between genders, and yet also a figure whose gaze into the mirror is doubled in the gaze of the reader.[141] The passer comes into being through the gaze of the reader witnessing her experience of de- and reassembling himself in the mirror, and of thereby participating in the 'transgender look'.[142] A key feature of transgender narrative and film,[143] the double gaze is also a structuring device in contemporary Barry biographilia, and lends itself with particular force to visual illustration[144] and dramatic juxtaposition on the stage (as in the mirroring effect produced by the two characters who embody aspects of the same person in Sebastian Barry's *Whistling Psyche*). Representations that take the form of caricature, however, subject the passer to the gaze of the viewer without enabling a circulation of gazes. The Victorian prototype of the unidirectional gaze that subjugates the passer to a heteronormative vision originates, again, from 'A Mystery Still':

> He would go about, bestriding his pony in strange fashion, with an umbrella over his head. His saddle was a curiosity. It was so comfortably padded and so safely shaped that, once wedged into it, it was a marvel how he got out of it. In uniform he was a caricature. His boot heels were two inches above the ground, and within the boots were soles three inches thick. Add to these boots very long spurs, crown the sandy curls with a cocked-hat, and complete all with a sword big enough for a dragoon, and you have the doctor complete. The pony was enveloped in a net from ears to heels, and swung the tassels about impatient of the gear. The black man attended at the beast's head, and Psyche tripped after them.[145]

This portrait had an extraordinary resonance that reverberated into the late twentieth century and beyond.[146] Its strong pictorial quality inspired illustrations to early twentieth-century representations of Barry, such as the cartoon that accompanied Marvell's 'The Mystery of the Kapok Doctor' in 1904, later reproduced in a 1929 article in the *Illustrated London News* (Fig. 3.6).[147] In conjunction with 'A Mystery Still', the caricature in turn appears materially to have influenced the representation of Barry at a pageant held in Cape Town in 1910, which subsequently left its mark on Olga Racster's imagination and in 1939 transmigrated into Rutherford's story-article 'Dr. James Barry'.[148] Text and image also had a bearing on twentieth-century biography; thus June Rose depicts Barry as 'trotting down the straight, tree-lined streets of the Cape on her pony, with a black servant carrying a sunshade at her side and a poodle yapping

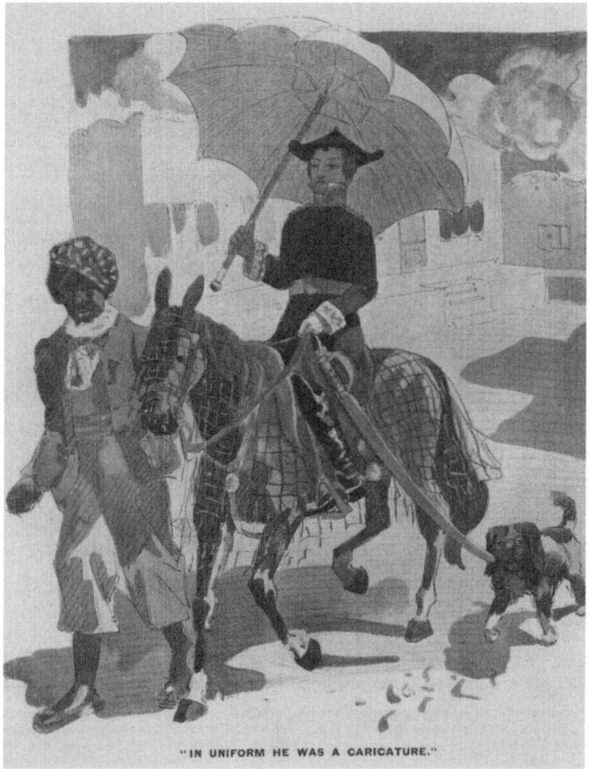

Fig. 3.6 'In uniform he was a caricature', cartoon accompanying George Edwin Marvell, 'The Mystery of the Kapok Doctor', *Cape Times Christmas Annual*, December 1904, p. 17, reproduced courtesy of the National Library of South Africa: Cape Town Campus

at her heels ... [and] with her sword and spurs gleaming, her tiny figure erect and proud, ... evidently enjoy[ing] the display and the comment her appearance provoked'.[149] That mnemonic of the Barry story, the black servant holding an umbrella over a diminutive officer figure, also features in Binnie's *Colours.*[150]

In its comic portrayal of the incongruities of a masculine self-construction that only resulted in making the subject's inherent femininity stand out more strongly, 'A Mystery Still' co-opts earlier references to the idiosyncrasies of Barry's military dress style (exaggerated spurs and an overlong sword are mentioned in Edward Bradford's account; the cocked hat is figured in the Corfu cartoon of the elderly Barry; the padded shoulders of the later 'Kapok Doctor', however, are missing) and adds conspicuous symbols of femininity (the umbrella) and otherness (the black servant, the pet poodle).[151] The netting that envelops and the tassels that adorn and feminize the pony, the 'strange' manner in which Barry mounts the animal and the choice of a womb-like saddle act as visual markers of the ineffectual masculine cover that fails to hide the female essence underneath. Especially in Barry's early career, of course, an extravagant outfit could signal the dandy's 'tireless application to costume' so much in vogue in the Regency period since Beau Brummel, or it could simply be adopted in compensation of a short stature.[152] Black servants were hardly uncommon at the Cape at a time of slavery; and dogs were frequently found in the company of the English gentleman à la Buchan or Somerset whom Barry sought to emulate.[153] The conjunction of all these aspects, however, establishes an overriding impression of femininity unmasked; a different version of the sexuality laid bare by Edouard Manet's *Olympia*, painted four years prior to 'A Mystery Still', in 1863. Olympia, too, is figured with a black (woman) servant and a pet (a black cat, albeit aggressively arched, to Barry's cuddly poodle).[154]

To twenty-first-century eyes, the 'Kapok Doctor' caricature resonates with drag and in its parodic excess and the 'selective mixing of elements from conventionally understood masculine and feminine repertoires' performs a version of what Rogers Brubaker terms the 'trans of between'.[155] If Victorian and turn-of-the-century representations satirized Barry as a freak and failed male impersonator, contemporary biofiction depicts freakishness as a strategic ploy which hides the female body in drag performance. Thus in Anne and Ivan Kronenfeld's *The Secret Life of Dr. James Miranda Barry* (2000), Pandora (Barry's fanciful birth name, probably inspired by his uncle James Barry's best-known painting) decides that exaggeration is the best disguise: given her petite shape, she 'would never convince anyone that she was a typical rough and tumble lad, a man's man. No, she would have to convince the world she was a youth of a highly strung countenance, tinged with eccentricities, captured in a small body.'[156] Consequently, she adopts all the accoutrements lambasted in the Barry caricature, and deliberately 'cuts a wild figure with her cockaded hats, her overly broad shoulders and lifted boots, as she walked ... about town, Psyche at her heel. Oftentimes Dantzen would follow holding an umbrella above her head to protect her from the sun.'[157] Her transformation from Pandora to James, however, is ultimately figured not as an assumption of (an odd) masculinity, nor as in 'A Mystery Still' as a comic excess of dual gender attributes that reveals rather than conceals Barry's femininity but, rather, as an act of symbolic castration, a loss of sex altogether:

> With quick and clean gestures she released one of the fasts holding her hair and before anyone really understood what she was doing she sliced off a handful. 'Lord Buchan,' she said, dropping the severed curls onto the table. 'You put forth your ideas behind another name. I will put mine forth behind another appearance.'
>
> The Earl of Buchan threw his head back with a roar of laughter, but when Pandora looked at Leander his face was ripe with disgust.[158]

The personal cost of her 'grand masquerade' is high as Leander (the man of her choice, Miranda's son) rejects her as a lover.[159] For Barry's 2016 biographers du Preez and Dronfield the price Margaret Bulkley paid was even higher than the mere loss of a lover. While biographers usually speculate about the historical Barry's sense of liberation and pleasure in donning the extravagant, dandified male garb of the time, the authors of *Dr. James Barry* conceive of their subject as a woman permanently psychologically maimed by her life as a man; dramatically, the moment of transformation is therefore marked as an act of mutilation:

> Then came the shears. Her red-gold hair was unpinned, unplaited and shorn, ropes of hair falling around her shoulders and slumping to the hearth rug. ... Now when she looked in the glass, Margaret saw a stranger who had stolen her face. ... Had she known that the dress [she had discarded] was the last she would ever wear, she would surely have rethought her plans ... [H]er identity as a girl, a woman and a person was bound up with the clothes she wore. ... [S]he could hardly imagine how painfully that dress, and others like it, would tug at her heart in the years to come.[160]

Instead of the comfortable, sensual shape and fabric that embodied her identity, Margaret feels badly constrained by garments that lock her into an alien male role: 'Every item ... irritated the senses: the woollen stockings chafed, the heavy tailcoat and surtout weighed the shoulders down, the high collar and tightly knotted cravat constricted the throat, and as for the breeches ... well, ... [they] were quite unspeakable.'[161] In Sebastian Barry's play *Whistling Psyche* (2004), Barry similarly finds that 'As that male jacket closed over my chest, and those trousers engulfed my thin legs, some other hidden blanket suffocated the fire of a conventional future, where … I would have enjoyed the love of another human person'; hence the importance of his dog, Psyche, as a companion against loneliness.[162] Cross-dressing here is tantamount to self-entombment.

While the protagonist of Ann Florida Town's Young Adult novel *With a Silent Companion* (1999) is also initially inconvenienced by her new clothes and (temporarily) forced to renounce romance, her love of medicine makes up for the sacrifice: once her masquerade is complete, she throws herself into her studies and, convinced that '[i]t was something she [was] born to do', she 'glowed with happiness' in the pursuit of her work.[163] Here, therefore, the transformation scene, played out in different stages in front of the mirror as Margaret turns herself into James, marks an experience of gradual empowerment, not loss, as she moves from initial bewilderment ('What a lot of bothersome flaps and buttons … skirts are a lot more comfortable') to a sense of adjustment ('I won't miss having to tie up all those petticoat strings') and a recognition of the arbitrariness of gender norms: 'I wonder why things button up differently on men's clothing than on women's clothing?'[164] (Conversely, Frederic Mohr's Barry realizes that dressing in trousers for a man means to choose a side.)[165]

At first, Margaret feels a 'scarecrow', with her flapping trousers and sleeves hanging down 'well below her fingertips'; but, '[l]aughing … at her reflection in the mirror', she sets about shortening the trousers, tightening the cuffs, and, overcoming her confusion about what to do with a long piece of cloth, wraps it as a tie round her neck: 'Some men, she knew, wore a long brooch to hold the ends in place. Others, the "dandies" who dressed in a more fanciful manner, looped the ends of the stock into a wide bow.'[166] The neck-tie, even more than the breeches, thus epitomizes Garber's notion of the transvestite 'foundation garment', the vestment that, like the cod-piece in Renaissance drama or the stage curtain that separates 'real' from 'unreal', simultaneously signifies presence and absence (the Adam's apple; male genitals).[167] This neck-tie or a starched collar are featured on all of the factual portraits as well as contemporary cartoons of Barry (see Figs. 1.1, 2.1, 2.4, 2.5, 2.6, 2.7, 3.1, 3.2, 3.4, 3.5, 3.6, 4.4). Having thus symbolically endowed herself with the markers of virility, Margaret must dispose of all visible reminders of her femininity.

The last stage in the process of becoming James is, here too, the cutting off of the long hair. ('A Mystery Still's' anecdote of the subversive haircut is thus given new meaning in the transformation scene.) At first 'Margaret looked in shock at her reflection … [and then] looked at the floor. The sight of her beautiful hair lying there in careless piles was devastating.' When she brushes her new hairstyle into shape and turns to face the mirror one more time, 'A stranger looked back at her – someone who might have been related, but certainly not the young girl she usually saw.'[168] Glancing at the stranger in the glass, however, does not constitute a moment of self-alienation, as is the case in du Preez and Dronfield, but rather an experience of agency and triumph in the knowledge of her powers of regeneration and self-staging. The visual transformation being complete, she is ready to perform her new self in the outside world: 'And now the play begins … We shall see … just how capable an actress you are'.[169] As James, the English medical student, she progressively feels 'more like [a] young man'.[170]

And yet, like du Preez and Dronfield's, Town's James never quite makes the full internal transition, which is the reason why, in later life, she degenerates into a caricature of himself: 'In an effort to reinforce her identity, she exaggerated masculine traits and unwittingly made herself into a comic figure.'[171] Freakishness, then, is not the result of crossing from female body to male costume, but the failure to complete the process from woman to man in psychological terms. In a narratological sense, this failure is overdetermined by the authors' persistency in their choice of pronoun and inner gender identity: Margaret can never 'really' become James since she remains identified as female. This is encoded paratextually on Town's book cover, where a male officer shown from the side, whose face is turned away from the viewer, looks at his likeness reflected in a handheld mirror. Unsurprisingly, it is a woman's (Fig. 3.7). The silent companion ever resistant to Margaret's transformation is her quintessential femininity.

In these texts, then, as in the Victorian foundation myth, the body is an essential entity that rules the mind and which no manner of performance will have the power to release from its control. What distinguishes the contemporary versions from the Victorian model is the protagonist's glance in the mirror, an act of self-reflection that opens the text up to a double gaze; this gaze, however, reaffirms heteronormativity. In their representation of a quasi-Lacanian 'mirror stage', modern and contemporary biographilia use the looking glass as a symbolic moment to depict the protagonist's mental and psychological experimentation with a male persona and the experience of self-transformation, an experience that can also, crucially, highlight the gender crosser's self-division.[172]

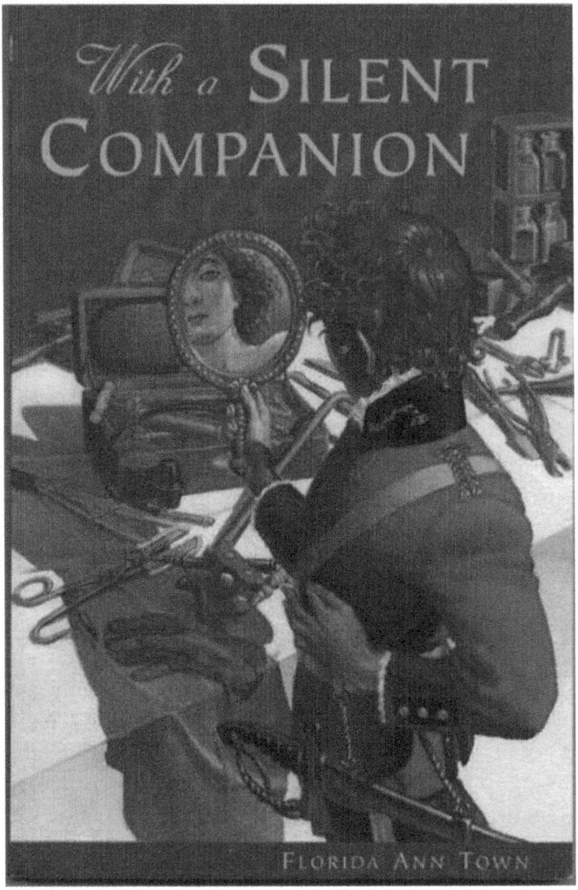

Fig. 3.7 Cover reprinted with permission from *With a Silent Companion* written by Florida Ann Town, cover art by Igor Kordey, published 1999 by Red Deer Press

In contradistinction to these texts, which dramatize the experience of an extraordinary heroine who feels compelled to impersonate a man by no inner desire but entirely because of social conditions, postmodernist fiction like Patricia Duncker's, discussed in more detail in the next chapter, seeks to reflect the ambiguity of Barry's identity through the fluidity of language and form. Barry's gender remains open for exploration in fluctuating first and third-person narrative. An intermediate example between

Barry as a gender passer and Barry as a gender crosser is Sylvie Ouellette's *Le Secret du docteur Barry* (2012). Here, the protagonist is introduced as a young man with a secret, who in order to study medicine has decided 'to turn his back on his childhood, his origins, and even his identity'; to achieve his aims, he knows that he must 'assume fully the role that had devolved on him': 'Il lui fallait … faire le grand jeu'.[173] His mother comments proudly that he plays his role to perfection: 'tu deviens vraiment un homme'.[174] This transformation to manhood, again, comes to pass through extended self-communication with his mirror image:

> Barry would deliberately place himself in front of his mirror for long minutes in order to practice the right kind of poses.
>
> 'I have succeeded, I'm exactly like them now,' he thought every time he was complimented on something …
>
> … Above all, the dandy had to astound and provoke envy in those who looked at him, a matter in which Barry took immense pleasure.[175]

The stability and inner consistency of his performance of masculinity is put to the test when Buchan, bringing news of Miranda's imprisonment, addresses Barry, for the first time in the text, by his female name. It is only now that Barry's secret, his female birth identity, is lifted for the reader. But Barry will have none of it: 'For me, Margaret Bulkley no longer exists. She died when James Miranda Barry was born.' When Buchan objects that 'you will never be able to deny your femininity', Barry protests (in unconscious echo of Sarah Grand's Angelica performing Diavolo): 'But in the eyes of the world, I am a man! … For a number of years now, I've been learning to speak like them, to walk like them and even to sit down like them! … I behave like a man, I think like a man, and I now consider myself altogether a man'.[176] When, in undressing, the woman's shape resurfaces in the mirror, he feels 'almost surprised'.[177] It is as a male that he attracts the attention and desire of Somerset. But in the ensuing affair Barry is refeminized: as he is trying on a highly eroticized dress, a gift of Somerset's, she 'finally caught sight of her face in the glass. She trembled violently, astounded to see herself a woman … Somerset placed himself behind her, embracing her'.[178] Now her female body is revealed also to others, such as Cloete, who promptly falls in love with her. But though reciprocating Cloete's feelings, Barry will not act on them since to fulfill her desire (and live with Cloete) would entail a formal return to femininity.[179] Years later, in Jamaica, Barry has re-internalized her manhood: 'Her gestures no longer had to be studied or borrowed; they came naturally.'[180] But do they, really? The complexities of a male identity that inhabits an anatomically female body is emblemized by the tropic island and its (manifestly racialized) topography:

> each was a world of its own, at the heart of which resided an enormous complexity. Despite their constrained dimensions, they could offer astonishing contrasts to those who knew how to discover them. In one sense, they very much resembled James Miranda Barry .... *Their beauty masks the horrors they enclose; their rigid geography and immutable borders stand in strong contrast to the freedom they can furnish at the same time.*[181]

In its representation of transgender as racial alterity, this passage captures the conflicted nature of the textual construction of Barry's sense of self: if his female body, 'immutable' in its contours, constitutes a 'horror', while the mask sets him free, this 'freedom' is always already circumscribed by the rigidity with which the narrative voice reasserts Barry's femininity by corseting him into a linguistic framework from which 'she' cannot disentangle herself. Oddly, after the shift from male to female pronoun at the initial disclosure of Barry's birth identity, the text persists in referring to Barry as a woman ('elle') throughout his life trajectory, returning to the opening male pronoun ('il') only after Barry's death in the Epilogue, precisely when he is revealed to his contemporaries as female. The narrative voice thus continues to exert Buchan's essentializing control that Barry so passionately contested at the start of his career.

Biofiction, in contrast to biodrama, rarely offers a sustained autobiographical account by Barry. Alongside Duncker's contemporary work, an early twentieth-century exception in the form of a diary narrative is Racster and Grove's 1932 novel adaptation of their 1919 play, *The Journal of Dr. James Miranda Barry.* As in Town and Kronenfeld, Barry's impersonation originates from external circumstances, not any internal wish for masculinity. Here it is not the desire to study medicine or lead an exciting and purposeful life but the need to find release from a violent marriage that, almost accidentally, leads Lady Barrymore to take up her disguise. After a particularly unpleasant altercation with her abusive husband, she retires to her room 'with the single intention of escaping, somewhere, somehow.' As she passes a door, she (rather conveniently) comes across a set of male clothes, remembers that she had once attended a fancy-dress party attired as a man, undetected, and realizes that she has found the solution to her problem: 'The sense of having cast everything away held me like the grip of Fate. Very quietly I took these clothes, put them on, and walked out of that poisonous abomination I had called my home'.[182] Initially uncomfortable in her male persona, it is through self-observation in front of a mirror that she starts to feel at ease with her new identity, gaining in confidence in the process: 'Repeatedly every day I stare at myself for hours in the looking-glass. I see myself growing masculine. It is curious how the mind affects the body. … I had large, tender blue eyes; they are still large, but have lost their look of timidity.'[183] Her mirror reflection assumes the role of a close confidant to whom she turns in a crisis: when, settled into her medical post at the Cape, she hears of her husband's appointment, a turn of events that will make a re-encounter unavoidable, and after a fit of hysterics behind closed doors that nearly gives her away, she seeks to reassure herself by inspecting her assumed self as if from an outsider's point of view:

> I stared at myself from every angle, anxiously looking for the change I expected to find. I tested how I appeared, serious, laughing, surprised. When I could see no alteration, my heart beat more freely. The realization of the victory I had publicly achieved took possession of me. By good luck I was safe, free, an honourable man (!); I might be tired and my legs might tremble, but *no one … knew*.[184]

Even Somerset, who does know, admits that 'there are times when I forget your sex'.[185] If the glance in the mirror is a means of continually reconstructing and reaffirming her fragile sense of self, a private rehearsal of her public performance, it is her masculine clothes that confirm her identity as a man. Decked out in the dandy's attire, a 'coat of the latest "Pea-Green Hayne," a satin waistcoat, a vast cravat fastened with many scarf pins, and a pair of tight-fitting "inexpressibles"', she feels herself reborn into a 'fine gentleman' – and a 'goodlooking' one at that.[186] Not only does she find the courage to 'strut past [her] husband's house' in broad daylight, she also discovers that her clothes invest her with considerable sex appeal: a housemaid hints at her availability, and the 'effect on Mary [a male friend's sister] has been of the extreme kind'.[187] So persistently is Barry incommoded by other women's desire that she comes to a realization of the ease with which femininity can be deployed to manipulate sexual encounters and, if unsuccessful, sexual slander; in this particular 'war between the sexes', men are 'repeatedly beaten.'[188]

While in Ouellette's *Le Secret*, Sebastian Barry's *Whistling Psyche* and Kit Brennan's *Tiger's Heart*, Barry is queered by the magnetism her dandified body exudes on bisexual and gay men, and a lesbian Barry is feminized by being recognized as one of their own by a group of black women in Duncker's story 'James Miranda Barry', in Racster and Grove's novel Barry's heteronormative sexuality and essentialized femininity are rarely in doubt. For however much she may exalt in her looking-glass performance, 'sw[i]ng[ing her] hips smartly, walking with squared shoulders and head lifted high above [her] stiff collar', ultimately Barry remains painfully aware that her show of masculinity conflicts with her irrevocably female-as-feminine sense of self: 'Though I may congratulate myself for *acting* like a man, *my own woman-self* is scandalized'.[189] This is illustrated vividly when her greatest triumph as a man – a quasi-sexual taming of a wild horse with the understanding of a tender lover – ends in humiliation, pain and exposure: having recognized her husband among the observers, she loses control over the horse (and her masculine performance); the ensuing accident kills the horse and returns her to her erstwhile victim position as the suffering wife under constant threat of spousal violence – until, that is, a 'real' man, Somerset, intervenes to rescue her.

The looking glass thus serves as a complex symbol both of the tentative, sometimes painful, mostly playful, experimental and self-affirmative transformation from woman to man, and thereby as an act of subject-(re)constitution, but also as a moment of crisis, a boundary marker between femininity and masculinity as well as between performance and (psychical and bodily) identity. This dual and conflicting function is also present in the second 'bodily relic' of the Barry narrative, the duel.

That Barry's career had involved active contribution to that most ritualized form of male-to-male combat, the duel, was a constituent component of the story from the start: the first posthumous account in *Saunders's News-Letter* drew attention to Barry having 'fought one duel, and sought many more' in the same sentence as discussing his medical education, talent and achievements, as if to substantiate the extent of the Inspector General's imposture in the professional sphere with reference to Barry's credentials in standing the test of masculinity in an ancient ritual.[190] Another early commentator, Edward Bradford, who had worked with Barry in Barbados, recalled his former colleague boasting of having 'shot one of his [fellow-duellist's] whiskers off' while at the Cape.[191] When a reader correspondence developed in the *Lancet* thirty years after Barry's death, Ebenezer Rogers described meeting Barry on a crossing to Barbados, where the 'doctor was going at the time to visit her old friend and enemy, General Sir [Abraham] Josiah Cleote, with whom, when aide-de-camp to the Governor of the Cape, she had fought a duel and was wounded in the leg.' Cleote (Cloete in today's spelling), he continued, later stepped in to prevent a duel with another officer, Colonel Shadwell Clerke; 'he, too, was challenged for some fancied insult, but …General Cleote pooh-poohed the idea and made them shake hands.'[192] In further elaboration of Barry's duel with Cloete, Rogers cited Sir William Macintosh, who had known Barry in Corfu, and who recollected Cloete (here spelled Cleotè) telling him that

> a buxom lady called to see [Lord Charles] on business of a private nature, and … they were closeted for some time … Dr. Barry made … disparaging remarks … 'Oh, I say, Cleotè,' he sneered, 'that's a nice Dutch filly the Governor has got hold of.' 'Retract your vile expression, you infernal little cad' said I, advancing and pulling his long ugly nose. Barry immediately challenged me, and we fought with pistols, fortunately without effect.[193]

Rogers quotes Macintosh quoting the 'very words' of Cloete, imparted during a dinner party and remembered years later, framing Macintosh's recollections with his matter-of-fact assertions that Barry 'was the daughter of a Scotch baronet, Buchan' and had been 'brought up in Malta': evidently, this narrative is heavily fictionalized.[194] Fittingly, the episode concludes with Rogers's gratified side glance at his own novel (a presentation copy?), which he finds (or, for publicity purposes, perhaps invents as being) displayed on Macintosh's table during their conversation. That the anecdote of the duel is recorded as documentary, first-hand evidence by all biographers with no reference to the double framing of the story accentuates the myth-making quality of all ostensibly 'biographical' information about Barry.[195] A second account, transcribed from Cloete's papers by the antiquarian bookseller R.C. Bellenger on behalf of Major-General A. MacLennan in 1969, gives the following version of events:

> At this time (1820) there was at the Cape a very remarkable Character in Staff Asst. Surgeon, Dr. James Barry, M.D., who combined in an extraordinary degree, the rarest qualities of Esculapian Talent, with the most mischievous propensities of a Monkey, and all the subtle wiles of the Serpent. – An altercation with this strange little Being, having caused the infliction of a personal insult on him, led to the necessity of giving him satisfaction be *[sic]* a hostile meeting in which he had his shot, which he subsequently declared had carried off 'The Peak of the *Captain*'s Cap'. (Captain Cleote)[196]

The understatement and detachment notable in the latter part of the extract, which stand in contrast to the satirically loaded language in its opening sentence ('mischievous ... Monkey', 'subtle wiles of the Serpent'), alongside the longer passage's reference to Barry's sex being discovered after a postmortem examination (a legacy of 'A Mystery Still' echoed in Marvell's story), offers further illustration of the fictionalization processes to which duels were subject: Barry 'declared' he had shot off the top of Cloete's cap, but Cloete does not verify this point, and indeed as a mere commentator he appears to be entirely dissociated from that 'other' Captain so remote from himself that the person involved in the duel becomes a cardboard figure whose sole function it is to serve as a target for Barry's aggression; there is no indication of Cloete himself having fired a shot in turn, perhaps because he did not wish to incriminate himself further in his participation in an outlawed act. If the description of the event is based on Cloete's words, it is quite possibly also an act of generosity, for, while fictional accounts tend to place considerable dramatic emphasis on Barry's superior duelling skills, as Rachel Holmes points out, Cloete was in fact by far the more experienced shot and may well have deliberately misfired in order to spare his colleague.[197]

These two framed first-person accounts of Cloete's 'altercation' with Barry exemplify the essential literariness of the duel. A highly stylized, formulaic, theatrical form of bodily engagement between men, the duel, as John Leigh has noted, 'belong[s] to the realms of fiction'; if duellists were 'always implicitly consulting previous duels', this placed particular significance on *literary* narratives of duels since the prevailing means of obtaining information on duelling etiquette was textual.[198] A rich source for biographilic exploration, Barry's duel has inspired book covers, such as the Bloomsbury edition of Duncker's novel. Here, the duel is co-opted for an additional context, with the sailing boat in the background pointing to a tale of adventure, possibly piracy (Fig. 3.8).

The cultural emergence of the duel as a male upper-class rite can be placed in relation to three specific contexts. The first is the eighteenth-century association of the duel with style, poise and aristocratic codes of honour.[199] While Cloete's second account dates the duel to 1820, the values embraced by Barry's titled mentors (the Earl of Buchan and particularly Francisco de Miranda, a nobleman by both birth and French military distinction) would have left their mark on his masculine self-construction in this sense as it did in others.[200] Although the new century saw an increasing embourgeoisement of the custom, the aristocratic tradition

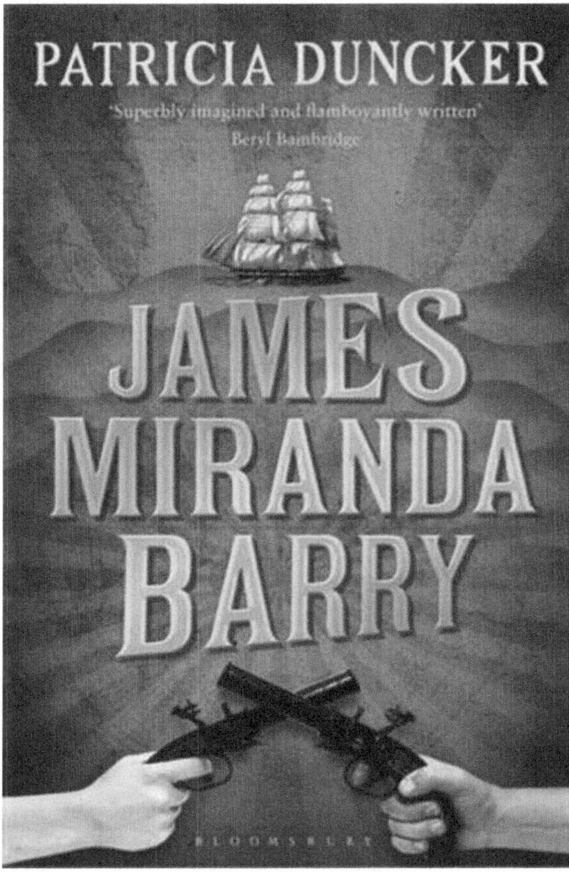

Fig. 3.8 © Patricia Duncker, 2011, *James Miranda Barry*, Bloomsbury Publishing Plc

continued into this period; the duel in 1829 of Barry's compatriot, the Dublin-born Duke of Wellington, turned Ireland in the public imagination into a hotbed of duellists.[201] Secondly, by 1816, Leigh observes, the duel had come to be seen as a means of self-affirmation for the 'modern democrat' and was now 'tied to notions of liberty', the 'sovereignty of the individual' and 'opportunities for self-expression'.[202] Duels could be fought on nationalistic as well as individual grounds. This, rather than the lady's honour, may have been the reason for Cloete, the son of an influential Dutch settler family, taking offence at Barry's remarks about Somerset's visitor, if indeed this is how the situation came about.[203] Thirdly, as a male rite of passage that had almost 'become an everyday occurrence', a duel may have been difficult to avoid, especially for a man who was as intent as Barry was on sustaining his credibility as an 'officer and gentleman'.[204] It was also the only time an army surgeon could make use of a weapon. The duel, in short, made a man of Barry.

If the duel, pace Leigh, was a 'set piece' in literature between the seventeenth and early twentieth centuries, this is doubly the case in cross-dressing narratives, where the ritual often features as an additional marker of the protagonist's masculine valour (or lack of it).[205] Binnie's *Colours* comically deflates Jane Barry's imposture when she finds herself caught out by a duel she has desperately sought to avoid; her reluctance to engage in manly combat instantly arouses suspicion that she is gay or even worse, a woman.[206] In Marvell's 'The Mystery of the Kapok Doctor', on the other hand, Barry proves his masculinity and *esprit de corps* by reining in his expert fencing skills and deliberately taking a blow in order not to harm his erstwhile adversary whom he has recognized as a brother in spirit: 'A dozen times I could have run him through and through. But … I had determined on the course I would follow, and … allowed his rapier to pierce the sleeve of my jacket, scratching my arm and drawing blood … Honour had been satisfied. No one had been hurt.'[207]

While in this case no harm has been done, the duel also offers an opportunity to explore the tricky affair of how to address more serious injury while avoiding exposure. Reginald Hargreaves's heavily embroidered history of women warriors references duelling among the heroines' most distinctive exploits. Thus Christian Ross 'had decidedly the best of it' in her confrontation with an opponent, while Mary Reid 'was no stranger' to the custom: 'twice she had had her man out'.[208] Barry's duel receives the greatest narrative attention and here serves as an illustration of the hopelessly 'irascible and umbrageous temper' of a woman who repressed her sexual instincts and sublimated them with acts of aggression. The duel is framed by two scenes in which Barry is disciplined for her unruly behaviour: an earlier argument with Somerset in the course of which Barry was 'picked up bodily by the justly incensed Governor and ignominiously dumped out of the study window' (an episode that Hargreaves purloined from 'A Mystery Still' and which also figures in Racster and Grove's play, Rose's *Perfect Gentleman* and Mohr's *Barry*); and a concluding passage that shows Barry being punished for picking a row in the officers' mess by being expelled and, as in 'A Mystery Still', subjected to formal arrest and forcible return to Britain.[209] The stoicism and restraint Barry displays at the duel is thus undercut by the two anecdotes that enclose it:

> Throughout the whole business Barry maintained her usual air of frigid self-control, and never by so much as the flicker of an eyelid betrayed the slightest qualm of fear. The second having placed their principals, the word to make ready was given. Turning her meagre frame so that it presented the smallest possible target to her opponent, the little doctor slowly raised her pistol arm and took steady aim. A word of command, and both weapons flashed almost simultaneously. For a moment there was absolute stillness; the figures of antagonists and seconds alike stood rigid under the hard sunlight as though carved out of stone. Then Barry was seen to take a hesitating step forward, almost to stagger. Running up quickly, the surgeon in attendance anxiously questioned if she was hurt. But this Barry most strenuously denied, and pulling herself upright with an effort, walked toward the carriage … The next moment she had disappeared in a cloud of dust[.][210]

Placed in the context of two corrective interventions, the duel presents not so much a vision of Barry's heroism as, rather, an illustration of her acceptance of the inevitability of chastisement. Rendered in archetypal fashion, the passage also carries intriguing resonances of the prototypical male-to-male encounter in the American Western, a then emerging genre on the movie screen. 'A Mystery Still', by contrast, accentuates not, as Hargreaves does, Barry's sex antagonism born from female sexual self-repression but the companionship that develops from the shared, profoundly galvanizing experience of surviving a life-threatening stand-off. This, too, is a trope of the literary duel, which, as Leigh points out, is 'always an affirmation of a common bond'.[211] The Barry of 'A Mystery Still' sets out to assert his masculinity and finds a friend: 'a quiet little duel took place. It ended well. Hands were shaken, and cornet and doctor became good friends for life.'[212] In modern and contemporary Barry biofiction, the duel's function as a 'conduit for male friendship' serves to explore not homosexual but heterosexual desire.[213] Thus Ouellette's *Le Secret du docteur Barry* dramatizes the erotic tension that arises when an opponent seeking to offer medical assistance instead makes a sexual discovery as 'une scène de vaudeville': '"But … but …", he stammered feebly, utterly staggered by the sight that greeted him. "But you are a woman!"'[214] That Cloete is instantly stricken points to the sexual undercurrents entailed by the physical intimacy of duelling; when the object of illicit desire is identified as female, that desire may be articulated. Barry is already involved in an affair with Somerset, but the deep emotional attachment that develops in the aftermath of the duel spawns an intensity of feeling that lasts a lifetime.

The sexual frisson inherent in narrative explorations of Barry's duel is also present in the Kronenfelds' *Secret Life of Dr. James Miranda Barry.* Pandora arrives armed with Miranda's pistol case, but rather than following Cloete's manly example and firing demonstratively over her head, she ungraciously shoots him in the leg. In its emblematic representation of Cloete's wound the text inverts the trope of Barry's injured body: as blood spreads in a 'long oval stain on Cloete's white breeches', he is symbolically deflowered by the experience, while Pandora is initiated into penetrative masculinity.[215] Though this Barry, too, is in a prior relationship (with Miranda's son), the duelling situation again generates desire; Pandora subsequently feels a distinct pang of jealousy when she sees Cloete, in close bodily contact, dancing with Somerset's daughter Georgina. Indeed, duelling appears to have an aphrodisiac effect that can implicate participants other than the main actors. In Racster and Grove's play, Cloete becomes Barry's (unacknowledged) love object, even though he is his second and not his opponent; Barry is, however, never able to disclose her feelings. In modern and contemporary biographilia, then, the trope of a fundamentally masculine ritual can be employed to jolt the cross-dresser into a recognition of her repressed sensibilities and desires, directing her reawakened femininity into 'proper' (heterosexual) channels while at the same time denying the heroine bodily fulfilment.

That straight passions are ultimately frustrated in these texts indicates that, fundamentally, the duel of a gender passer always entails a slippage of hetero and homoerotic encounters. As a narrative device the duel therefore lends itself with particular force to the exploration of sexual tensions between men. In Duncker's *James Miranda Barry*, Captain James Loughlin (a character modelled on Cloete) is suffused with an intense sense of attraction to Barry after their duel, at which Barry had spared his life after 'neatly slic[ing] off one epaulette and a dark curl of hair' and, suddenly indifferent to the eligible young lady on whose account he had engaged in combat, presents his love offering of wild orchids to Barry instead. He never conceives of Barry other than as a man and after his death vigorously protests that 'No woman would be capable of such a deed'.[216] What he means is that his lifelong admiration and affection are so profound (because not acted on) that they could not have been inadvertently devoted to a mere woman. Where Loughlin is filled with a love he dare not name, Brennan's Cloete finds his unarticulated desire for Barry turn into revulsion when he discovers not only that Barry is a woman but that she has an affair with her black servant. The discovery of the couple's cross-racial transgression brings home to him the magnitude of his impulse toward sexual transgression. His subsequent murder of Dantzen, an act of racial hatred, is also a violent displacement of his self-loathing.

In other texts, heterosexual desire is queered at the sight of Barry's 'true' body. When in Juta's *Cape Currey* the Governor's daughter, Georgina Somerset, unbuttons the unconscious Barry's jacket to ease the flow of blood from the wound he has sustained in his duel with Cloete, she is horrified to discover layers of towels covering the body of the man she loves. After half-unwrapping the body, she faints, overcome by 'ghastly waves of heat and horror', as the recognition dawns on her that her object of desire might be other than she thought: 'This creature was not for her or for any woman'.[217] And yet, while she cannot fully acknowledge what she has seen, cannot even express her disgust at the thought of Barry's swathed body other than in French ('épouvantable! – chose dégoûtante! – abominable!'), her sense of abjection is curiously commingled with dawning desire aroused by the sensual atmosphere of sweltering summer nights:

> during the days – one forgot. But then there were nights. And it was during the nights that remembrance came: the hot still nights when one sheet as a covering seemed an unbearable weight upon her slim, hot little body: nights when the cicada sang and hummed unweariedly among the gum trees outside her window, and the small green frogs in the water … croaked in chorus: nights when she tossed and turned, tired yet sleepless, the pillows growing hot beneath her restless head, turned and turned again with eyes half closed in weariness; and always the relentless memory wide awake and remindful: then great unrest would seize her: limbs refused to remain extended, and brushing aside the entangling mosquito curtain with hot hands she would feel the cool hard floor under her naked feet and grope her way to the moonlit world outside the window; her body pressed against the cool plaster wall, arms wide apart and the warm breeze, heavy with sea moisture from the dark bay, playing round the frills of her nightdress: as in Nature flowers unfold in graceful strength new petals during the night and are ready to greet the sun, fresh with the dews of night yet upon them, so after one of these 'awaking' nights and hours passed at the windows, facing the half-opened wonders and facts of her sex and her world, … she would summon her maid, and … would canter down … to the white sands of the Bay … But here … to be obliged to face these night ghosts … was too overcoming to be supported.[218]

Georgina's 'awakening' to the 'facts of her sex and her world' follows the half-revelations of Barry's body and a public placard's anonymous denunciation of Barry's and her father's shameful misconduct. In her night visions, vague insinuations of sexual relations between men intermingle with the memory of Barry's body and her growing awareness of her own body's arousal: faced with this onslaught of queer desires (for Barry the man, who is accused of entertaining an affair with her own father; Barry the woman who, engaged in the same affair, is symbolically placed in the position once held by her mother; Barry the quasi-Frankensteinian 'creature' of composite sex), small wonder if Georgina feels bewildered. Under the impact of this experience, however, she finds herself galvanized into action, at the same time as Barry is progressively disempowered. While, prior to his duel, he had taken a heroic stand in a bar fight, once he is wounded he becomes vulnerable to private and public voyeurism and scandal. If the duel thus precipitates the collapse of Barry's masquerade, it marks the start of Georgina's agency – and of a cross-dressing escapade of her own. Barry's emasculation acts as the catalyst for Georgina to come into full possession of her own faculties. The 'pink and cream' girl whose hyper-femininity exerts a tantalizing, perilous allure on men ('wild cambering briar roses that entangle you in their delicate meshes') reconstitutes herself as a swashbuckling hero when, after stealing into his bedroom to purloin his uniform while he is asleep, she impersonates Barry to remove the offending placard from the marketplace in the middle of the night.[219] A 'fetching little mannikin', she feels proud of her bravery as much as of her performance: 'I did look my part … It is really not a hard thing to look extremely like a man.'[220]

Georgina's gender imposture appears more successful than Barry's because, conceived as a passing adventure rather than a lifelong chore, it is more pleasurable. For, as the reader learns after Barry's second duel, when, in an echo of the earlier scene, he is again wounded and his sex is discovered by Cloete, his assumption of a male persona originates from a disappointment in love. Like Barry, however, Georgina too, after assuming the guise of masculinity, is overcome by sudden bouts of sleepiness, as a result of which the placard is read by a passer-by and her plan to protect the family is only partially realized. Ultimately, then, female masquerade is forever at risk of exposure during moments of unconsciousness, whether these are caused by injuries inflicted in duels or derive from simple exhaustion. The trope of the duel here combines with that of the bedroom revelation scene to subject the gender passer to the voyeuristic gaze of other characters as well as that of the reader. Just as Juta's novel disintegrates into generic confusion and excess as one sensational disclosure is followed by another, so the Barry mythos more generally is at its most spectacular when it focuses on the primal scene: the bedroom/deathbed discovery.

The bed(room), as Garber has noted, is a key site of detection and revelation in cross-dressing narratives, for this is where '"[t]ruths" about gender and sexuality' and thus about the body of the cross-dresser are (thought to be) uncovered.[221] Such 'bed scenes' displace sexual into detective energy as the '"crime" of impersonation' is unearthed.[222] They rely on the suspension or even cessation of the gender passer's agency, usually at times of sleep, unconsciousness, or death. If the 'ur-locus' of discovery is the deathbed, Barry biographilia shifts the role of detective from the doctor (who is here doubly disempowered as the body under investigation and as the undiscerning colleague) to a female subaltern figure, the charwoman who laid out the body.[223] This has the effect of bringing the female cross-dressing plot full circle: the woman who assumed male garb to escape poverty is stripped of her disguise by another woman who, because of her inferior sex and class, is denied compensation for her labour.[224] A variant of the dramatic circumstances of the unnamed layer-out's discovery and the disregard she experienced was published by a contemporary officer's wife, Elizabeth Fenton, after Barry's death.[225] Fenton's journal records the account of a nurse who claimed to have 'been driven from the Cape by Dr. Barry' after discovering his sex when in a medical emergency she had 'made an unceremonious entrance into his room':

> Thereon he flew into a most violent passion. She declares and steadily maintains, that the nominal Dr Barry *was* and *is a woman*. From this time he displayed the most implacable dislike to her, even to making it a condition not to attend in any family where she was employed. The truth of this strange tale I cannot pledge myself to uphold, but well I remember listening to it one tedious night ...[226]

When Fenton met Barry in Mauritius, in 1829, she found that there was 'certainly something extraordinary' about him.[227] She had cause to distrust him and accused Barry of 'malice' in bringing formal charges against the two medical officers who had attended her when she experienced complications during childbirth. Given her involvement in a public inquiry that, after the officers were cleared of any wrong-doing, resulted in talk about the 'removal' of Barry, her nonchalant comment that 'under these circumstances ... a tour of the island together seemed both agreeable and natural' casts some doubt over the reliability of her account.[228] Her reference to the nurse's 'strange tale' told 'one tedious night' in India lends the episode a self-consciously story-telling edge.

Mrs. Fenton's anecdote of the involuntary spy, combined with an episode adapted from Rogers's *A Modern Sphinx* in which a fellow-officer comes to be cast as an adversary, is integrated into the duel story in Rutherford's 'Dr. James Barry'. Barry's second, Surgeon Foss, is rudely sent on his way when, on realizing that Barry has been seriously injured after his stand-off with Cloete, he insists that 'I must dress the wound. Get into your bedroom. ... I will undress you and soon get you right.' To his bewilderment, Barry flies into a rage and '[f]rom that day ... kept out of Foss's way and avoided any intercourse ... If Foss happened to be of the same company Barry made a point of ignoring him, and even failed to recognize him when they met.'[229] The figure of the nurse makes an explicit fictional appearance in Racster and Grove's *Journal*, in two different incarnations. The nurse's working-class position is racialized, with Barry/Lady Barrymore expressing profound suspicion of an Indian Ayah: 'I find this strange Eastern person disturbing. She has alarmingly observant black eyes. ... Can these Eastern people .... distinguish sex in this manner?'[230] Ironically, it is not the Indian nurse but a white Western woman, Mary, the wife of a fellow-officer, whose gaze proves even more disconcerting after Barry wakes up one morning realizing that the night before she forgot to pull the blinds of her bedroom window and could therefore have been observed undressing from Mary's window.[231] Her fear of exposure by a woman whose advances she had previously rejected prompts her to block her husband's promotion to ensure that the couple remain at a safe geographical distance from her – a variant of Mrs. Fenton's nurse finding herself 'driven' from the Cape. Ultimately, Racster and Grove's Barry fails in her medical duties when she ignores Mary's desperate pleas to attend to her during a difficult pregnancy: Mary dies in childbirth, and there is no indication that she had spied on Barry and discovered her secret.

A more positive outcome of the nurse detection trope is featured in the Kronenfelds' *Secret Life*, where the Irish nurse McNamara bursts into Pandora's room while she is resting after delivering a baby by Caesarian section. When the nurse is persuaded by Barry's enemies to go public with what she has seen, Barry has a constructive 'woman-to-woman talk' with her, upon which McNamara withdraws her accusations and Barry in exchange sails for Britain, never to return to the Cape.[232] What is striking in all these narratives is that even though the reader is fully aware of Barry's impersonation, the credibility of the nurse is still undermined by crude racial, ethnic or gender stereotyping (the sinister Ayah, the tippling and slatternly Irish nurse, the sexually profligate and femininely deceitful Mary), as if the factual layer-out had to be chastised again and again for her disclosure of Barry's sex, even though it was this act that made biographilic exploration possible in the first place.

If the layer-out is discredited in narrative representations of the discovery scene, the figure of the doctor is afforded a greater measure of respect. While in their factual accounts, David McKinnon and G.W. Campbell conceded that they had overlooked the 'crucial point' of Barry's sex because they had not examined the body in any detail (McKinnon because he 'could positively swear to [Barry's] identity', having known him as Inspector General for 'eight or nine years', and Campbell because Barry's room was always cast in darkness), the fictionalized doctor and officer is equipped with a detective's impetus and acuity in lifting the impostor's cover.[233] In his *Lancet* contributions Ebenezer Rogers cited an officer's confidential communication to garner reader interest in and authenticate his novel:

> I met the colonel commanding a northern sub-district at mess shortly after the publication of 'A Modern Sphinx' in 1881, and taking me aside he gave me the following startling information, ...which, so far as I can remember them, I will tell in his own words: 'I was quartered as a subaltern in Trinidad while Dr. Barry was serving there in the capacity of principal medical officer. One day a friend of mine, an assistant surgeon, asked me to walk with him into Port-au-Prince. "The P.M.O.," said he, "is down with fever at the house of a lady friend, but has given strict injunctions to us not to visit him. Nevertheless, I feel bound to call and see how he is. Will you come with me?" On arrival my friend entered Barry's bedroom, while I remained on the verandah. In a few minutes he called me excitedly into the room, exclaiming, as he flung back the bedclothes, "See, Barry is a woman!" At that moment the P.M.O. awoke to consciousness and gazed at us bewilderingly. But she quickly recovered presence of mind and asked us in low tones to swear solemnly not to disclose her secret as long as she lived. "As a matter of fact," added the colonel, "I have never till now mentioned the subject."'"[234]

The assistant surgeon's deliberate disregard of Barry's express interdiction turns the scene into a version of the allure of the forbidden chamber of fairytales and anticipates his excitement at unmasking Barry (a different kind of Bluebeard): that this is an act of chastisement is suggested by the triumphant brutality with which he exposes the unconscious body to his fellow-officer's gaze. The anecdote, which follows the same narrative logic (and aggressive promotion of his book) as Rogers's other 'witness' statements, was disputed both by the officer in question, J. de Montmorency, and by Surgeon-General Sir T. Longmore, who knew the family where Barry had lodged: 'It was not discovered that he was a female.'[235] The scene is reworked in Binnie's *Colours*, where the doctor in question expresses his profound admiration for Barry's achievements.[236] Similarly, in Ouellette's *Le Secret*, Barry is reassured that his secret will be protected 'at all cost', and he continues to be addressed as a male; 'See, Barry is a woman!' turns into 'I see you as a pioneer ['un pionnier' not 'une pionnière'] of medicine, in more than one way since this evening.'[237] Rogers's own novel trebly displaces the episode, by having it take place off-page, turning the doctor figure into an officer's wife (Mrs Elrington) who tends to Barry (Fitzjames) during an illness, and by including an earlier satirical version of a near-discovery. When accommodation is scarce on a crossing, a fellow officer is assigned Dr. Fitzjames's room (in adaptation of Rogers's experience of sharing a cabin with Barry).[238] Accidental discovery is pre-empted by Barry's dog Psyche protecting his master's bodily privacy when the other man gets too close for comfort. Though Barry assures the assembled company that 'the little brute was harmless as a mouse', '[p]oor Burke's bleeding arms and legs told a different tale'.[239]

This story is adapted in Rutherford's 'Dr. James Barry', whose protagonist, flanked by dog and goat, succeeds in persuading the Captain to grant him a room of his own, on the grounds that his 'little dog … was trained to resent the entrance to Barry's bedroom on shore of any stranger and would be just as truculent in a ship's cabin.'[240] Ouellette's novel adds a further quota of parody to the plot device of building suspense by subjecting Barry to the imminent danger of bedroom exposure, a crisis that is then averted at the last moment by the intervention of a friendly pet. When in *Le Secret* Barry is badly incommoded by an amorous officer's wife who has already stripped herself to the waist and is in the process of launching herself at him, Barry is saved from assault by the sudden and startling appearance of the goat she keeps in her cabin: 'Seeing the disgust on the woman's face, she [Barry] knew that she would not have to worry about her again.'[241]

The sensational element of the bedroom discovery scene can thus be exploded through comedy. As in the duel trope, it can also serve to queer heterosexual desire. Thus in Racster and Grove's *Journal*, Barry faints from exhaustion after a sleepless night of ministering to countless patients during a smallpox epidemic and awakes on the shoulder of her best friend, the nurse Sophie:

> My face was so close to hers, I kissed her. Sophie promptly turned me over … and smacked me. Round us were the sounds of heavy breathing and moaning, and through the window came the eternal whiffs of nitrous fumes and burning wool. We had experienced such an orgy of pock-marked faces, of sunken eyes and grunts of pain. … We suddenly burst into laughter!
>
> 'Ye'd be spelding with me in the gloaming would ye?' Sophie giggled …
>
> 'I'm struck with ye,' I retorted almost smothered.
>
> 'I'll have none of that, sir,' from Sophie, with another smack on the seat of my breeches.
>
> 'Ye're a bonnie lass. Peety ye're married,' I answered.
>
> 'You and your nonsense!' from Sophie … 'Why don't you marry and keep chaste?'[242]

Sophie and Barry's banter, conducted in the medium of Scots, the dialect of their home country, does little to camouflage the sexual tension that has developed between them. Sophie does not know Barry's secret and takes her for a man. The epidemic subsides and 'Life is [soon] normal again', but the fact that Barry registers the anger of Sophie's husband indicates that she is well aware of the undercurrent of hetero and homoerotic desires that underprop her close friendship with Sophie.[243] That Barry's diary entries nonetheless conclude with her undisclosed love of Cloete is the textual/sexual equivalent of her gender masquerade. The actual passion Barry can never own up to is for Sophie.

Duncker's *James Miranda Barry* offers the most self-consciously and ironically queer adaptation of the bedroom discovery trope. Here Barry is at the height of his career and utterly at ease with his identity and body; his charismatic personality exerts an irresistible pull on both women and men. As in Ouellette's novel, one of his female admirers, the governor's daughter Charlotte, attempts to bring matters to a close. When after a feast he helps her intoxicated brother back to his room, she induces Barry to extend the service to her, and he obliges in order to ensure her safety, for she too has indulged in too much drink. Once in her room, Charlotte begins to undress, dragging him on the bed, and Barry is able to disentangle himself only by taking the initiative:

> There was only one way to end this. He pulled her face round towards him and kissed her ferociously on the lips. Lotte sank back with a gasp. … She flung herself against him. He kissed her again, harder this time.
>
> Lotte let out a ravished sigh … She had all her desires at last. She had captured the alluring, the enticing, the mysterious Dr Barry.
>
> Not quite.
>
> With his left hand Barry pulled her skirts right up to her thighs and beyond, then reached down into her most secret places. She cried out, startled and amazed. The doctor's expert knowledge of anatomy came into play. She was soaking wet with involuntary excitement. He found out the source of her pleasure and rubbed her gently into ecstasy, his mouth hard against hers, stifling the little screams which poured forth … He waited until the soft electric shocks subsided, then began to liberate himself, with some difficulty, from her octopus petticoats. …
>
> … Listen to me, Lotte. Don't ever get so drunk again with a man you don't know. Someone will take advantage of you. …
>
> … She did and did not hear him. She failed to understand. She did feel the fatherly kiss, which he at last bestowed on her damp curls. … [She] fell asleep feeling nothing but the warmth and dizziness of satisfied and completed love.
>
> Barry let himself out through the front door, well aware that he was observed by dozens of admiring eyes, and strolled home beneath an aureole of stars.[244]

Here, then, a text subverts the bedroom trope by conferring ultimate sexual control on Barry rather than stripping him of agency and by enhancing rather than resolving the textual play with the mystery of the 'truth' of his body. To observers, Barry has established his prowess as a lady killer when he is seen walking away from the Governor's house in the middle of the night. The potential cause of discovery, Charlotte, never questions his sex; convinced that she has had penetrative intercourse, she maintains even decades later, after Barry's death, that she can '*quite positively affirm* his masculinity'.[245] Nor is the reader – the invisible voyeur in the bedroom – any the wiser. In highlighting Barry's 'expert knowledge', the novel engages us in an elaborate tease, for does this knowledge derive from his anatomical studies, his long-standing relationship with the actress Alice Jones, his own bodily experience, or all of these in conjunction, thus affording him the means of transforming a situation of threatened exposure into an experience of sexual gratification for his companion if not for himself? Does Barry really only want to extricate himself from Charlotte's grasp or does he, too, derive pleasure from the encounter; and are his 'fatherly' kiss and admonishing words just another game with the reader? In sexualizing the bedroom revelation plot, the text offers an illustrative answer to the question that was so often asked after gender passers' death, of how (and if) they had misled their sexual partners (an issue that Barry's lover Alice faces on the concluding pages, when the retired actress is shown preparing for her last and 'best performance', an interview with probing female journalist Henrietta Stackpole, a character transmigrated from Henry James's *Portrait of a Lady*: a textual play with the posthumous legacy of two different gender/sex variant Jameses).[246] Here, then, the novel's metadramatic foreclosure on the bravado finale that takes place beyond the drawn curtains of the text ironizes the sensationalist theatricality of the Barry story.

An engagement with sensation is constitutive of Barry biographilia because the Barry mythos is inextricably tied to Barry's contested body. The secrets, transformations and performances of this body are explored through the central tropes of the textual corpus that developed from the Victorian foundation myth. This myth largely builds on the two modes established by 'A Mystery Still' and Rogers's *A Modern Sphinx*, humour and sensation, sensation tinged with melodrama in its Victorian and with sex in its modern and contemporary variants. The vivid and witty narrative dramatization of Barry's eccentricity and bravado in 'A Mystery Still' inspired caricatures, which in their turn, alongside key passages from this first story and sensational periodical press anecdotes stoked by Rogers, became mnemonic relics that found their way into twentieth and twenty-first-century biographilic work. The use that biographies in particular have made of the foundation myth and its key constituents, sometimes un-self-consciously, reverberates in contemporary biofiction and, as will be examined in more detail in the next chapter, has also left its mark on biodrama. The regularity with which the central components of the myth circulate in Barry biographilia establishes an element of consistency through intertextual blurring within a genre that is marked by instability of form.

Three narrative relics predominate as set pieces of the Victorian story and its afterlife: Barry's self-constitution through a bodily make-over in front of a mirror; the assertion of this new self in a duel in which models of masculinity are tested in physical encounters that spawn queer friendships; and the threat of exposure in unguarded moments in the bedroom:

moments of crisis as much as they are moments of transformative performance. The primary focus of this chapter on narrative tropes and their co-option and subversion across Barry biographilia has served to investigate the circulation and transmigration of the 'bodily remains' of the foundation myths and their representations of Barry's 'real' and imagined gender and sexuality. In their adaptive appropriations of the mythos and their playful explorations of its spectacular aspects, these texts all partake in what I have conceptualized as 'sensation biographilia', a category extended from Kohlke's 'appropriated biofiction' to the wider genre of Barry life-writing. Essentially, all Barry biographilia is appropriative in the sense that it is grounded in an intertextual engagement with the (textually or pictorially inflected) bodily 'remains' and remediations of the Barry story.

What is striking about Barry biographilia across all inflections of appropriative and sensation modes and beyond the shared exploration of body plot structures is that, with the exception of Duncker's novel and Holmes's biography, the expectation of a teleology in interpretative approaches to gender variance is not fulfilled. The critic or reader who anticipates a conceptual progress narrative, from the Victorian 'woman in man's garb' through the twentieth-century 'feminist male impersonator' to the twenty-first-century transgender individual will be disappointed. One of the most probing questions Barry life-writing raises, therefore, is why even in the present century, which has seen ever increasing levels of interest in and cultural, social and political discourses on transgender, Barry continues to be cast, uncritically, as a woman. Barry biographilia's emphasis on performance may yield some insights into this conundrum. Just as the Barry character is depicted as experimenting with the transformation of the body and the performance of selves, so too is Barry biographilia profoundly concerned with the performance of transformative acts. The next chapter will pay focused attention to the biographilic performance of gender through the performance of genre and genre subversion in contemporary biodrama, biography and biofiction.

CHAPTER 4

Performances in Gender and Genre: Barry in Contemporary Postmodernist Biodrama, Biography and Biofiction

> When I was a boy I was told that when I began a story, to begin at the beginning and continue to the end …
>
> James Barry, speech at court-martial (1836)[1]

> I was much less interested in the 'why' … this seemed to me self-evident – than in the 'how' …
>
> Kit Brennan, Foreword to *Tiger's Heart* (1998)[2]

> [G]ender proves to be performative – that is, constituting the identity it is purported to be. In this sense, gender is always a doing, though not a doing by a subject who might be said to preexist the deed … [T]here is no gender identity behind the expressions of gender: that identity is performatively constituted by the very 'expressions' that are said to be its result.
>
> Judith Butler, *Gender Trouble* (1990)[3]

> The error of the willful biographer lies in her refusal to be changed by her encounter with the ghost she chases; the method of the transgender historian must be encounter, confrontation, transformation.
>
> Judith Halberstam, *In a Queer Time & Place* (2005)[4]

In its exploration of the key constituents of the Barry myth, the last chapter pointed toward the performative aspects of Barry life-writing. Whether Barry is depicted as the swaggering hero of a duel or the comical spectacle of a 'miniature man' decked out in full uniform, with a grotesquely over-

A. Heilmann, *Neo-/Victorian Biographilia and James Miranda Barry*, https://doi.org/10.1007/978-3-319-71386-1_4

sized sword that always threatens to trip him up, the textual and pictorial *mise-en-scène* of Barry's gender performance always also offers an illustration of the performative acts of biographilic works themselves.[5] If, in the Butlerian sense, gender is produced and naturalized by ritualized acts that perform the idea of a 'gendered essence' (consolidating the notion of an essential concurrence of gender and the body), and if performativity denotes the 'ways that identities are constructed iteratively through complex citational processes', the portrait of James Barry that originated from 'A Mystery Still' and the early anecdotes and caricatures have shaped all subsequent representations, prompting echo effects either through direct replication (as in most of the works discussed in Chapter 3) or through ironic subversion (as in Duncker's novel).[6] Just as Barry is shown posing in the mirror, so each text 'performs' Barry performing gender in the looking glass of previous performative turns. To borrow Kit Brennan's words, what is at the heart of this chapter it is not so much 'why' but 'how' Barry has been performed, and how this enactment of an enactment has affected the generic structures of biographilic texts. For Butler's conceptualization of gender as a performative act of 'doing' rather than an ontological state of 'being' can with equal force be applied to genre.[7] Max Saunders's concepts of 'autobiografiction' and 'biografiction' (in my use of the term adapted to 'biographiction') will serve to examine the – conflicted or self-conscious – blurring of generic boundaries between biodrama, fiction, biography and fictional autobiography.[8] This will involve paying close attention to the self-reflexivity and revisionist strategies which Ansgar Nünning identifies as key features of such works, and which effect a 'shift [of] emphasis from the mere writing, or rewriting, of an historical individual's life to the epistemological and methodological problems involved in any attempt at life-writing itself'.[9] Ultimately, to what extent and in what ways have postmodernist life-writers responded to Halberstam's call to embrace transformation in the encounter and confrontation with Barry's transgender ghost?

This chapter, then, returns to the questions raised at the start of the book in considering how gender and genre might interact in the (metatextually refracted) construction of the figure of the historical gender crosser in life-writing. While the focus of previous chapters has been on determining the key features of Barry biographilia as an umbrella genre and tracing the modulations of such shared features across the corpus of works, this chapter seeks to scrutinize the particularities of the forms themselves in the context of their respective biographical, biofictional and biodramatic paradigms. If the last chapter was largely concerned with Victorian and earlier twentieth-century life-writing and with the adaptive processes that the original motifs and key images underwent in later works, this chapter's emphasis is on contemporary postmodernist texts and the way in which the stories they tell take their cue from Barry's own strategies of self-creation. To draw on one example, Barry's courtroom reminiscences of his boyhood (as referenced in the opening epigraph) signal a performance of self that was predicated on the conceit of linearity, continuity and straight(forward)ness to mask radical transformation and self-invention. How is this fabrication of gender and identity reflected in the self-enactment and play with form in Barry life-writing? In order to gain closer insight into the textual specificities of biographilic forms while attending to their boundary blurrings, this chapter is organized into separate sections on biodrama, biography and biofiction.

That the cultural 'memory' of James Barry was from early on marked by a distinctly theatrical quality is indicated by Ebenezer Rogers's reference to the ease with which the story that he had spun would lend itself to the stage: 'How the Adelphi pit, or the Surrey gallery, would roar with laughter and shudder with sympathy at possible complications!'[10] The burlesque and melodramatic treatments Rogers invoked were notable in the first stage production, by Olga Racster and Jessica Grove, but later twentieth and twenty-first-century dramatizations have developed the material in new ways. The first section in this chapter therefore examines contemporary biodrama, a type of play that, in Benjamin Poore's definition, 'aims to tell the life story of a historical individual from birth (or early youth) to death, supposedly narrated by that individual, and featuring him or her stepping into role as protagonist as well as narrator'. The form is distinguished by the way in which it 'weav[es] together documentary evidence from letters and other writings with direct audience address and, usually, a self-conscious theatricality'.[11] In Barry biodrama, gender performance is underpinned by the theatrical resonances of a character doubling that, by externalizing the protagonist's inner crises, encourages a response of 'empathetic unsettlement' in the spectator.[12] Here, then, the Barry story crosses over into trauma narrative.

'The Mourner of Myself': Duality, Conflict and Redemption in Biodrama[13]

Authored in the 1980s, 1990s and the first postmillennial decade by playwrights whose national identities (the UK, Ireland and Canada) relate to key locations in Barry's history, Frederic Mohr's (David McKail's) *Barry:*

Personal Statements (1984), Jean Binnie's *Colours* (1988/89), Kit Brennan's *Tiger's Heart* (1996) and Sebastian Barry's *Whistling Psyche* (2004) problematize questions of duality and (self-)division, performativity (the iteration of acts) and performance (the *mise-en-scène* of Barry's self-construction). While these also feature in Olga Racster and Jessica Grove's *Dr. James Barry* of 1919, a significant difference between this stage play and contemporary biodrama is that external action is internalized; conflict and strife move inward. Concerned with mapping moments of spiritual crisis, postmodern Barry plays tend to dispense with the larger cast of Racster and Grove's production, reducing the number of actors to five (*Tiger's Heart*) or two (*Whistling Psyche; Barry: Personal Statements*).[14] With a minimum cast of fourteen playing forty-five characters with thirty-two speaking parts, Binnie's *Colours* diverges from the other contemporary dramas, but here, too, the focus is on the inner development of the protagonist, who recollects and comments on crises and turning points, during which the characters enacting scenes from her life freeze into stills. The bare stage represents Barry's mind; all furniture is carried on by the actors to set the scene for Barry's memories.[15]

The transformative agency that in biofiction culminates in experiences of triumph is in contemporary plays transmuted into the dramatic exploration of a tragic personality and his internal dilemmas. That these plays depict Barry in the process of reviewing his life at the point of (or, in the case of *Whistling Psyche*, after) death aligns biodrama with biofiction; as Ina Schabert notes, metatextually inflected biographical fiction typically engages with the protagonist's '"last days" and the death-bed meditation' to 'enable the author to represent the reality of the individual … with an extraordinary force.'[16] However, where biographies and biofictions draw attention to the remarkable achievements of Barry's life, bioplays are more likely to shift the emphasis to the irony and tragedy of an identity forged from exceptional will-power and self-discipline that in death is subjected to an absolute loss of control. As the Barry of *Whistling Psyche* bemoans, 'so my story is reduced to this, a drunken old woman fumbling in the parts of a helpless, dead personage, and anything I did to redress the unforgivable imbalances of this pretty world is as nothing, swallowed up in the Leviathan of this revelation.'[17] Here Barry is summoned as a spectre of the past who haunts the present in search of an enlightened community: 'though I long to go, I cannot go, for there is no approbation, no love … to release me'.[18] While intradiegetically, Barry's interlocutor, present or implied, serves to proffer redemption, extradiegetically the audience assumes this cathartic role. When Barry sighs, 'I wish I were a person in an age when my achievements might be seen as mighty things', the words are calculated to resonate with spectators and readers.[19] As David Cregan suggests, the secular space of the theatre here takes on the transcendental quality of a 'ritual of longing, reconciliation, and transformation' in a process that, in Poore's terms, turns dramatic entertainment into 'epiphany plays'.[20] Harnessing the double vision of neo-Victorianism, a genre whose backward glance always serves to address modern-day concerns, biodrama thus seeks to reclaim Barry as a precursor figure whose internal conflicts are of direct relevance for us today.

The doubling effect resulting from the associations drawn between past and present is enhanced by the format of a one or two-person show which throws into relief the act of impersonation by making the spectator aware of 'the *extraversion* of the actor [and] the *introversion* of the signifier' (the role).[21] In *Tiger's Heart* all but the actor playing Barry are assigned two roles, thereby highlighting both the duality of characters and the disjuncture between act and actor. Doubling is also a prominent feature of Binnie's larger-scale *Colours*, where all actors bar Barry are performing multiple parts and the tension between the protagonist's female self and body (Jane) and male role (James) is represented by two separate actors. The play itself performed a doubling act in being produced in the same month in two countries (Ireland and England), each a significant setting for the Barry story, with two separate stage aesthetics, Jude Kelly's Dublin-based 'Regency romp' being juxtaposed to John Harrison's 'Brechtian' interpretation in Yorkshire.[22] (This difference in approach is encouraged by the generic hybridity of a play that blends together elements from a multiplicity of forms: comedy, the farce, romance, melodrama, psychodrama and hagiography.)

The emphasis on duality draws attention to the internal self-division of the Barry character in terms of gender or age: paired with Florence Nightingale in *Whistling Psyche* and mirroring her/himself in the juxtaposition of recollecting and recollected/re-enacting selves in *Colours*, Barry is split into a younger and older personality in Mohr's monodrama. In his 'Preface' Mohr compares the solo play's emotional 'intimacy and intensity of the [protagonist's] need to unburden' to psychotherapy: 'a solo should be something dragged out of the subject by the need to impart an understanding to another person, rather in the manner in which people trapped in old fashioned railway compartments were buttonholed by other passengers, whom they would never meet again after the journey, and so could be treated as a free psychiatrist'.[23] Mohr's railway carriage is reconfigured as a waiting room in a Victorian railway station in *Whistling Psyche*, where the soliloquizing Barry comments that 'A person tells stories because he does not wish the wave of silence to drown him'.[24] Conjuring up the spectre of Coleridge's 'Ancient Mariner', Barry's 'buttonholing' of a reluctant listener turns biodrama into a confessional narrative of self-mourning.

The intimate first-person perspective that these plays unlock on Barry's internal conflicts can be placed in the context of Max Saunders's concept of autobiografiction. In his definition of autobiografiction as 'fiction impersonating life-writing', in the sense that '"real" autobiographical experience' in the form of 'spiritual experience[e]' is turned into fiction, Saunders draws on Stephen Reynolds' early twentieth-century coinage of the term as denoting a form of life-writing that provides 'a record of real spiritual experiences strung on a credible but more or less fictitious autobiographical narrative'.[25] Notably 'it isn't just the form that is fictionalized', Saunders explains, 'but the autobiographical experience itself'; this 'fictionalization is presented in what is therefore pseudo-autobiographical form'.[26] Autobiografiction thus marks the interface between 'autobiographical fiction and "unreliable autobiography"'.[27]

Given that plays are not fiction and theatrical production processes move well beyond textuality, how can Saunders's concept be co-opted for drama; and why should it in the first place? Arguably, while Saunders establishes auto/biografiction as a 'model for modernist engagements with life-writing', the concept lends itself to a more comprehensive application across twentieth-century and contemporary biographilia.[28] Saunders's definition is broad enough to permit consideration of a wide variety of self-conscious and playful forms of biographilia, including those that mimic aspects of biography (the 'imaginary portrait') and drama (the dramatic monologue). If the category is extended both temporally and conceptually, to what might be called contemporary 'autobiodramatic texts', then bioplays can be considered to form part of a wider paradigm of 'autobiografictional' life-writing. Including biodrama in this concept adds to our understanding of neo-Victorianism's textual and conceptual experimentation with multiple forms of life-writing and the way in which 'autobiography, biography, fiction, criticism' and also other types of biographilia 'begin to interact, combining and disrupting each other in new ways'.[29]

While Barry biodrama can thus be conceived as embracing an autobiografictional mode, it also engages with other literary forms. The troubled soliloquies particularly in Mohr and Sebastian Barry's plays are evocative of the dramatic monologue. A form that came into its own in the Victorian period (most prominently in the poetry of Tennyson and Browning), the dramatic monologue is, like biodrama (and neo-Victorian biographilia more broadly), distinguished by generic diversity.[30] Featuring individuals in crisis, it privileges speakers who belong to a community of outsiders: 'iconoclasts, individualists, misfits, and rebels'.[31] This certainly applies to Barry and Nightingale in Mohr and Sebastian Barry's plays; in *Whistling Psyche*, Barry refers to his 'lifetime of resistance and revolution', and Nightingale recalls being told that 'I should have been born a man, because I was like a man and worse than a man, in my ambitions'.[32] As Glennis Byron points out, contemporary revisionist versions of the dramatic monologue often 'draw upon characters from literature [or] history', are 'frequently marked by an overt feminist politics' and tend to 'represent an incongruous "I"' whose 'divided consciousness' calls attention to 'questions of representation'.[33] This is reflected in the blurring first-person perspectives of *Whistling Psyche*, the doubled and thereby merging character roles in *Tiger's Heart,* and the disruption of any sense of a 'unified' first-person account in Mohr's play, where the identity of the middle-aged Inspector-General of the second part who keeps cracking officers' mess jokes is only gradually revealed to be the older version of the heavily pregnant woman awaiting delivery in the first.

The theatrical attributes of the dramatic monologue are a further context for the use of this form in Barry biodrama. As Cornelia Pearsall remarks, dramatic monologue, or 'monodrama', 'seeks to dramatize, as well as to cause, performative effects'; in staging a 'dramatic transformation of a situation or a self', both speaker and poet are 'attempting to create reactions and larger social transformations in the world outside'.[34] Whether either dramatic monologue or Barry biodrama may lay claim to bringing on social and political change is debatable, but the relevant connection between the two forms here is that both address an extradiegetic spectator: 'allied to drama', dramatic monologue, like biodrama, 'requires an audience' and seeks to interact with it.[35] Contemporary plays on Barry thus both draw on and revitalize the lyrical form of the dramatic monologue. This is most notable in Mohr's solo play, where Barry's interlocutors are implied but not physically present. Binnie's *Colours*, by contrast, populates the stage with the materialized recollections of the heroine's inner life. In *Whistling Psyche* the monologic structure of Barry's soliloquies and Nightingale's self-reflexive responses gradually develop into a fragmented dialogue. Brennan's *Tiger's Heart* is at the furthest remove from the dramatic monologue proper, but its short, clipped scenes predominantly organized around dialogic sequences between two speakers retain traces of the form. In their dramatization of the fissures in Barry's performance and internal sense of self, the postmodernist plays by Mohr, Sebastian Barry and Brennan revolve around three main themes: the conflicted nature of Barry's gender identity, as revealed in the precariousness of a life spent 'always proving' over and beyond the social/cultural performance of masculinity; Barry's duality, reflected in the juxtaposition of younger and older selves in Mohr and male and female medical reformer and rebel in Sebastian Barry; and the intersectionality of gender, ethnicity and race, which, in *Tiger's Heart*, is explored through Barry's relationship with his black servant Dantzen.[36]

The first of the contemporary biodramas, Mohr's *Barry: Personal Statements* draws attention to the motif of self-division both structurally and sartorially with two solo plays that together make up Barry's composite identity. The audience is introduced to a pregnant young woman 'near her time', dressed in a 'loose-fitting white cotton shift' that gives her the appearance of a 'freshly scrubbed healthy child'. The speaker of the second part is an older gentleman (as soon transpires from his words, a senior military officer) who wears a 'frock coat over a black waistcoat and striped trousers'; his elegant pocket watch and cravat held in place by a 'jewelled pin' signal material comfort and a secure social position.[37] Here autobiodrama as theatrical production and autobiodrama as text create different effects, for whereas the reader will immediately identify both characters as James Barry on the basis of the opening blurb and the stage directions, which set the two monologues forty years apart, in two different locations (1819, Mauritius and 1859, Montreal), and refer to the aged Barry as a general, the theatre audience may place the scenes as contemporaneous and not make the connection between the two actors playing the same person at different ages until the older Barry recapitulates the story of his youth.

The two Barrys' identities are fractured by gender, age, and clothing, even sartorial colour schemes (the manicheistic contrast of white and black perhaps hinting at the starkness of the gender binary). Outer garments also indicate inner frames of mind: as a state of undress, the young Barry's loose and unrestricting chemise not only reflects the practical needs of a woman about to give birth but also suggests a greater psychological openness; certainly this Barry shares her secret with the (invisible, presumably native Mauritian) midwife who stands in for the audience. The insouciance of the 'female' Barry who, notwithstanding the fact of her having lived as a man for a decade, 'regards her very obvious pregnancy ... as just another surmountable hurdle in some exhilaratingly challenging adventure' was considered unconvincing by reviewers of the original UK production.[38] The elderly Barry, by contrast, is carefully buttoned up and gives little away; clothes evidently make the man. The play's subtitle points to the divergence in the nature of the two 'personal statements', with the spirited reminiscences of the first part being set against the guarded doubletalk of the second, in which Barry's 'clipped syllables' and crude jokes signal the habits and self-presentation 'acquired in a lifetime of officers' messes'.[39] In this military context the titular reference to 'personal statements' assumes a more formal, legal dimension that, to the initiated reader/spectator, may recall Barry's court-martial. Are Barry's 'personal statements' his deposition, his legal and moral defence, for being, or for failing to be, 'an officer and gentleman'?[40]

The dramatic device of splitting Barry in two offers a practical demonstration of the impersonator's strategy to '[h]ide in the open, where no one thinks to look'.[41] While the medical student plays at being 'one of the boys', admitting that 'My performance is still far from perfect, the woman in me shows through for those with eyes' (such as the Scottish Highlands herbalist Auld Janet, whose healing skills inspire Barry to take up medicine), the older Barry has perfected the mask to the point of having internalized it.[42] Thus, in telling us that 'I might well have married ... but the mother of my child was a free spirit', he is both playing a game (hiding in the open) with his interlocutor (and the audience) and at the same time is manifesting a sense of self-division.[43] Is this a sign that Barry 'has begun to blur the truth of his/her [sex] even when alone' or, rather, that what began as impersonation has grown to be 'the truth' of lived experience, 'the mask [having] become the face' (as Patricia Duncker's Barry puts it)?[44]

In Part Two Barry crudely refers to Queen Victoria's 'cunt-stricken son', recalls another officer telling him that in the hot climate of India the soldiers tend to take up buggery, and recounts a lengthy anecdote about a soldier whose persistent erection while on parade failed to subside even after he was given time off to be with 'his woman' because it was the commander he fancied. Is this macho-homophobic discourse with its anxiety about homosexuality that is masked as smutty banter a clever performance (who would detect a woman in this guise?), or does it represent Barry's inner identity as a military man who can crack a dirty joke (even if – or because – his private life is unusually chaste)?[45] That the latter story directly follows the recollection of Somerset's death, and is succeeded by a reference to his son's demise from leprosy, implies that an excessive exhibition of a particular type of masculinity might serve to conceal – or repress – the resurgence of acutely painful feelings and the recognition of his lifelong loneliness. It is this pervasive sense of loneliness that connects the two personas across the gulf of time. (The paralyzing prospect of a life spent in separation from others is conveyed in Mohr's script for a television adaptation; the manuscript markedly breaks off at the precise point when the young student recognizes that he will have to 'add loneliness to my curriculum'.)[46]

That solitude is the keynote of his experience is implied by both the young and old Barry's protestations of having led a full (sexually at least temporarily fulfilled) personal life. Masculinity here serves as a screen to cover up an overpowering sense of futility and loss. A subsequent anecdote suggests that Barry has internalized the masculinity he displays, but that this identity is so fragile that any reminder of what he once was and can no longer represent poses a serious threat to his self-perception: the woman professional. Thus the achievement of the first 'lady doctor', Elizabeth Blackwell, is mocked with another innuendo, this time about straight sex, an allusion that Blackwell promptly fails to comprehend – 'that's spinster doctors for you'.[47] Barry's intensely conflicted gender identity culminates in his affirmation of difference: 'All I will say is that while I have not married, I have not denied myself experience. But throughout I have behaved responsibly and, I hope, like a gentleman.'[48] Ultimately, it is Barry's over-identification with a deeply misogynist brand of masculinity that freezes him into a perpetual state of self-division. For the play ends on the revelation that the reason for the duel he is about to fight (and in which he may lose his life) is that he has been called names, 'Old-Womanish' being the worst insult he can imagine.[49] His self-alienation and fear of femininity are most prominently reflected in his loathing of Florence Nightingale.

The terms on which Mohr's Barry dismisses Nightingale are pointedly gendered: her 'scheming petticoteries' rely on pulling strings in high quarters and 'bullying and nannying the officers in pursuit of some crazed destiny she had marked out for herself'; Nightingale is embarked on a grandiose project of self-glorification that denies recognition to actual reformers like

Mary Seacole and Barry himself.[50] Hysteria, autocracy, megalomania and cattiness: Nightingale epitomizes the stereotype of narcissistic and power-hungry femininity. Implicitly, what Barry finds most objectionable about Nightingale is that her aggressive deployment of femininity invalidates his own sacrifices and achievements; hence his over-performance of military masculinity. In a similar gesture, the Barry of *Whistling Psyche* lights a cheroot. As Claire Gleitman comments, 'can there be any prop more masculine than a cigar …? Precisely as he arrives at what is so profoundly galling to him – that Nightingale did not need to dissemble her gender and was lionized for the work that she did as a woman – he engages in the most overtly male behavior … [and] clings to a masculinity that is in fact not natural to him'.[51] Arguably, of course, that particular expression of masculinity is a cliché that never can be 'natural'. Moreover, as Freud is said to have quipped, '[s]ometimes a cigar is just a cigar'; (Sebastian) Barry here plays with his audience's post-Freudian self-awareness.[52]

Whistling Psyche echoes many of the sentiments of Mohr's protagonist. In its dialogic structure, however, it offers insight into both characters' interiority, thus establishing crucial connections between them. Here the dramatic monologue is co-opted for what Pearsall calls 'monologic conversations': sequential soliloquies that in their speakers' self-absorption throw into relief the alienation and isolation of each.[53] Gradually, the monologues start to intersect and overlap in theme, motif and language. Gleitman notes the echo effect in Nightingale's 'dailysome' responding to Barry's 'noisome', just as Barry follows Nightingale's harrowing account of the horrendous conditions of the Crimean war caused by indifference and the petty rivalry of commanders with a tale about Major Barnes, a pioneer of engineering with a vision of utopian progress who, when faced with the failure of his dreams, sank into depression and fell victim to the neglect and physical abuse of the asylum system.[54] It is not only their emotional responsiveness to 'the extraordinary music of human pain', anger about the unnecessary suffering inflicted by those in power ('the gift of the mind of those that rule is to engender miseries') and the desire to bring relief through reform that unites them.[55] (This mirroring effect is also represented in Kate Milsom's re-imagination of the Barry–Nightingale encounter in her 2017 portrait of *James Barry 1789–1865*.)[56] Though they are set up as contrasts in the opening (Barry's diminutive size and 'anxious' expression being juxtaposed to Nightingale's imposing height and supreme self-confidence), in the course of their monologues it becomes clear that they are mirror reflections of each other.

For all their difference in nationality, class, upbringing and gender identity, Barry and Nightingale are impelled by the same spiritual needs, have made similar sacrifices, conceive of themselves in parallel ways as 'soldier[s] of medicine', and suffer alike from loneliness and a sense of futility and self-mourning.[57] In their need for companionship, they have turned to animals (Barry to his poodle Psyche, Nightingale to her owl Athena, forgotten and starved during Nightingale's hectic preparations to leave home in order to escape domestic suffocation). Both draw on animal metaphors in the depiction of self and other: while Nightingale's satirical conflation of Barry with his goat recalls Barry's reference to the 'Meadow Lady' and 'Cow' in Mohr's play, her self-comparison to a giraffe signals the visionary power of the rebel and reformer that will always make her stand apart, just as Psyche's 'heart of a lion produced by nature in miniature' encapsulates Barry's 'own human soul' as well as of course his petite build.[58] Significantly, Psyche, the titular heroine of Sebastian Barry's play, though heard barking on several occasions, remains absent from the stage, as she does in Mohr's biodrama, as if to indicate the spectral nature of Barry's suppressed femininity.[59]

Barry's self-repression is pinpointed not only by the elusive Psyche but also by his prolonged resistance to his alter ego Nightingale's attempts to engage him in a conversation. That Nightingale is figured not with a lamp but a music box signposts her desire to escape silence or the exclusive sound of her own voice. When she first comes across Barry in the otherwise eerily empty waiting room and starts listening to his self-ruminations, she is intrigued; then, struck by the unexpected affinities in their experiences and feelings, she progressively becomes more frustrated with his introversion and refusal to interact with her. It is only when she expresses her revulsion at his disclosure of his affair with the married Somerset that, for the first time, he addresses her directly: 'You hate me now?' If their conflicting stance on sexual morality threatens to break the rapport that has developed, it is Barry's memory of his stillborn child that brings them together again: '*Against her will, Miss Nightingale is moved*.'[60] The play maps a spiritual journey from psychic trauma to self-reclamation and reconciliation as the two characters progress from their initial positioning as strangers, through confrontation as adversaries, to a recognition of their emotional kinship. *Whistling Psyche*'s monologic conversation has strong psychotherapeutic undertones since, in that they bear witness to their own pain, and, by listening, relieve the pain of the other, Barry and Nightingale make peace both with each other and with their inner selves. *Whistling*

Psyche thus ends with the transformation of selves that Pearsall identifies as a feature of dramatic monologue: '*There is the quality of a daguerreotype about them – a strange marriage, an unexpected couple. The owl calling softly. Their nearest hands just touching, perhaps by accident. And the dark retrieves them.*'[61]

The lyrical finale connotes cathartic closure, but readings of the play are crucially dependent on how this final scene is produced; as in Mohr's *Barry*, the dramatic effects of text and performance may well diverge. Significantly, as noted by Gleitman, the original production concluded on a much more explicit vista of physical intimacy, with Nightingale 'remov[ing] Barry's jacket, his shirt, and his bindings to reveal, just for an instant, his breasts', and the curtain falling on the couple's embrace.[62] I concur with Gleitman that the embodiment of what is so essentially a transcendental moment can only dilute the intensity of the spiritual coming together of the two characters.[63] It also undercuts the possibility opened up by the play that we read Nightingale not as a separate individual but as a psychic part of Barry: the embrace of two women would then point to the rebirth, in death, of the formerly divided self. Where the emphasis of the text lies on the reconciliation of dual (transgender) selves and spiritual epiphany, a performative focus on the 'truth' of the body posits a resolution to Barry's self-mourning in the companionship and shared experience of women. More problematically, the stripping of Barry's torso to reveal the woman underneath invokes the biographilic trope of the bedroom discovery scene discussed in the last chapter, placing Nightingale in the position of the officers who in Ebenezer Rogers's anecdote lifted Barry's bedclothes for the enlightenment of the reader, here the play's audience: 'See, Barry is a woman!'[64] Shifting the attention from Barry's psyche (the titular focus of the play) to the material body, a body violated by the 'despicable, horrible' exposure to which he was subjected after his death, returns the play to Barry's traumatic, Caliban-inflected sense of defilement: 'I am nothing... A filth, a darkness. My own history hurts me.'[65] Nightingale's baring of Barry's body also recalls Barry's earlier account of how this body became the object of women's erotic fantasies of 'unclothing me, revealing me, opening me like a parcel hidden long underground, like a box said to contain jewels' – prompting a very different type of rapture to the transcendental experience suggested by the closing tableau of the text.[66]

Whether embodied or spiritualized, the finale offers cathartic release to Barry's and Nightingale's existential anguish. In the surrealist context of the play, both characters are of course already dead, the waiting room with its stopped clock (arrested time) a site of purgatory. As Gleitman observes, the chronological specificity of the setting – 'around 1910', the year of Edward VII's death, the year Virginia Woolf identified as the birth of modernity – marks this liminal space out as a suspended moment of transition between the demise of the extended Victorian world to which the two characters belonged and the killing fields of World War I that engendered modern consciousness.[67] Like the Victorians in Matthew Arnold's 'Stanzas from the Grande Chartreuse' (1855), Barry and Nightingale are trapped 'Wandering between two worlds, one dead/The other powerless to be born': rebels, visionaries, pioneers and yet rooted in the ideological paradigms of their time.[68] Thus, while Barry identifies as 'that other sort of creature, neither white nor black, nor brown nor even green, but the strange original that is an Irish person', attributing his instinctual commitment to the plight of the dispossessed to his ethnicity and childhood experience of poverty and colonization, he is nevertheless a representative of the British empire.[69] His spiritual renewal (via Psyche and her successors, all imported from England) is, Gleitman points out, 'sustained … [by] the imperial center'.[70] The most manifest example of his conflicted position as both insurgent and servant of empire is his relationship with his black servant.

From the inception of the myth, Barry's African servant was constructed in biographilia as a confidant who knew and loyally protected his master's secret even beyond death. In 'A Mystery Still', 'Black John' is Barry's last and prototypically 'faithful' attendant, a companion to whom Barry, a man 'always considerate to his dependents', speaks 'almost tender[ly]' of his 'lonely life' shortly before he dies.[71] Variants of the 'companionate servant' paradigm that airbrushes the power structures of the master/servant relationship, especially complicated in the early part of Barry's career, a time of slavery, can be found across biographilic works; as Rachel Carroll notes, 'colonial subjects and spaces are often made to serve as metaphorical vehicles for Barry's experience, their own historical reality obscured or erased as a result.'[72] That Dantzen/Danzer was in fact indentured to Barry at the age of twelve and ran away twice, to be recaptured and punished with confinement to Robben Island, has only recently been brought to light by Michael du Preez and Jeremy Dronfield.[73]

Binnie's *Colours* bestows considerable agency on Barry's servant Joseph that moves beyond the loyal companion trope. The play inverts the mirror scene, merging it with the bedroom discovery plot: when Barry undresses in front of a mirror, Joseph observes the woman being born from the slipping clothes; he subsequently responds to his employer's duality by addressing Barry simultaneously as Sir and Madam.[74] In his role of protector he assumes parental function, replacing Barry's mother (by tending to Barry's physical wounds after the duel with Cleote and her psychological trauma following her rape) and competing with his father (with whose ghost he quarrels about whether or not to withhold news of Jane's daughter Marion's death). Prominently, it is Joseph who concocts the cocky story of the haircut to mitigate Barry's desertion of his post and bail him out at his court-martial. Ultimately, however, Joseph remains beholden to his status as best supporting actor; the end of the play sees him pay an emotional tribute to Barry's valour.[75]

By contrast, Sebastian Barry and Kit Brennan's biodramas problematize the contemporary desire to project notions of modern political correctness into Barry. Thus, confronted with the abject conditions inflicted on the empire's 'destroyed and enmired peoples' in the colonies, the Barry of *Whistling Psyche* finds his 'white heart blackening secretly' with rage, and takes personal action when he rescues a black boy from the leper colony; but it never occurs to him to examine his own instrumentalization of Nathaniel as 'a fine heart ... at [my] side', always 'to hand' when needed and otherwise happy to sit 'patiently [and out of sight] in the third-class waiting room'.[76] In his capacity of homemaker, Nathaniel takes on the function of an undemanding and solicitous quasi-wife; he can be relied on to 'arrang[e] all things with his domestical genius, buffing both house and master till we shone'.[77] It is 'my good Nathaniel' who delivers Barry's child, 'as tender and strong as any midwife, laboring in the shame and mystery of his master'.[78] In feminizing his servant, Barry is able to reaffirm his own sense of masculinity while at the same time turning a service relationship into an affective family bond. Consequently, Barry has no conception of Nathaniel wishing for any other life; but to Nightingale, his state of subjection and condemnation to a half-life are self-evident when she recalls the 'dejected African serving man trotting after like a shadow'.[79] Flanked as he is by Barry's poodle and goat, the figure of Nathaniel serves to mock cultural tropes, raising questions about our contemporary responses to Barry's conflicted sexual and racial politics.[80]

This conflict is key to Brennan's *Tiger's Heart*. The most extended and complex treatment of the master/servant dynamic, the play anachronistically endows Barry with a proto-modern consciousness to reflect on the way in which equality discourses are invariably inflected by power imbalances. A humanitarian reformer and egalitarian, Barry acquires a servant-slave by default when he witnesses a brutal beating and buys the slave to save him from further violence. On discovering that Dantzen can read (a punishable crime in a slave), he reassures him that he wishes to help, drawing analogies with the support he himself received from his former mentors. The character of Barry serves to illustrate to a contemporary audience the dangerous naïvety of an egalitarianism that disregards the weight of historical power differentials. Barry's assertion that 'I don't believe in master and servant. I've hired you, to do a job' is countered by Dantzen's statement of facts, 'in the law you own me'. When Barry is hurt by what he perceives as Dantzen's rejection of his advances of friendship, protesting that 'I want to *save* you … You'd think you'd be grateful!', Dantzen rejoins by reminding Barry of the parallels to his own life: 'Were you grateful, to your patron?' Their first sustained dialogue as master and servant, in a scene entitled 'To Learn', thus acts as an object lesson, to both Barry and the spectator, about the limitations of liberation discourses that do not take account of the way in which self-identified liberators themselves are implicated in the power structures they seek to break down. While to Barry, 'Knowledge is power', Dantzen warns that 'Knowledge will kill me.'[81]

Although initially knowledge offers Dantzen a level of protection (familiar with subterfuge, he intuits Barry's mask), ultimately he is proved right: 'White woman now man. You are still like them.'[82] In attempting to help Dantzen trace his wife and son, Barry unwittingly becomes the cause of their further enslavement. But Barry, too, is locked into the master/slave economy. In a sophisticated play with doubling devices, *Tiger's Heart* establishes Barry's own entrapment in his relationship with Somerset. An autocratic aristocrat with unrestrained and abusive habits, Somerset expects sexual services in exchange for career advances. Enthralled by Somerset, Barry enters her servitude willingly. In both relationships the power dynamic is undercut by the mutual threat of exposure. Though he is Dantzen's legal owner, Barry is dependent on him keeping her secret; but, as Dantzen remarks, 'Who would believe me. Doctor sir.' As her employer and as a lover who knows her sex, Somerset holds double power over Barry, who could, however, reveal Somerset's homosexual practices, a 'hanging offense'; yet, as Somerset points out, 'This colony is mine. No one will listen to your little voice.'[83] The fates of Barry's sister, murdered in pregnancy, and of one of Barry's patients, a syphilitic prostitute, are a stark reminder of the bleak prospects for women to survive the heterosexual power economy. Cast off by Somerset when she falls pregnant, and with the thought of her sister in mind, Barry cannot see a future for her child and induces an abortion.

Barry's belief in the power of human agency, that 'Life is what you make of it, what you can do with it' is invalidated with the rape and death of Dantzen's wife and the sale away of his son at the very moment when Barry is attempting to obtain their freedom.[84] When in the aftermath of their traumatic experiences, Barry and Dantzen become friends and then lovers, the single human relationship in the play that is grounded in genuine and shared affection is still shown to affect them in drastically different ways. Discovered by Cloete, they are exposed to the force of the law, but it is Dantzen who pays with his life for their racial transgression. In the course of the play, Barry's Enlightenment philosophy is repeatedly challenged by Dantzen and later his son Galawa, who offer indigenous wisdoms as a counter-discourse that is more suited to the realities of their lives under slavery conditions. Dantzen seeks to teach Barry the combined tactic of dissimulation and continuous vigilance which he visualizes as 'the Two-Faced': the person with two faces, 'no back, only front, on both sides, always on guard', who '[c]an see them coming both ways' but 'hide[s their] true sel[f], inside.' The only danger is to 'wear [the mask] too long' lest 'you'll forget who you really are'.[85] Ironically, of course, this is a strategy which Barry the gender passer has long embraced, although she has not always been able to sustain it, as in her affair with Somerset. In her relationship with Dantzen it is because they become unguarded and fail to watch 'both ways' that they are discovered.

That Dantzen's 'Two-Faced' is neither fully achievable, nor the best means of survival, is suggested by Galawa's tiger stories. In the first story, the tiger, unware that he is 'safer when they [are] friends', is destroyed because he leaves the forest; safety thus lies in companionship.[86] But because this companionship is always under threat from outside forces, the only way to survive is to 'ride the tiger': to face the fear and meet the danger head-on: '"*Xa uqabela ingwe, mlungu, uyiqabela unom'phela.* When you ride the tiger, white man, you ride it forever." – (…BARRY laughs – a wry laugh filled with recognition. It releases her.)'[87] Now an old man about to die, who has mourned Dantzen and blamed himself for his death all his life, Barry is released from guilt by Dantzen's son, the embodiment of his conscience, memory and trauma. In his turn, by extending forgiveness, Galawa is released from his own 'tiger', his fear and hatred of the man he had wrongly identified with the regime.

Like *Whistling Psyche*, the play ends on a conciliatory, cathartic note. Here, too, there is a sense of transcendence, spiritual and also, importantly, in racial terms. In closing on Galawa's words, in both his own and Barry's language, the play moves beyond exploring the parallels between gender and race crossing to adopt a transracial vision. Rogers Brubaker has drawn attention to the way in which 'Thinking about race through the prism of sex and gender reverses a longstanding tradition of thinking about sex and gender through the prism of race. The irony in the reversal is that in this trans moment it is the increasingly sophisticated understanding of the *fluidity and artificiality of gender* that can be leveraged to highlight aspects of the fluidity and artificiality of race'.[88] The spiritual coming together across race, gender and age that enables Barry's release is such a 'trans' moment.

Tiger's Heart offers a substantially different engagement with the Barry myth from the other plays. Like *Whistling Psyche* and Mohr's *Barry: Personal Statements*, Brennan's drama grounds Barry's gender subversion in his capacity to challenge wider social and political regimes of power. But more explicitly than in the other dramas, this Barry's experience illustrates that gender/power relations are inexorably imbricated with questions of race and empire. *Tiger's Heart* is focused less on Barry's self-division than on his sexual/racial politics – and on his sense of guilt. In this respect, the play constitutes not so much a dramatic monologue as a dramatic dialogue with a contemporary postcolonial audience. If Mohr's play concludes with Barry attempting to reaffirm his fragile male identity by overplaying his participation in hyper-masculine discourses and rituals, and *Whistling Psyche* culminates with the reconciliation of Barry's dual gender identities, *Tiger's Heart* problematizes postcolonial concerns about empire, collective responsibility, and the politics of resistance. What all these plays have in common is their self-conscious *mise-en-scène* of the postmodern condition – gender, race and trans identity, sexual dissidence, the legacy of colonization and slavery – projected back onto the historical figure of James Barry. This refraction of Barry in the mirror of postmodern identity categories is also key to the narrative strategies and self-enactments of biography.

The Biographer's Tale: The Authorial Self-Staging of Biographiction

In adaptation of Saunders's definition of biografiction as the 'interaction between biography and fiction' in biographically-inflected fiction, my use of the term 'biographiction' places the emphasis on the imaginative acts of biography (biography that draws on the methods of fiction).[89] Biografiction, in Saunders's conceptualization, is biographical fiction (biofiction) that plays with 'invented narrative' to counterfeit biography, either for satirical effect ('mock-biography') or to enhance the appearance of authenticity ('pseudo-biography').[90] Examples from Barry biographilia are 'A Mystery Still' (satire) and Marvell's 'The Mystery of the Kapok Doctor' (an unimpressive attempt at faking verisimilitude). At the other end of the spectrum, Florida Ann Town's *With A Silent Companion* presents a contemporary instance of what might be called 'pseudo-biografiction': nominally a work of fiction, the book illustrates, if anything, the need for the interpenetration of 'fictional' and 'factual' components to produce an organic text, irrespective of whether the intended outcome is to be biofiction or biography. In an early conceptual juxtaposition of biography and biographical fiction Schabert noted the dangers of 'contamination' in commingling ostensibly disparate forms of biography: 'fictional elements destroy the reliability of the text as a source of factual information whereas the factual narrative interferes with the imaginative vision'.[91] The inner life of Town's Barry is indeed atrophied when the novelistic is superseded by the biographical account; but it is the lack of cross-pollination between the two narrative modes, not their co-existence, that splits the work apart.

In contradistinction to pseudo-biografiction, the prototype of self-conscious postmodern biografiction is 'metabiographical fiction': in Saunders's words, 'fictional works with biographers as central characters'.[92] This metafictional form is related to Laura Savu's 'postmortem postmodernist' category of 'author fiction': biographical fiction that takes historical authors as its focus.[93] While neither type of biofiction is represented in the Barry archive, A.S. Byatt's *The Biographer's Tale* (2001) with its biographer-narrator and biographer-subject offers a compelling metafictional commentary on biography as a medium that is defined by the convergence of autobiography and fiction. For to make sense of the fragments of biographical data, the biographer must invariably weave 'his own lies and inventions into the dense texture of collected [and selected] facts'.[94] As Byatt's protagonist comes to recognize, 'the compulsion to *invent* was in some way related to my own sense that in constructing *this* narrative I have had to insert facts about myself, and not only dry facts, but my *feelings*, and now my interpretations. I have somehow been *made* to write my own story.'[95] These observations are echoed in life-writing scholarship: the biographical portrait, Schabert affirms, 'is, inevitably, a self-portrait as well.'[96] In Barry biography, the biographer's acts of self-portraiture, involuntarily or intentionally, repeat the biographee's own prior processes of self-invention, in the same way in which Barry's hybrid and indeterminate gender identity is mirrored in the blurring of generic conventions.

In her differentiation of 'fictional' and 'factual' forms of life-writing, Schabert pits biofiction's impulse towards 'essentiality' against biography's drive for 'authenticity'. Thus biofiction

> expresses what its author feels to be the characteristic, essential qualities of a particular individual in a particular historical situation ... The criterion of poetic essentiality demands a creative use of the evidence. ... The historical facts ... are thereby transferred to metonymic or even symbolic status.[97]

Applied to Barry biographilia, this metonymic function is fulfilled by the three plot elements discussed in the last chapter that constitute the 'body parts' of the Barry story: the mirror-transformation scene, the duel, the bedroom/deathbed revelation. These are indeed the main narrative building blocks of Barry biofiction, but as Chapter 3 indicated, they also feature in biography; the sensational disclosures after Barry's death in particular are key to biographical explorations.[98] Are these (ostensibly) fact-based, fiction-inflected stories narrated in different ways in biography than in biofiction, then? 'Factual' biography, Schabert affirms, must present 'a record of what, according to the evidence, must have happened ... No factually false statement may be introduced for the sake of essentiality'.[99] Biofiction or, in Ira B. Nadel's words, 'verifiable fiction',[100] does, nonetheless, share with biography a 'respect for the evidence'; both make use of historical sources to 'develop ... clues into significant moments, imagined from the inside'.[101] The difference is therefore one of degree more than kind and resides in how the material is 'shape[d] ... into a life story': biography places greater emphasis on documentary evidence, while biographical fiction seeks to bring us closer to the 'truth' of an individual through invented narrative.[102] This is supported by the way in which biographers draw on the correspondence and periodical press reports following Barry's death, whereas biofiction dramatizes the death scene and its aftermath, focusing on the subjectivities of those involved (Barry, his servant, the layer-out, friends, his lover).

However, the juxtapositional relationship between fact and fiction that Schabert posits, even in the closer relationship between 'imaginative biography' and biographical fiction, is ultimately not substantiated by Barry life-writing, which sees an intertwining of fact and fiction in both biofiction and biography. Biographical reconstructions of Barry draw on the narrative conventions of fiction, while novels based on Barry's life (like neo-Victorian biofiction more generally) engage with the factual contexts both intradiegetically and extradiegetically, the latter typically in the paratextual form of a preface, afterword or appendix. In some instances, biographilic texts collapse genre conventions altogether, as is the case in N.J.C. Rutherford's 'Dr. James Barry', an article published in the *Journal of the Royal Army Medical Corps*. Ostensibly presented as a 'biographical' piece (and read as such by some later biographers), Rutherford's text is a compilation and fictionalization of Victorian newspaper reports interspersed with anecdotes and passages from (mostly unacknowledged) prior biofictions, in particular 'A Mystery Sill', *A Modern Sphinx* and 'The Mystery of the Kapok Doctor'.[103]

If contemporary biofiction usually credits its sources, biographies often dispense with footnotes, references and other scholarly conventions, thereby undercutting the historical facticity and authenticity of the material.[104] Expectations of facticity are further destabilized by the choice of overly sensational or melodramatic titles evocative of fiction: *The Strange Story of Dr. James Barry: Army Surgeon, Inspector-General of Hospitals, Discovered on Death to be a Woman* (Isobel Rae); *The Perfect Gentleman: The remarkable life of Dr. James Miranda Barry, the woman who served as an officer in the British Army from 1813 to 1859* (June Rose); *Scanty Particulars: The Mysterious, Astonishing and Remarkable Life of Victorian Surgeon James Barry* and its titular variants, as discussed in Chapter 2 (Rachel Holmes); *Dr. James Barry: A Woman Ahead of Her Time* (Michael du Preez and Jeremy Dronfield).

The story-telling impetus invoked in biographies' titles is reinforced by the use of fiction to enhance the exposition and interpretation of facts. This is a feature of du Preez and Dronfield's *Dr. James Barry* (not surprisingly so, given it is the collaborative product of a scientist and a novelist). Chapters often start with a narrative dramatization of the hero/ine's outlook, sometimes by giving insight into her/his perspective, more often by directing the reader's gaze to Barry and the changes s/he is about to experience or has just undergone. Thus our glance moves from the 'little girl with red-gold hair' watching an incoming cutter at the quayside in Cork to the 'fair-haired young man' on deck of a vessel 'gazing down at the oily water' in the London docks and then the 'young officer with red-gold hair' standing on a cliff overlooking Portsmouth Harbour pondering his future; fifteen years later the middle-aged officer is pictured back at the London docks after postings in the Cape and at Mauritius, and a further five years on Margaret Bulkley is shown returning to the Cork waterfront from the West Indies, in search of the past and a destitute parent. Five decades after setting out from London, and exhausted from the long sea voyage back from Canada, Barry finally comes to rest in the city.[105]

Typically, Barry is captured at moments of inner departure or crisis, looking out at sea from the shore, or inland from an incoming vessel. The English war ship Bellerophon (named after the Greek mythical figure) which attracts the young Margaret's interest at the start and then becomes a means of transport for the officer, stands metonymically for Barry and his military career: the daring of a hero who, supported by his winged horse (his medical expertise), sets out to slay the Chimera (disease, prejudice, bureaucracy, ignorance). The journey motif is further highlighted with section headings that locate Barry in shifting geographical and temporal settings. Fictionalized passages thus serve as vignettes that introduce readers to key passages in the life of the biographical subject.

Holmes's *Scanty Particulars* offers a particularly skillful, metatextually refracted example of creative-critical interpenetration. The chapter that deals with Barry's medical reform projects at the Cape places his championship of the weak and marginalized in the context of his quotidian social interactions. It begins with Barry starting out on his regular morning visit to a local coffee shop where, relaxed and sociable, he treats Psyche to her favourite sugar buns, to the amusement of the owner, Mrs. Saunders, who will later prove 'one of Barry's most steadfast allies'.[106] This glimpse into his private life and integration into the local community act as a counterpoint to the chapter's concluding observations on Barry's 'obsession with the exact enforcement of rules and regulations': if in the pursuit of duty, 'his identification of his own person with his institutional office' came close to 'pedantry', this was to a large extent due to the stake he held in official documentation as a source of authentication for his self-fashioned identity; but he also had a personal investment in communal relations.[107] The fictionalized opening brings us closer to Barry as an empathetic character while also providing a backdrop to his humanitarian mission.

The impression that a fictional scaffolding helps unlock a multidimensional vision that enriches biographical narrative is heightened in Holmes's work by a Preface that, in its first UK edition, positions the text in explicit contravention of the 'convention amongst those who attempted to provide factual accounts of Barry's life to begin its telling at the end' – to begin, in other words, with the deathbed revelation.[108] This biography, then, emphatically proclaims its departure from the established model of essentializing Barry through the facts of his body, raising questions at the same time about the reliability of these 'facts'. The wording (previous biographers '*attempted* to provide factual accounts') suggests the failure of such an endeavour, so that this 'new' biography is introduced as being both more of an imaginative reconstruction *and* more authentic than its predecessors. (Ironically, the US and second UK editions of Holmes's book omit the first two and a half pages of the conceptual discussion, thereby discarding the self-referential claim to exceptionality.)[109]

In further illustration of the constructedness of all biographical narrative, the Preface is headed by an epigraph that reproduces Barry's court-martial pun on beginnings and endings, itself a model of slipperiness and an intriguing anticipation of Lewis Carroll's *Alice's Adventures in Wonderland* (to tell a story by beginning at the beginning and continuing until the end).[110] The first chapter (in all three editions) starts pointedly not with the prototypical opening of the Barry story (the aftermath of his death, an inflection of Derrida's 'closure without end', the personal apocalypse that spells new life),[111] but with the symbolic coming into being of 'James Barry' in a manner that is informed by precisely the kind of 'creative use of the evidence' that, according to Schabert, privileges biofiction's 'poetic essentiality' over biography's factually recorded historicity.[112] Significantly, Holmes begins with a fictionalized narrative, related for greater immediacy of affective impact in the present tense.[113] Readers are introduced to Barry's inner world, motivations and impulses in a dramatic *mise-en-scène* of his first dissection lesson, the initiation rite for the newly born medical student. It is worth quoting this passage at length:

> He recalls the scene like a demonic dream. A room of instruments and shadows, the temperature of a meat-safe. A place between the artist's studio and the butcher's shop. The air clammy with malodorous condensation. Mr Fyfe's three greenhorn students huddle in a group, uncertain of the etiquette of approaching the dissecting table on which a body is laid out beneath greasy sheeting. ... James Barry has a particular fascination with the study of anatomy, with the folds and secrets of the flesh. He breathes hard through his mouth, fighting back panic as Fyfe lifts the sheet. ... Barry struggles to translate the clean and figuratively precise lines of his anatomical textbooks into the irregular landscape of the purplish swollen body laid out before him. ....
>
> Heart thumping, temperature rising with the bile in his throat, in this claustrophobic space the only heat he can feel is his own. Yet in Fyfe's chilly candlelit rooms James Barry's cold sweat of dread anticipation turns to the flushed rush of heated fascination.

> … Barry's startled attention is drawn to the face of the corpse. Stripped of the animation of everyday life it is a face unsexed … Barry is looking at the inverted mirror of a woman's body. A life anatomized. The scalpel cuts a swathe through the history of this corpse, revealing its physiological secrets to the students … discovering things unknown to the woman during her recently ended life.[114]

Holmes seeks to establish Barry's profound personal interest in probing the 'physiological secrets' of anatomy and 'grasping' the transformations and metamorphoses of the human body. She later discusses the subject of his medical thesis in much detail, drawing on historical case studies to illustrate the close resemblance between the symptoms of female hernia and the intersexed body. In the quasi-primal scene of Barry's first dissection, the corpse is identified as both female and 'unsexed', a radically ambiguous and intermediary entity, as indeterminate a body as Barry, it is implied, would have experienced his own anatomy. Holmes's biography is carefully organized around this first chapter, significantly entitled 'Betwixt and Between', which sets the scene for subsequent authorial commentary about Barry's perplexing condition, moving full circle in the concluding chapters, which explore his case through the lens of intersex – the hermaphroditism to which Staff Surgeon McKinnon, when pressed, had referred in his letter to the Registrar General. It was because he was aware of the irregularities of his body, Holmes argues in 'Habeas Corpus' (her final chapter), that the young Barry was drawn to his academic discipline: 'he studied medicine to learn more about himself.'[115] Not only that, but how except in the guise of the gentleman physician could he protect himself: 'Safer by far to become a medic himself… than run the risk of becoming a specimen … It was the perfect disguise.'[116] *Scanty Particulars* is thus marked by the meticulously patterned, circular structure and aesthetic self-referentiality that Schabert defines as chief attributes of biofiction:

> The introductory section of a fictional biography often anticipates the curve of the life which is going to be related; the last pages tend to resume … the major scenes, the dominant themes … grouping them into an impressive finale. The outer world of biographical fact is seen in reference not to history but to an inner world which is the creation of the novelist: the external events find their counterparts in acts of expectation, planning, foreboding, of recollection and interpretation. The facts are thus made to operate as the constituent parts of an aesthetic structure; their function as factual information is suspended.[117]

Scanty Particulars both exemplifies and disproves Schabert's relational model. The factual foundations of the biographical narrative are here not suspended, but heightened by the fictional element. Whereas other biographers like Rae, Rose, du Preez and Dronfield start with the factual afterlife, the revelation of Barry's 'true' sex, the discovery of the female body, Victorian periodical press reports and private communications of Barry's contemporaries, Holmes chooses the subject constitution of 'James Miranda Barry, medical student' as the central axis of her story: 'As a student, the young Barry was obsessed by midwifery, obstetrics, anatomy, and morbid dissection. The career of James Barry began with the search for truths about human metamorphoses – the journey of the body into life and death. In 1865 Barry's own body passed into history as one of the most disputed corpses of the modern age.'[118] The incorporation of biofictional elements into the biographical superstructure of *Scanty Particulars* serves to construct a persuasive argument for reading the documentary evidence as a case of intersexuality. The shift of emphasis from the posthumous discovery of Barry's anomalous (female) body to the young Barry's experience of studying the idiosyncrasies of the human anatomy, thereby taking possession of the peculiarities of his own, grants the biographical subject an agency that the other biographies neutralize by beginning with the exposure of Barry's secret following his death. This is an agency that is more commonly found in fiction; indeed, in its use of the dissection scene, Holmes's text is closer to Patricia Duncker's novel than to preceding biographies.[119]

What is of interest here is not so much the question of Barry's 'essential' or 'real' self or body that has so invariably exercised biographers, fiction writers, playwrights and critics. Rather, the crucial concern is to examine the way in which gender ambiguity – in Jacques Derrida's categorization, 'impurity, anomaly, or monstrosity' – is constructed in biographilic narratives, and how this ambiguity is inscribed into, enfolded by or, as Derrida and Avital Ronell put it, 'invaginated' in their textual compositions.[120] Notably, Barry's blurred and unstable gender and body infect the writing of the story itself, engendering the textual blurring and breaching of genre boundaries even where this is at odds with the expressly professed intention of the author. Thus Rae starts *The Strange Story of Dr. James Barry* by juxtaposing fact (biography) and fiction (the novels by Ebenezer Rogers, Olga Racster and Jessica Grove): 'in the light of [the] facts' that her biography will establish, she asserts, 'the old romantic figure of James Barry disappears'.[121] Notwithstanding her affirmation that

'This biography contains no fiction', she subsequently draws on fictional sources – 'A Mystery Still', *A Modern Sphinx* and Racster and Grove's *Journal of Dr. James Barry* – to support her factual account.[122] Her description of Barry's appearance is heavily influenced by the *Cape Times* cartoon accompanying Marvell's 'The Mystery of the Kapok Doctor' (Fig. 3.6): 'Dr. James Barry ... trotted down the street on her pony, wearing cocked hat and long sword, and followed by the usual retinue of large black servant and small black dog'.[123] All later biographers follow Rae's lead in kitting Barry out in Racster and Grove's dandified attire of 'pea-green Haynes' coat, satin waistcoat and close-fitting 'inexpressibles'.[124] Rae, Rose, du Preez and Dronfield render an (in Rose unsourced) passage from 'A Mystery Still' (the hyperbolic narrative of Barry's arrest on St. Helena) as documentary evidence.[125] Rose adopts the Victorian story's comic statement about Barry's vegetarianism and his fictional denouement, incorporating Rae's story of the black box and adding a second footman. Du Preez and Dronfield adapt 'A Mystery Still's' normalization narrative (the disappointment in love that prompted Barry's gender imposture) into a version of the deathbed disclosure scene by conjuring up glamorous fashion plates kept under lock and key in Barry's travelling trunk, revealing Margaret's tragic longing for her lost womanhood.[126]

Narratives circulate across biographilic works and transmigrate from one form to another: when Rose speculates about the backstory to the two rings that according to a family legend told by J. C. M'Crindle Barry had presented to his parents alongside other gifts, one 'a signet ring with a crest on it', the other a 'memoriam ring' with an engraving ('Sacred to the memory of Marion', or 'Mary Anne', as suggested by du Preez and Dronfield), how much is the anecdote, related over eighty years after the event, inflected with fictional material, such as Ebenezer Rogers's *A Modern Sphinx*, in which a ring passed down the generations as a heirloom plays a central role in unravelling the heroine's origins?[127] Or were the two rings of family lore conflated with the 'diamond ring' Barry mentioned in his 'humble memorial' as having received from 'Arch Duke Charles for services to one of His Imperial Highmen's men'?[128] The memorial ring makes another quasi-spectral appearance in the 'Foreword' to *Tiger's Heart*, where Brennan, in implicit reference to Rose ('Was Marion perhaps Barry's own name before she became "James"?') remarks that 'Barry's real name *may* have been Marion'.[129] In Binnie's *Colours* the ring is a lover's gift from David Erskine, and Marion the name of Barry's daughter.[130]

This drive, in Barry life-writing, towards the fictionalization of factual contexts is highlighted in Holmes's biography in the self-conscious play with fictional paradigms. Thus Holmes records one twentieth-century account in which the layer-out's name (which she, too, mistakes for that of Sophia Bishop) was confused with Dickens's Mrs. Gamp; indeed, this is an analogy that is not lost to other biographers.[131] In further exploration of the productive tension between 'fact' and 'fiction', the title of her biography, *Scanty Particulars*, is derived from an 1895 letter to the *Lancet* in which a Janet Carphin reminisced about the stories her friend John Jobson had told her about his fellow student Barry, thus playing with the factuality of historical hearsay.[132] Documented correspondence carries symbolic and literal weight in both biofiction and biography. In Duncker's novel transcriptions of original documents (such as Barry's letter to General Miranda of 7 January 1810) are adapted to fit the narrative context and interspersed with fictive letters by invented characters.[133] Holmes draws on correspondence to authenticate Barry's identity as the elder of the Bulkley sisters, born in 1789/90. As she points out, the handwriting in Margaret Bulkley's letter to James Barry R.A. in 1804 bears strong resemblance particularly in the rendering of individual letters to Barry's signature as pupil dresser at Guy's and St Thomas's (1812) and to the aged Barry's handwriting in his 1859 'Memorandum'.[134] Yet no documentary evidence of the handwriting is provided in the otherwise richly illustrated book, which in the pictures section, besides portraits of the various protagonists, features the title page of Barry's thesis and Barry's registration at St Thomas's (but not his signature). In the absence of any conclusive evidence such as would be furnished by reproductions of letters (or the citing of earlier work that established Barry's birth identity), the reader is expected to rely on the 'truthfulness' of a biographer who elsewhere playfully engages with the fictionalization of her subject. Is this all a clever authorial masquerade, then, a tongue-in-cheek performance that mimics James Barry's self-representative acts through textual parameters, creating a paradigmatically postmodernist approach to the story?

This postmodernist approach manifests itself in the self-reflexivity and intertextuality that both Holmes the biographer and Duncker the fiction writer embrace, and which relies on readers' prior knowledge of earlier texts. The lack of handwriting samples, for example, may appear less puzzling to readers familiar with William Pressly's scholarly work that in 1985 first established the connection between Margaret Bulkley and James Barry; that Pressly is not mentioned in *Scanty Particulars*, on the other hand, has the effect of inadvertently conferring the credit for this discovery on the biographer herself.[135] In a different inflection of this textual strategy Holmes repeatedly refers to the previous biographer June Rose's speculations about mysterious events in Barry's life without, however, giving precise clues as to the nature of the supposition. Rose posits the possibility that Barry's abrupt departure for Mauritius in late 1819, where he stayed (as Holmes claims, on his own initiative) until 1820, might have served to conceal a pregnancy.[136] Holmes mentions a 'mystery' 'hinted at' by earlier biographers but in order to sustain narrative misdirection does not explain the context,[137] and only much later into her book discounts speculation about Barry's pregnancy with reference to the likelihood of his intersexed condition. Likewise, she refers to the mysterious pillows Barry had designed for himself (a biographical version of the towels that are so prominent in the Barry mythos) and whose loss he deplored in 1836 without indicating their potential function; Rose suggests they might have been used during menstruation.[138] Holmes thus stimulates curiosity in her readers by pointing to an unspecified enigma, only to withhold further information:

> The purpose of the 'three pillows of a particular description' seems baffling. Barry did not clarify their use, nor the nature of the 'severe accidents' that made them necessary, but the vehemence of his long letter of protest makes it clear that whatever their function, these mysterious pillows were crucial to him.[139]

It is only in the concluding part of her book that Holmes returns to the pillows as a possible means with which Barry might have addressed physical discomfort arising from an intersex condition.[140] The effect of this strategy of invoking and yet always frustrating the desire for spectacular revelations is to turn the text into a detective story: there is a mystery the reader is invited to ponder and if possible solve; prior knowledge of other texts may be helpful, but it may also deflect from the direction of the narrative shaped by Holmes.

Detection, as Marjorie Garber has noted, is a key trope in cultural narratives of female transvestism and sex/gender transgression: the crosser always materializes only to disappear, leaving behind 'a trace, or, rather, the record of a trace'; in this way 'the trace left by the woman in man's clothes, by the construct of cross-dressing, becomes the impetus for detection'.[141] In Holmes's biography the generic conventions of detective fiction are crossed with those of the mystery tale. As the back cover intimates, 'Barry was not what he seemed ... [H]e concealed a secret that went right to the heart of his identity'.[142] In gesturing at while hiding (what she considers to have been) Barry's 'real' condition, the biographer emulates Barry's gender masquerade (hiding the female body behind a show of dandyism). As I noted in Chapter 2, the 'Preface' supremely circumvents the question of Barry's gender by bypassing the use of pronouns. Given the nineteenth-century medical and military context, the reader unfamiliar with the story is likely to take 'James Barry' for the man he (and Holmes) set him up to be. Barry is explicitly referenced as male from the first chapter. Rather than his masculinity, what is at stake, the text insinuates, is his sexuality: in the 'Preface' Holmes's reference to Havelock Ellis's *Sexual Inversion*, in which Barry's case is treated as a '"distinguished instance" of dissident sexual psychology' is a ploy to misdirect readerly attention to what appears to be a story about homosexuality.[143] This inference is supported by the subsequent portrayal of Barry's flamboyant dandyism in chapter 3 and seems fully substantiated in chapter 5, which recounts 'the gravest crisis of Barry's young life', the sodomy libel:

> Barry had flown close to the wind in his flagrantly intimate relationship with Somerset ... It is easy to imagine the extreme degree of inner turmoil and fear of exposure this crisis caused in Barry. For Barry had secrets. These were not the ordinary secrets of petty irregularities and youthful indiscretions that most people carry with them. Barry's secrets were of a nature that placed him beyond the understanding of the society in which he moved. They were also the secrets of the impostor.... Somerset was, Barry says simply and suggestively, 'my more than father – my almost only friend'.[144]

Having previously established that it was at the Cape that Barry 'fell truly in love for the first time', Holmes leaves little doubt about a sexual relationship with Somerset, Barry's 'highly eroticized paternal protector and, probably, initiator in the rites of sex'.[145] In a deft double-entendre the text surreptitiously points to Barry's gender crossing ('impostor'), only to shift attention to the reputed double infamy of gay sex with a man alleged by some to be his own father.[146] All is, however, not as it appears. The narrative climax – the disclosure of the secret – follows in chapter 10, aptly (and ironically) titled 'Beyond a Doubt'. This chapter effects a dramatic caesura in the text: introduced with an epigraph by Herculine Barbin (1838–1868), a prominent historical intersex individual, it finally lifts the mystery of Barry's origins and circumstances, positing that the ostensibly female body the charwoman thought she had found may have been intersexual. Ironically, as Rachel Carroll points out, Holmes subverts biographical tropes of Barry only to reaffirm them in a different way: 'Instead of conducting a post-mortem over Barry's death, … Holmes positions herself as a key actor in his birth' by 'reinstat[ing] the biographer as the knowing subject who authors the transgender life retrospectively'.[147] In support of her case, Holmes draws on Barry's thesis and research on intersexuality to establish the close link between intersexuality and (misdiagnosed) hernia, arguing that Barry chose his dissertation topic for good reason.

And yet, while the entire text has been building up to this revelation, the 'Epilogue' problematizes the emphasis on Barry's anatomy as an exclusive marker of his identity: 'Barry himself did not seem to think that his sex was the most important thing about his own life … it did not finally determine who he was or what he achieved.'[148] In this philosophical approach to sexual difference Holmes's closing representation of Barry appears a good deal closer to our own time than his. This is of course a trope of neo-Victorian fiction, which typically imagines its Victorian characters as our precursors and psychological contemporaries. Hence the retro-nostalgic desire that Barry might have wished for rediscovery by the afterworld: 'In my pursuit of James Barry', Holmes writes, 'I wondered often whether or not he wished ever to be discovered'; did he 'hope that he might be understood better' by a future society?[149] Just as Barry fashioned a new identity and life for himself, so, Holmes implies, her biography fashions him a spiritual afterlife in our contemporary period. Having 'left plenty of clues for us to find if we look hard enough', Barry must have been 'in search of the spirit of the age, now or in the future, that can accommodate his difference'.[150] Clearly, the implication is that this age is ours. In her retro-prospective project of recovery Holmes casts herself in the character of a conjuror crossed with the resurrection woman, while at the same time admitting to an 'uncanny feeling of plundering Barry's grave'.[151] This conflicted sense of biographical identity is projected into a dramatic finale, set in Cape Town, in a fictionalized scene that summons Barry's spirit in the symbol of a sudden gust of wind that takes hold of the manuscript pages:

> I sit writing the end of Barry's story at the southernmost tip of the world – from where Europe looks turned upside down. A winter wind is blowing across this distended peninsula appended to the bottom of Africa, stirring up a storm where two oceans meet and mingle indistinguishably. … Barry never truly belonged anywhere, but it was in his progressive desire to struggle against injustice and inequality that Barry finally can claim his belonging.

> With a sudden and unexpected force, this wind catches these pages, lifts them out of my hands and disperses them down the mountain to the ocean. ... I bid adieu to Barry. My journey is over.[152]

In the geographical juxtaposition of two continents, each of which looks 'upside down' when viewed from the other angle, but which ultimately overlap and blend into each other, the way their surrounding oceans do, the passage invokes a powerful vision of Barry himself, always engaged in transcending boundaries: of geography, politics, body, and temporality. The journey is completed, it is implied, because Barry has been reclaimed – for himself and for us. Invoked first in the 'Preface', the journey motif as an emblem of the biographical project brings the work full circle. The role that on the closing pages is accorded to affect and metaphor offers a reflection on the authorial self-staging processes involved in biographical work; for, as Schabert asks, 'where is the line to be drawn between the novelist's imagined facts and the biographer's imaginative use of the facts?'[153] *Scanty Particulars* displays all the features that Schabert identifies as constitutive of biofiction: self-referentiality, essentiality (with the story being informed by aesthetic considerations and the use of symbol and leitmotif to pattern the text), novelistic structures.[154] Conversely, the text also meets one of the criteria included in Max Saunders's definition of biografiction, metabiographical 'fiction [that is] in some way *about* biography and biographers'.[155] Barry biography, then, like Barry biodrama and Barry life-writing more generally, self-consciously and playfully engages with its own performance, and crossing, of generic conventions, typically by drawing attention to the performative strategies of the subject of its enquiry.

Hence the prominence of the mirror motif in biographilia: when Barry is portrayed scrutinizing his newly transformed self in the looking glass, an implicit invitation is issued to readers to project a version of themselves into the image. The text itself, then, assumes a mirror function, reflecting back to us an illusory glimpse of ourselves, as we might (imagine ourselves to) have been, with our modern consciousness transported into the past. In its first, most basic manifestation, this mirroring effect is intended to enhance reader identification (especially in works that present the historical personality through a contemporary lens, with the subjectivity, thoughts and vocabulary of the author's time). At a second, more metafictional level, it may serve as a self-referential commentary, as in biodrama or in Holmes's image of the scattered pages of her not-yet printed text (which of course we read in its perfectly assembled published format). In an earlier scene Holmes depicts Barry working on his dissertation at home, so absorbed in his research that he is 'unaware of the figure framed by the full-length cheval-mirror standing in the corner of his room'; the shadow figure invoked here is that of the author.[156] Thirdly, the mirror metaphor implicitly summons the power of time-travel for Barry himself, enabling the historic subject to see into the future, scrutinizing *us* in the looking-glass at the same time as we are embarked on re-envisioning him. Barry's gaze is explicitly directed at us on the cover of the Penguin edition of Holmes's biography (see Fig. 2.3); similarly, at the close of Binnie's *Colours*, he takes his leave from the stage of his life by scrutinizing the audience, pondering how many other successful passers there might be beside him.[157] This sense of Barry looking back at us, turning us into an object of study ourselves signals a fourth inflection of the motif, for mirror imagery can also serve as a means to establish ironic distance between reader and text.

In illustration of this latter usage, the opening page of Patricia Duncker's postmodernist novel, *James Miranda Barry* (1999), presents us with a child's gaze at the kaleidoscopic surface of water:

> I am now peering over the side of the balustrade. What can I see? A torrent of yellow flowers, falling, falling into a large basin. A stone dolphin with two putti astride, laughing forever, their faces turned in different directions. A little spurt of water. And circle upon circle of reflections. My face, far below me, shimmers, vanishes, shimmers, gone.[158]

Like the reader glancing down the page, the narrator-protagonist looks from a height at a fountain below, registering the shifting images of the face reflected in the water blending, dispersing, reforming, dissolving. The flowers whose impact disturbs the surface, creating the swirls, represent the plot that is about to unfold. Flanked by two effigies of Cupid – figures evocative of the promise of a gratification that may be enjoyed only ever in darkness, beyond the world of vision – the face that is forever changing shape stands for the mutability of gender, identity, and narrative that is at the heart of the text. That the figurines are placed in such a way that, mischievously (laughing), they direct our gaze away from rather than towards the centre of vision conveys a powerful impression of the fundamental dissociation of observer and image, reader and text. On its very first page, then, the novel stages its own (and its protagonist's) coming into being in the friction between authenticity and illusion, 'truth' and 'lies'.

'There Are No Truths, There Are Only Layers of Lies': Performing Barry in Postmodernist Biofiction[159]

Holmes engages readers in a game of detection by simultaneously summoning and withholding key information about Barry and earlier biographical works. Conversely, Duncker's two biofictions, both with the same low-key title, assume that readers can place 'James Miranda Barry' and will be attracted to the narrative play with a real-life character. Like the bioplays discussed earlier in this chapter, Duncker's story and novel illustrate Saunders's concept of autobiografiction, in particular the ways in which the different forms of life-writing interact to create new critically and biographically inflected fictional versions of their (semi)autobiographical narratives.[160] While the novel's alternation of first and third-person perspective and discontinuous chapter structure fractures the text and thereby keeps the reader at arm's length, in the short story (originally published in 1989 and reproduced in Duncker's 1997 collection *Monsieur Shoushana's Lemon Trees*), by contrast, the reader is positioned as a privileged insider, either because she is already initiated into Barry's secret or because she will be able to read between the lines and grasp what remains hidden to the outside world. This outside world, significantly, is the world of men; implicitly, the story thus constructs the knowing reader as female.

Narrated in the first person by a protagonist who is depicted in the act of writing, the text can be placed in Saunders's sub-category of '*unframed pseudo-autobiographical* works' such as epistolary fiction and fictional diaries or letters without a frame narrative.[161] The mature Barry is depicted working at his desk, late at night and in an exotic location. The official report on which he is engaged leads to self-reflection and a review of his most significant experiences: the moments which 'made' James Miranda Barry. The first two glimpses we are given into the personality single Barry out and situate him at a distance from his British fellow professionals. An ambitious scientist, he is working tirelessly for 'the archives, posterity, history'; like Holmes's, this Barry, too, has a sense of and writes for the afterworld.[162] Confident in his difference from and superiority over his military colleagues, he knows that his success relies on his innovative spirit and his readiness to breach barriers of convention, class and race. In contradistinction to the other expatriates, who 'keep a fine wire netting between themselves and this … island', he has gone native, sharing his food with his local cook and, when necessary, eating with his hands.[163] Evocative of the dramatic monologue of Barry biodrama, the direct address to an invisible interlocutor – 'Does that shock you?' – heightens the impression that Barry is reaching out to the contemporary reader, while at the same time hinting at an impending revelation of a more serious transgression.[164] That this disclosure is likely to be connected with women is implied by the third piece of information: at pains to protect the black nurses who work in his hospital from sexual harassment by his fellow officers, Barry always 'believe[s] what the women say': women's speech, women's feelings, women's insights are of paramount importance.[165] This passage leads to a flashback that identifies the 'originary scene' of transformation, the moment of Barry's self-constitution.

If Holmes pinpoints the young student's equation of femininity with abjection in the professional context of the dissecting theatre, Duncker locates a similarly negative response to adult femininity at a much earlier stage in the protagonist's life, in the world not of science but of art and culture. When the child stole in on a visiting painter and sought to make sense of the details in his oversized historical painting, what stood out were the 'huge, fleshly thighs of the Sabine women'.[166] Again the female body is associated with abjection, in the form of a chain of thoughts that connects female flesh with male desire, male desire with violence, violence with marriage, and the collective male violation of women with the building of empires (in a similar scene in Duncker's novel, the protagonist's uncle, the painter James Barry, explains that 'all societies are based on the seizure, slaughter and slavery of women').[167] Revolted, the girl declares that she will never marry. 'Then, child,' the painter replies, 'you must become a man. Learn to live in this world. Earn your own money. And stay out of debt.'[168] Just as the painter's work triggered off the girl's rejection of the female condition (subjection in marriage), so his response prompts her self-constitution. Textually her coming into being is indicated by a change of pronouns, from 'she' (the girl) to 'me', James Barry.[169]

The consequences of Barry's decision to assume a male identity appear unrewarding: solitude, homelessness, peripatetic displacement, and an absence of romantic love: 'I have spent my life in exile, ferociously guarding my privacy, travelling the world, searching out hot climates, courting danger, discovery, court-martial, disease. I have never been wealthy. I have never been loved.'[170] This disclaimer, however, is followed by the second hiatus in the story, the recollection of a passionate affair, conjured up by Barry's glance at 'a small old-fashioned miniature' that sits on his desk, 'a silhouette of a woman with her hair piled in curls'.[171] This beautiful indigenous woman self-confidently courted the officer; because she recognized him for what he was, he was able to reveal himself to her:

> [T]hen came the moment of exhilaration, recognition, joy. Holding the candle to my face, her eyes gleamed like fireflies in wet guinea grass.
>
> 'What are you?' she said.
>
> 'You know,' I replied. And I covered her damp breasts in kisses, all of which she repaid in full.[172]

The affair ends melodramatically, with Barry killing a rival in a duel and being 'posted elsewhere'.[173] However, the loss of the lover does not entail the absence of a community of like-minded spirits. After his reminiscences Barry walks outside, to find black village women smoking in a group. They invite him to join them: '"Siddown. We know what y'are." ... I sit among them, contented. Here, at last, I am no longer misunderstood.'[174] This is the community of which the reader is encouraged from the start to become part (significantly, the story was first published in a collection of lesbian feminist fiction).[175] Given the frequent slippage, in late-twentieth-century critical discourse, between cross-dressing, female masculinity and lesbian identity (prompting Halberstam to caution against the equation of female masculinity with lesbian sexuality), it is notable that Duncker's story is the first (and, together with her novel, only) instance in the Barry canon explicitly to place Barry on a lesbian continuum.[176] In contradistinction to Holmes's representation, it is not biological difference but a proto-feminist consciousness that determines Barry's gender crossing. And it is other women, women othered in terms of race or sexuality, who have the sensitivity and insight to acknowledge Barry as one of their own because they too must perform in a world governed by white heterosexual men. Each of these women shares Barry's experience of duality, inner and outer identities, self-representation and self-realization.

In its metafictional self-awareness, play with narrating ('I') and narrated ('she') protagonist, invitation to the reader to picture herself as part of the community ('we') that is invoked by the ending, and in thereby positing that 'the resolution of the autobiographical dilemma comes not through the desire to say "I know myself" and "I am that one", but the ability to say "I am all those ones"', Duncker's story is a rare example, in Barry biographilia, of what Lucia Boldrini terms a 'heterobiography': autobiofictions, narrated by historical characters, that display 'self-consciousness, in their structure, thematic texture and intellectual premises, of the implications of the autobiographical in the construction of subjectivity, in the operation involved in assuming another's voice, of the gap – historical and philosophical – inherent in the "double I" they stage.'[177]

This heterobiographical play with a 'double I' that draws together first-person narrator and narrated protagonist, intradiegetic interlocutor and extradiegetic reader into an illusory communal identity has its counterpoint in the perspectival vacillation of Duncker's novel: the shimmering, blurring 'face' of the narrative as it is depicted in the opening image of the child's glance into the reflecting surface of the water. Here, the illusion of a continuous and unitary sense of self (and gender) is deconstructed not through converging singular and plural autobiographical perspectives (I/we) but by shifting first and third-person narrative (I/he) – a juxtaposition of (gendered) viewpoints that is reflected paratextually on the Serpent's Tail cover of the novel, with Ingres's *Grande Odalisque* looking speculatively over her shoulder, at us, while an androgynous, gun-wielding figure, featured in profile in the background, is apparently oblivious to the reader (Fig. 4.1).

In its complex choreography of structure and point of view, Duncker's novel exemplifies Schabert's conceptualization of metatextual biofiction: 'multilayered and multiperspectival' texts that deploy 'different angles of view' and 'different stages in time' to call attention to the 'contradictions and inconsistencies' within the source material; such irregularities and 'missing evidence' are of 'structural importance too' since narrative fissures reflect on gaps in the historical record and thus on the elusiveness of the individual who is in the process of being re-imagined.[178] When that individual is a trans person, textual instability serves to problematize the trebly intangible nature of gender, identity and documentary material. The reconstruction of such a resisting subject can pose considerable difficulties, as noted by Duncker herself, who found that it was only by setting aside her manuscript and writing another novel, a metafictional tour-de-force on the slippage of textual and authorial body and the passionate, haunting, hallucinatory intensity of the reader-writer relationship, that she was able to return to James Miranda Barry.[179] The novel was thus shaped into being out of gaps: 'the space between texts … where every writer can take risks' and the 'space between the writer and the reader'.[180] The resulting text constitutes a composite body of creative-critical, intertextual and documentary sources whose structure problematizes the continuity of voice and point of view, chronology and plot. Changes in narrative

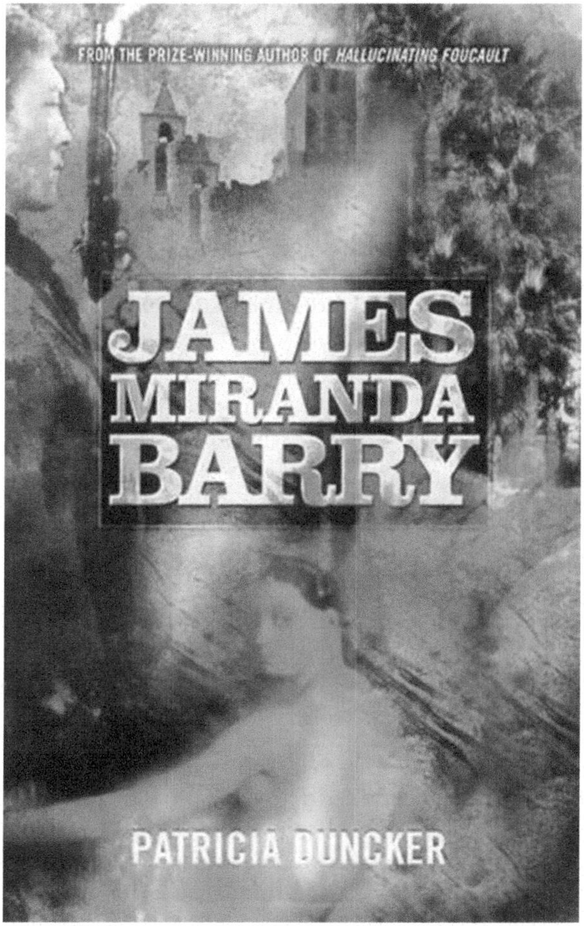

Fig. 4.1 Cover of Patricia Duncker's first UK edition of *James Miranda Barry*, Serpent's Tail, London, 1999, courtesy of the publisher

perspective effect a shift in focus. First-person narrative, often in the present tense, mostly marks the emotional life and moments of crisis experienced by the narrated I, whereas third-person narration, in the past tense, tends to provide a broader sweep of the events, usually but not exclusively from Barry's angle. Barry's gender duality is mirrored by the use of dual narrative perspectives, a duality that is doubly refracted in the novel's first extended chapter by the juxtaposition of first-person thoughts and third-person references which frame the child's transition from girl ('she') to boy ('he').

The novel begins with the toddler's sensory impressions and imaginative play-acting, in the course of which the girl imagines herself a boy soldier in the likeness of his adoptive father, General Miranda, protecting his 'Beloved' (the mother), suggesting that gender is both performative and wrought by familial relationships and affective role models. The journey on which the reader is invited to embark in following the text's unstable and fluctuating first to third back to first-person narrative resembles the child's endeavour to make sense of the world. The dreamy glance into the fountain is followed by the discovery of another object that presents itself to the child's gaze, a Gothic version of the first, which replaces the impressionist reflections of water with the spectral vision of a buried 'other' self that is conjured up only to be lost again. As the child explores the garden of Lord Erskine (Buchan's) 'House in the Country', s/he stumbles over a grave:

> The earth sarcophagus is cracked across. There is a huge fissure in the lid of the grave, as if the last day had already been announced and the spirit had escaped. I peer surreptitiously into the crack, but see only lichen, earth and broken stone. I sit staring at shining wet oceans of green and a trembling grave. This is a child's grave … [S]he is coming back, struggling under the weight of earth. I lean forward to help. … She descends back into the grave with a flurry of wet, crumbling earth.[181]

The actual child buried here is Erskine's: a marker of his personal loss and the backstory to his willingness to 'father' (the as yet unnamed, still submerged) Barry. On a secondary level, the hallucinatory revenant prefigures the later Barry's entombed femininity, just as the child's longing to embrace and thereby release the phantom anticipates the elderly Barry's desire at the end of his life to retire from masculinity and resurrect his dead female self. In a third inflection of this multifaceted metaphor, the aged Barry when visiting his mother's grave will experience a repetition of this early scene.[182] The use of identical prose in the two passages highlights the uncanny influence Mary Ann has always held and continues to exert over Barry's life: as Barry learns from Miranda, it was she who, in submerging herself, brought 'James Miranda Barry' to life.[183] It is no accident, therefore, that the first references both to the three-year-old toddler's female sex and to the ten-year-old's make-over into a boy issue from her mouth.[184]

The centrality that is accorded to symbol and leitmotif in Duncker's novel matches Schabert's description of the key features of biographical fiction. A further instance of aesthetic patterning is the use of paintings as a plot element. James Barry's *Jupiter and Juno on Mount Ida* (1804), dominating the landing in Miranda's London town house, unsettles and frightens the child who recognizes his mother and Miranda in the figures. Just as he discovers his mother's face in all of his uncle's mythical goddesses, so later will he be unnerved to come across the likeness of his lover Alice in Barry's *Birth of Pandora* (c.1791–1804).[185] The paintings direct attention toward a recognition of the painter James Barry's sexual jealousies and desires, hinting at a potential affair with Alice and, more momentously, at the incestuous relationship with his sister that might have produced the child who bears such resemblance to his uncle and carries his name. The towering figure of James Barry the elder and his impact on the identity formation of James Barry the younger is thrown into relief in the cover of the German-language (Berliner Taschenbuch Verlag) edition of the novel, which is adapted from James Barry's *Self-Portrait with Paine and Lefèvre* (c.1767, Fig. 4.2).[186] Just as the uncle's youthful artist identity was shadowed by painter friends, so the nephew's sense of self is forever haunted by him. (Such haunting is the dramatic frame for Binnie's *Colours;* here, too, Barry Junior is the direct issue of the painter, whose larger than life personality and hunger for 'colours' keeps the 'son' enthralled even beyond his father's death).

In Duncker's novel, while the depiction of the elderly painter's fraught mental state and dismal living conditions at the time of his demise are informed by biographical scholarship, the factual contexts of the younger James Barry's life are subordinated to the literary transposition of the material.[187] As a literary re-imagination rather than reconstruction of Barry, the novel bestows on Barry a childhood that, as Holmes notes, is necessarily absent from biographies, but in exchange erases his teens.[188] Similarly, the selective focus on symbolic sites of Barry's career ('The Colony', 'Tropics') blanks out crucial stages and locations that were instrumental to the historical Barry's professional (and personal) development. The opening vista of the cracked tomb, then, stands as a symbol for a narrative structure that is marked by gaps and fissures, boosting the expectation that the body that lies within can be glimpsed (and understood), yet always thwarting the desire for full

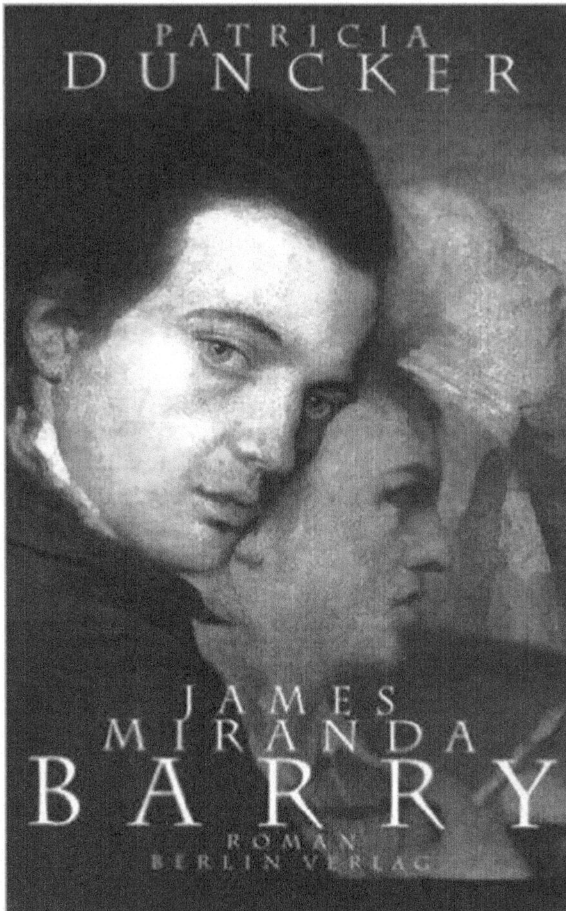

Fig. 4.2 Cover of the German edition of Patricia Duncker's *James Miranda Barry* (Berliner Taschenbuch Verlag, 2002), reproduced courtesy of Rothfos & Gabler

(in)sight while encouraging imaginative encounters. This is particularly the case once Barry has served his apprenticeship (both masculine and medical) and set out on his professional journey abroad; the text markedly shuns settings that might be inflected with too many prior associations, such as the Cape Colony.

His first and longest appointment overseas, Barry's twelve years at the Cape make up a significant part of biographical narratives and are core to early biofictions such as René Juta's *Cape Curry* and Olga Racster and Jessica Grove's *Journal of Dr. James Barry*. This was the posting where Barry enjoyed his greatest triumphs and suffered his greatest defeats. It has also furnished ample material for considerable speculation about his relationship with Somerset (Rose conjectures about Barry being the granddaughter of Mrs. Boscawen and therefore Somerset's niece; a rumour arose during the 'placard affair' that Barry was Somerset's son; Rose and Holmes speculate about the likelihood of a relationship between Barry and Somerset, with Rose implying that the child the layer-out claimed Barry had borne was Somerset's).[189] Duncker's novel, by contrast, entirely circumvents this period by contracting it to a few years that are excluded from the text, setting the action instead in Edinburgh, on Malta/Corfu, Jamaica and in London.[190] Instead of the Cape voyage into heterosexual romance – the trope so often explored in Barry biographilia – the text aligns the hero's trajectory as 'a passage through space, a journey from one location to another', thus adopting the same structure as transsexual autobiography.[191] However, whereas the journey script of transgender autobiography, as conceptualized by Jay Prosser, follows a distinct teleology (from suffering through medical recognition to transition and the new life), this motif is undercut in Duncker's narrative by the fact that Barry's journeys out of and back to Britain are motivated by his love of Alice Jones (as Eveline Kilian points out, he leaves for his first foreign posting when Alice refuses his offer of marriage and returns to London when, having retired from public performance, she is ready to settle down).[192]

The original place of departure that remains a constant as a spiritual home in Barry's peregrinations is Lord Erskine's Shropshire estate, which features in all but two parts of the novel. In this way the reader's attention is guided to Barry's relationship with the fictional Alice, a kitchen maid in Erskine's employ who, after a spell as a painter's model, attains fame and fortune as the distinguished Mrs. Jones, an actress celebrated most particularly for her unparalleled performance of cross-dressing parts, and who in middle age, when playing boys in breeches is no longer becoming, takes up another type of acting as a spiritualist medium. Alice's own trajectory indicates that it is the performativity of identities and not so much the protagonist's sexuality that constitutes the focal point of Duncker's novel.

As in the case of the journey plot that leaves out key milestones in the historical Barry's life, readers who expect to find the realist narrative of development that a title named after a single character suggests, or who come to the novel with knowledge of the historical subject, may feel confused by its chronology and textual fractures.[193] Georges Letissier points out that the text's '[s]patial displacement … initiates an experience of defamiliarisation' that serves to draw attention to the hero's 'Nomadic Transgender Identity', resulting in a 'skewed or queered version of the *Bildungsroman*'.[194] The novel's spatial ruptures are complemented by temporal ruptures; while we are introduced in great depth to a gender-fluid toddler aged three, we next meet the protagonist as a ten-year-old boy, having missed seven crucial years of emotional, psychological and mental growth. The text moves in breathtakingly rapid progression from the newly constituted boy to the (still under-age) medical student undertaking his first dissection and writing his doctoral dissertation. Jana Funke rightly argues that *James Miranda Barry* deliberately 'favour[s] obscurity over historical truthfulness and specificity' in order to 'defea[t] the use of transhistorical identity categories'; in doing so the novel seeks to 'call into question the epistemological validity of any identification with the past', most particularly by problematizing 'the desire to pin down past sexualities using present-day identity categories'.[195] Halberstam's concept of 'queer temporality' sheds further light on what Letissier has called Duncker's 'poetics of obfuscation'.[196] By upsetting 'straight' notions of progression, the novel adopts the 'queer temporality' that Halberstam identifies for transgender narrative. Such a text 'disrupts the normative narratives of time'; this serves to challenge 'the conventional binary formulation of a life narrative divided by a clear break between youth and adulthood.'[197] In this sense, then, the novel anticipates 'translit', a twenty-first-century category for 'fragmented narrative structure which shifts, not only between different time periods and places, but also between different genres' in order to 'set up expectations of certain rules only to break with them'.[198]

James Miranda Barry certainly resists and queers readerly desire for a 'straight' and unbroken narrative flux. Instead of conventional chapters the text is divided into six lengthy parts that represent way stations in Barry's emotional and professional lives (the child and the start of boyhood; the student trying to find his feet; the young doctor in the crossfire of dying uncle and elusive lover; the Colonial Medical Inspector at the height of his powers; the ageing Deputy Inspector General on his last posting; retirement, personal fulfilment and death). These parts are organized into a temporal and thematic structure with the use of asterisks, but the ostensible surface order is disrupted with a-chronological sequences. An example can be found in Part Four, 'The Colony', set in the 1820s on an island location inspired by the historical Barry's postings to Mauritius, Malta and Corfu (where he served in the late 1820s, 1840s and early 1850s).[199] The linear progression of the plot is dislocated abruptly with a reference to an earlier date – 'The year was 1817'.[200] This rupture to the sequential order of the narrative, however, marks a critical turn in the plot, for Barry's island idyll is brought to a sudden halt by the outbreak of cholera (an epidemic that first erupted in the wider region a decade earlier). The large casualty rate in the local population and the implementation of quarantine law establish a radical break from the island's past fortunes, just as they unsettle Barry's professional and affective relationships. The metaphorical death of his old life is confirmed when news reaches him of his mother's decease. Homeless again, Barry is propelled on to his next posting; Part Five of the novel sees him, years later, in 'The Tropics'.

Each part starts with a change in narrative perspective and at its close establishes a caesura, presenting a cameo of a particular stage in Barry's life, but withholding insight into his inner development across time.[201] While the first three parts follow a closer chronological sequence, the second half of the novel offers disjointed vistas, each ten or twenty years apart. It is as if the Barry of fiction much more than that of biography existed only in fragments, always at a distance from us, ultimately unknowable. While biographers like Holmes and du Preez and Dronfield take great pains to imagine an inner life for their subject in order to establish a fuller character and thereby encourage reader engagement, Duncker deliberately foils readerly identification processes, instead splintering her narrative as a marker of the patchy and erratic nature of the 'evidence' of Barry's life and the futility of attempting to confine Barry to an orthodox textual/sexual framework.

In its hybridity of form, the text bears some relation to Ansgar Nünning's biofictional categories of 'revisionist fictional biography' (which 'revise[s] the formal conventions of traditional biofictions, but … lack[s] … elements that break the aesthetic illusion') and 'fictional meta(auto)biography', that is, novels 'concerned with the recording of history and the problems of biography' which 'highlight … the process of biographical reconstruction' through 'juxtaposition of heterogeneous fragments'.[202] By presenting the reader with shifting vignettes, from fluctuating perspectives which signal that 'there is not one truth about [Barry's] life, only a series of versions', Duncker's novel, however, does not so much disturb the aesthetic illusion as prevent it from becoming fully established in the first place.[203] The text engages metafictionally with its own literary constructedness through multiple intertextual references (including German 'Sturm und Drang', the painters James Barry and Benjamin Robert Haydon, Joanna Baillie's *Plays on the Passions*, Richardson's *Pamela*, Shakespearean comedy, Elizabeth Gaskell's *North and South*, Henry James's *The Portrait of a Lady*). However, *James Miranda Barry* does not manifest the other key components of Nünning's concept of 'fictional metabiography': it does not focus on the interplay between the biofictional subject's past and the reader's present, it is not set in the contemporary period, nor does it foreground a biographer/narrator figure.[204]

Instead, Dunker's fiction guides reader reflection to its central exploration of gender (and genre) performance by interrupting the plot narrative at crucial moments with lengthy descriptions of stage plays, popular entertainment and private theatricals. Thus Part Two, titled 'North and South' in an intertextual pun on his rather different experience from Gaskell's Margaret Hale, places Barry's painfully guarded and self-conscious, yet gradually more confident self-presentation in a dissection theatre in relation to the complex machinery required for producing spectacular Gothic effects on the stage, and juxtaposes the attendance of a play in Edinburgh to Barry's participation in a communal Shakespearean extravaganza at Erskine's Shropshire country house. Since '[e]veryone was involved in the performance ... the division between spectators and players ceased to exist':[205] an invitation to the reader to participate in the performative project. Part Three sets James Barry 'The Painter's Death' against the backdrop of London melodrama and fairground burlesque. The dramatic device of the 'play within the play' of a novel about performance focuses attention on the self-reflexive nature of Barry's act: so engrossed does he become with the rousing contribution of a new actress in a breeches part whose heroic exploits are reminiscent of the fantasies of his childhood that he forgets about the primary purpose of his theatre visit, the discovery of Alice's whereabouts. Since Alice is rumoured to have taken up cross-dressing roles, the expectation is raised that she will be revealed as the heroine in male garb, only to be undercut when nobody among the theatre staff has 'ever seen or heard tell of her'.[206] The metadramatic aspects of such scenes are highlighted in the US edition of the novel, which depicts a fencing match between two opponents adorned in extravagant headdress, while a Medusaesque female face is suspended beneath the plank on which they stand, revealing the setting to be a stage and the contest but a 'Comedy of Masks', an act for the entertainment of an audience (Fig. 4.3).[207]

The *Commedia dell'Arte* motif and figures are adapted from one of Jacques Callot's seventeenth-century series of etchings of Neapolitan

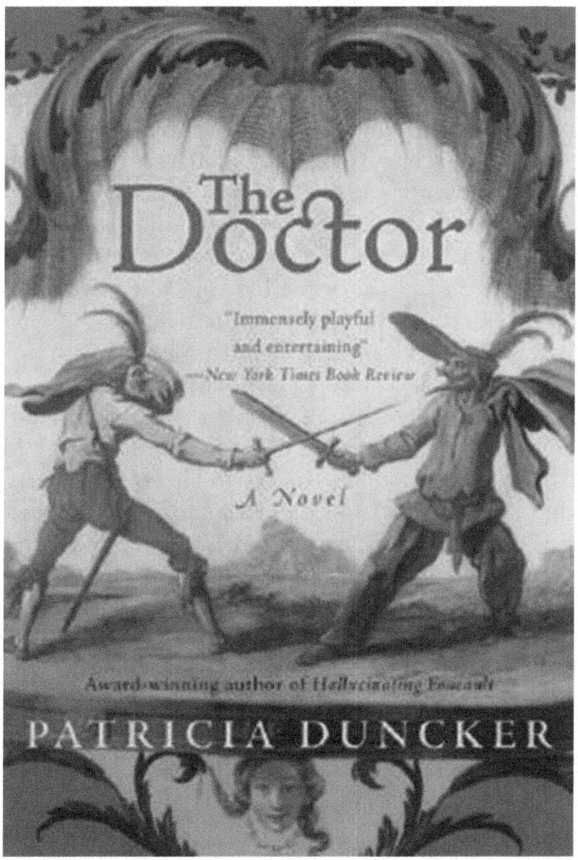

Fig. 4.3 Book cover (Harper Perennial edition) from THE DOCTOR by PATRICIA DUNCKER. Copyright/s 1999 by Patricia Duncker. Reprinted by permission of HarperCollins Publishers

dances, *Balli de Sfessanio* (c. 1622), which features a pair of dancers, Scaramucia (Scaramouche) and Fricasso.[208] In the original engraving, the figures are placed back-to-back, stepping away from each other as if to mark out the requisite space in preparation for a duel; the Harper Perennial image captures them at the point of head-on engagement. In either case the scene depicts a theatrical act, a performance. Performance as the central plank of Barry's subject constitution and self-construction is at the core of Duncker's and also Holmes's postmodernist texts; both present performance as the stabilizing factor of an otherwise ambiguous and shifting identity. Indeed, Holmes reminds us that performance formed a crucial part in the execution of medical responsibilities in the early nineteenth century: 'To be a surgeon was to live a life of performance under daily public scrutiny'.[209] A physician who was also an officer was bound to stand out even further: 'Much has been made of Barry's exaggerated dress … but it needs to be remembered that military dress for officers was calculated to distinguish and set its wearer apart' (a point also made by Rae).[210] Male fashion in the Regency period favoured an ostentatious feminine style, with clean-shaven faces adorned by wigs, and with 'stockings, stays and make-up' considered to be the paraphernalia of the gentleman (see Fig. 4.4).[211] It was only in Barry's later years, in high Victorianism, that his extravagant appearance (and lack of facial hair) seemed out of place in an age that demanded a more austere, somber and voluminously bearded presentation of imperial masculinity.[212] In the initial stages of his career, the public display and enactment of his medical and military identities facilitated rather than complicated Barry's gender performance.

That the earlier grandiose style came to be perceived as pompous and obsolete is highlighted in Duncker's novel when Barry challenges fellow officer Loughlin (loosely based on Josias Cloete) to a duel: 'Please tell Captain Loughlin that I shall discharge my obligations to the letter. Who on earth talks like that nowadays? It's as if he's repeating lines that have already been written.'[213] Similarly, when the opponents meet, the duel 'was played out like a formal piece of music.'[214] The formulaic nature of this performance is indicative of the heavily textualized foundation of a ritual that, as John Leigh notes in *Touché*, 'even at the height of its prosperity' already constituted an anachronistic, 'antiquated practice'.[215] The excess of ceremonial that shaped rules of deportment in a duel may well over-determine Barry's rigid attitude, but the script that he follows is clearly also that of his stepfather, the charismatic General whose name he carries and with whose duelling pistols he learned to shoot.

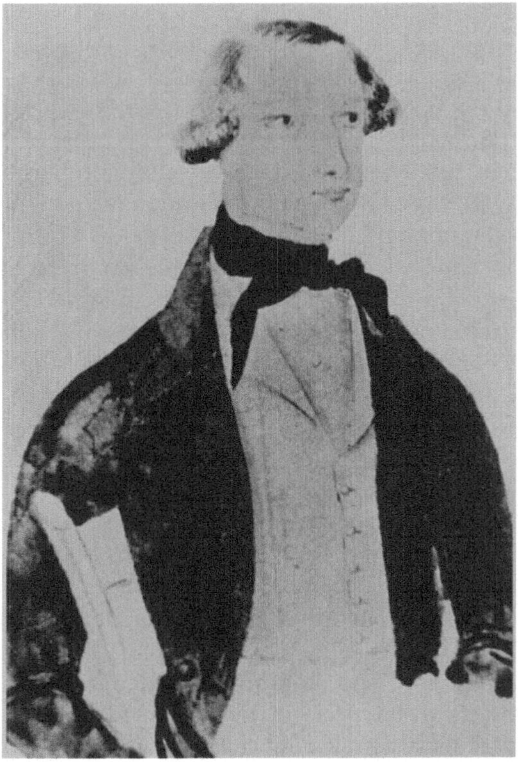

Fig. 4.4 James Barry; portrait (L0022268), reproduced courtesy of the Museum of Military Medicine[216]

Ending as it does with Barry's spectacular performance of his gunmanship and generosity in sparing his adversary, the duel proves to be the turning point in his identity formation. Agonizingly uncomfortable in his indeterminate and, to his mind, grotesque body at the outset of his journey and 'terrified of sex', he now begins to revel in the *mise-en-scène* of his masculinity, projecting a quasi-replica of the man who from childhood has fascinated and mesmerized him, Miranda.[217] Small wonder if Loughlin starts to feel that 'The man was like quicksilver, fluid, indeterminate, yet utterly beautiful ... he too had succumbed to Barry's magic and was, knowingly, a little in love with this man who had been tempted to kill him.'[218] Loughlin, 'confused and bewildered', is transformed by the erotic tension 'simmering in the air between them', but has no deeper understanding of his feelings; Barry does. When, in the wake of the cholera epidemic, Loughlin's regiment is about to be moved to the mountains and he arrives at Barry's quarters, distraught, to make a declaration, a 'look of exquisite pain passed over the doctor's face. Suddenly he reached up to James and embraced him tightly.'[219] Poised as Barry is in the space between genders and sexualities, Duncker allows her 'trans'gender protagonist to develop a sense of deep passion for both a woman and a man while infusing Loughlin, otherwise the prototype of 'straight', non-introspective masculinity, with romantic love for another man.

Not only Barry, but also Loughlin and especially Alice serve to explode the notion of an essential self or body. From the outset Barry is presented as a hybrid personality, 'outside every system'; at their first childhood meeting, Alice speculates that he might be 'a boy that's got enough girl for it not to matter too much either way.'[220] Funke suggests that Alice here seeks to deflect attention from her interest in another girl; and, indeed, the elderly Alice will make her aversion to public scandal explicit. But Alice is by far the most defiant character in the novel. Secure in her supreme self-confidence, she cares nothing about the 'truth of the body'; what matters, she affirms, is not the illusion of 'essence' but the material benefit of appearance: 'The truth, as far as she was concerned, was what you could get away with.'[221] As Eveline Kilian points out, the text here plays with (readers' recognition of) Judith Butler's deconstruction of Lacanian conceptualizations of female masquerade. Refuting Barry's nostalgic and, in light of his own career, paradoxical idea that there could be 'a "being" or ontological specification of femininity *prior* to the masquerade', Alice excels in the 'performative production of a sexual ontology, an appearing that makes itself convincing as a "being"'.[222] If men act as initial role models, patrons and financiers of Barry's crossing into masculinity, it is Alice whose support sustains Barry's performance. Indeed, Barry's transformation from female to male was entirely engineered by women: Erskine's sister Louisa and above all Barry's mother. Women, Barry recognizes, were 'the source of the plot'.[223] Rachel Carroll argues that Barry's 'identity is authored by others' to such an extent that 'his gender expression … emptied of personal agency' turns into a 'channel through which other women's narratives can be acted out'. If, as she notes, Alice's interventions into Barry's life present a comic counterpart to the sway that another working-class woman – the layer-out – exerted on the historical Barry's afterlife, Mary Ann's desire for self-empowerment is realized through displacement by steering Barry on his path (Duncker's emphasis on Mary Anne Bulkley's agency in driving events is echoed in Holmes's biography as also in Florida Ann Town's *With a Silent Companion*.)[224]

Even after his mother's death, Duncker's Barry is still subject to her plans. At the end of his career, in an anachronistic echo of Simone de Beauvoir, Mary Ann's younger and more successfully independent incarnation, Alice, succeeds in dissuading him from lifting his cover by coming out as a woman: 'You can't suddenly become a woman. It takes years of practice.'[225] After a lifetime spent as a man, Barry cannot simply switch identities. As Alice reflects later, '*He knows nothing about clothes, manners, gestures. He wouldn't even know how to walk up and down a staircase; let alone climb in and out of a carriage.*'[226] It is not only gender, but our very sense of self that is an act rather than an essence: 'what is your real identity? And what is genuine? ... Nothing's absolutely genuine. You aren't the same person with everyone ... You act out different roles. I've acted every minute of my life. I'm always on stage. We all are. It's all a performance.'[227] (In Binnie's *Colours*, Isabel responds in very similar terms to Barry's longing by telling her daughter that returning to womanhood would merely mean swapping one life of pretence for another).[228] Ultimately Barry comes to accept Alice's message. Gender and identity are like the maze on Lord Erskine's estate, the place where Barry's fate was originally decided in a meeting with the 'triumvirate' of men propelled into action by Mary Ann. In Barry's childhood the heart of the maze held a statue of Diana, but when he returns as an adult he finds nothing but 'an unmarked paved square' waiting to be repossessed.[229]

If the historical character of James Barry serves to illustrate that gender is an empty category until 'marked' through performance, later twentieth-century and contemporary postmodern biographilic constructions of Barry pinpoint the *textual* performances of gender as it is, in turn, enfolded and unwrapped, clothed and disrobed, revealed and concealed by the genre of neo-Victorian life-writing. The texts I have discussed in this chapter elude easy classification as fiction, biography or drama, vacillating as they do 'Between and Betwixt', borrowing from, intersecting with and blurring into each other. Like the face shimmering in the water of Duncker's fountain or the leaves blown apart by the wind and reassembled into the pages we read in Holmes, like the pairs of alter egos in Mohr, Sebastian Barry and Brennan, each copy and original at one and the same time, they blend, merge, disperse and reform in their adaptive interaction and self-conscious experimentation with the conventions and possibilities of life-writing. The multiple boundary crossings they enact are reflected in the diversity and (often) linguistic opacity of the categories proposed to conceptualize their play with form: (revisionist) fictional biography;

fictional autobiography; autobiofiction; autobiodrama; auto/biografiction and auto/biographiction; heterobiography; (fictional) meta(auto)biography. To adapt Judith Butler's opening dictum about gender, there is no genre identity behind the expressions of the genre of neo-Victorian life-writing: that identity is performatively constituted by the very 'expressions' that are said to be its result.

Like genre, gender is in these texts shown to come into being in the act of 'crossing' or, in Jacques Derrida and Avital Ronnell's words, in breaching 'line[s] of demarcation'.[230] The neo-Victorian and postmodernist play with transgender is, this chapter has argued, a prime example of both Derrida and Ronnell's 'law of impurity' and Hayden White's 'metageneric' 'paragenre'.[231] But – and I want to end the chapter on this questioning note – since critical theorists concur that hybridity is a defining feature of literary genre and of life-writing par excellence, and since feminist and transgender criticism have long established trans/gender as fundamentally unstable and fluid categories, neo-Victorian games with historical gender bending and crossing may not be so subversive, after all, but just an illustration of the norm.

CHAPTER 5

Trans*Form*ations: Transgender and Transgenre in Victorian and Neo-Victorian Life-Writing – A Conclusion

He had himself become the book. Now I was asking the book to yield up all its secrets.

Patricia Duncker, *Hallucinating Foucault* (1996)[1]

The more often generic borders are crossed and the less secure habitual categories stand, the more important it becomes to identify the genre conventions that a given work adapts, transforms and subverts.

Ansgar Nünning, 'Fictional Metabiographies and Metaautobiographies' (2005)[2]

'What do I do now with this pile of paper, impossible to neatly classify as an essay, novel, or allegorical memoir?'

Anne Garréta, *Sphinx* (2015)[3]

The 'third' is that which questions binary thinking and introduces crisis … The 'third' is a code of articulation, a way of describing a space of possibility. Three puts in question the idea of one: of identity, self-sufficiency, self-knowledge.

Marjorie Garber, *Vested Interests: Cross-Dressing and Cultural Anxiety* (1992)[4]

[T]ranshirstory is a story waiting to be told.

Jack Halberstam, *Trans* (2018)[5]

A. Heilmann, *Neo-/Victorian Biographilia and James Miranda Barry*, https://doi.org/10.1007/978-3-319-71386-1_5

This study has sought to respond to Halberstam's call by investigating the way in which the cultural history of James 'Miranda' Barry brings to light notable parallels in the category definitions, textual enactments and boundary transgressions of nineteenth-century trans/gender performance and the genre of neo-/Victorian life-writing. If, in application of Patricia Duncker's narrative exploration of reader/text/author relations, James Barry has become 'the book', this cultural amalgam of the 'archive' or corpus of texts that reconstruct (or creatively counterfeit) the figure enables significant insight into Victorian to contemporary gender/genre configurations. That in the memorialisation and remediation of James Barry the imaginative spaces opened up by the concept of the 'third' are given expression only to be closed down again is testament to the ongoing challenge posed by thinking through trans when the subject of enquiry is an historical personality. Just as Barry's gender crossing provoked, and continues to provoke, textual affirmation of his female body, so the biographical, biofictional and biodramatic play with genre conventions has prompted the critical impulse to redraw the generic borders and conceptual paradigms disturbed by the blending and intermixing of forms. The transgeneric practices of neo-Victorian life-writing – the impossibility to 'neatly classify' biographilic work (as affirmed by Ann Garréta's trans-narrator) – thus raise similar anxieties to Barry's transgender identity and are addressed by corresponding regulatory discourses.

It is striking that the prevailing representational model in Barry biographilia across the 150-year time period in question is that of the woman in disguise, impersonating a masculinity that does not, or never entirely, reflect her inner life, and whose primary driving force is not her gender identity but the desire to escape female oppression, draw economic benefit from her work, fulfil her professional potential, and/or lead a life of adventure and self-empowerment. This discourse of 'rationalization' is one of three strategies (alongside trivialization and pathologization) that Halberstam has identified as serving the project of stabilizing and normalizing transgender.[6] Faced with the possibility of the 'third', texts (and authors) predominantly circumvent the opportunity to write 'transhirstory' by re-inscribing the heteronormativity unsettled by the non-convergence, in Barry's life, of anatomy and identity. In this script the corporeal 'truth' comes to stand for the truth of Barry's story; in the process, Barry's female body is made over into a fetish. If, as Trev Broughton has noted, 'Victorian Lives … come down to us not so much shapeless as a particular shape: the coffin', Barry's corpse is condemned perpetually to be un-coffined for the sake of being reshaped into femininity.[7]

This emphasis on Barry's identity being grounded in a female body is not altogether surprising in texts authored in the late nineteenth to early twentieth century, a halcyon time for first-wave feminism which saw widespread anxiety about gender relations, competition in the professions, the purported unsexing of women and attendant attenuation of masculinity. In returning the gender outlaw to biological rule, cultural commentators, writers and playwrights sought to contain the social and political threat posed by the 'march of the women', while also at times articulating feminist concern at the stark choices women were compelled to make.[8] It is in this context that Barry is feminized as a (reluctant) Amazon who takes up her masquerade for the love of a man, or to escape one, and who, while proud of her medical achievements, laments her emotionally unfulfilled life. In the mid to later twentieth century, Barry is depicted in less conflicted terms as a female pioneer energized and empowered by an unconventional life; here, too, however, Barry is presented as a passer, not a crosser, and as a mournful figure shrouded in loneliness. Given the prominence of transgender discourse since the 1990s, one might expect a shift of focus to trans experience; and, indeed, crossing, intersexuality and aspects of trans identity are explored in some texts, most prominently Rachel Holmes's *Scanty Particulars* and Patricia Duncker's *James Miranda Barry*. But the majority of contemporary responses, even when they queer Barry (and Barry's sexual relationships), ultimately cast Barry as a (heterosexual) woman. To date, there has been no work of biography, biofiction or biodrama authored from within the trans community. Juliet Jacques's point about trans authorial absence from literary fiction holds true for Barry life-writing too.[9]

The biographilic impetus to feminize Barry can be attributed to a number of interrelated contexts. Just as the pre-Victorian female transvestite and woman warrior's threat to gender/power structures was diluted by returning her to traditional libidinal parameters (the 'follow your man' trope so deprecated by Victorian feminists like Ménie Muriel Dowie, as discussed in Chapter 3), so the nineteenth-century crosser is today often placed within an economy of queer desire that finds its resolution in a shift back to heteronormative romance. Romance (according to Julia Novak the 'dominant generic model' underpinning early to mid-twentieth-century remediations of the Victorian 'notable woman in fiction') then serves to domesticate gender-variant identity in the postmillennial era.[10] In conjunction with adventure and sensation, romance has been the prevalent mode of biofiction, from the inception of the Barry myth ('A Mystery Still' and Ebenezer Rogers's *A Modern Sphinx*) through early twentieth-century novels like Réné Juta's *Cape Currey* and Olga Racster and Jessica Grove's *The Journal of Dr. James Barry* to contemporary popular culture (Anne and Ivan Kronenfeld's *The Secret of Dr. James Barry*). As Chapter 4 examined, however, postmodernist biographilia undermine the conventional romance plot by turning it into a temporary phase that Barry outgrows as he gains in inner maturity (Frederic Mohr's *Barry*), by disrupting and fragmenting it (as in Duncker's two versions of James Miranda Barry) or by problematizing cross-racial desire at a time of slavery (Kit Brennan's *Tiger's Heart*).

The transgender potential of Barry life-writing is also constrained in the process of what Marie-Luise Kohlke has pinpointed as the contemporary neo-Orientalist fascination with Victorian sex – the cliché that Victorian sexuality was repressed, yet always straining for release, exhilarating in its harvesting of forbidden fruit, titillating in the depravity of its underworlds. In its obsession with the sexual lives of the Victorians, Kohlke argues, 'neo-Victorianism … has become the new Orientalism, a significant mode of imagining sexuality in our hedonistic, consumerist, sex-surfeited age.'[11] The inscrutability of the figure of Barry acts as a stimulant to the sexual imagination; as the protagonist of Sebastian Barry's *Whistling Psyche* comments, 'There is something provocative … about a person locked in mystery', inciting 'a kind of hidden lust' to unravel and take possession of what lies underneath the mask.[12] If in *Whistling Psyche* the mask does not yield up the truth, and sexual exchange takes place (as in the Greek myth) in the realm of dreams, beyond gender and temporality, elsewhere the fantasy of disrobing the man to uncover and resurrect the woman beneath has the effect of collapsing Barry's gender performance into mere sexual foreplay. Sylvie Ouellette's *Le Secret du docteur Barry* invokes the idea of queer subversion, depicting the protagonist's flouting of the constraints of custom, costume and corporeality, only to contain Barry's transgressive acts within a heterosexist economy of self-subjection. Though Barry eventually learns to reject fetishization, and even sacrifices romance to sustain his masculinity, the narrative voice consistently overwrites his self-definition by privileging anatomy over identity. Jean Binnie's *Colours* similarly bestows a measure of sexual agency on the protagonist but at the same time locks her within a male framework of references; Barry is and remains the father's daughter, never maturing to become the mother's son.

A third context for the feminization of the Barry figure is the feminist project of reclaiming women in history. It is not surprising that twentieth-century biographies by Isabel Rae and June Rose, written in the wake and at the peak of the second-wave Women's Liberation Movement, should have invoked Barry as a female pioneer, breaking through the academic, medical and military glass ceilings over half a century before the first 'official' British woman doctor completed her studies; nor that Edinburgh University should lay claim to having been the springboard for the UK's 'first female graduate's' distinguished career.[13] The intersecting nature of these modalities – romance, sex and sensation, and the reclamation of historical women – is reflected in Olga Racster and Jessica Grove's early twentieth-century play *Dr. James Barry*. In the postfeminist period Florida Ann Town's novel-biography *With a Silent Companion* seeks to serve a similar purpose in providing young adult readers with an historical sense of one woman's path into self-liberation at a time when, collectively, women lacked educational, professional and political rights. Likewise, Michael du Preez and Jeremy Dronfield's *Dr. James Barry: A Woman Ahead of Her Time* commemorates Barry as a ground-breaking female figure in medical history, but this objective is neutralized by the emphasis on Barry's painfully frustrated femininity and failure successfully to perform in either gender: 'it was an imposture that was ... impossible to perfect.'[14] Ultimately, if Barry's anatomy and birth identity are taken as determinants of his identity across the entire span of his life, the portrait that emerges is that of a sad and lonely figure of despondency.

Essentialist readings of Barry are, finally, assisted by the identification processes cultivated by the neo-Victorian invocation of the past as a commentary and reflection on the present. These identification processes, however, also facilitate transgender approaches. Of the three biographilic forms discussed in this book, stage drama sustains the greatest level of audience detachment in the physical separation of actor and spectator, a division that also underscores the temporal disjuncture between nineteenth-century character and contemporary viewer and that viewer's metadramatic awareness of the performative nature of identity. Biodrama thus encourages empathy while maintaining distance: 'the truth', Brennan proposes, 'she did not want us to know'.[15] Since not knowing means not being in a position affectively to over-invest in the character, spectators are encouraged to ponder the question of Barry's gender identity at one remove; without a narrator's pronomial steer, they are more likely to be swayed by the character's self-presentation. Given that a biopic is in planning, it will be interesting to see how the medium of film accommodates proximity and distance to the Barry character.

Biofiction, by contrast, fosters close emotional affinity with the protagonist; since readers can understand and empathize with Barry, they are seduced into believing that 'Barry was like us'. In biography, the novelistic slippage of reader into character is inhibited by the historicizing narrative even as the fictionalization of critical moments brings the protagonist and his experience to life. Barry here assumes precursor function, distant from us in time and yet in spiritual proximity; in his difference from his contemporaries, his insistence on self-determination and his professional and humanitarian convictions, he prefigured relevant aspects of our time and the way we think now: hence Barry's representation as a quasi-feminist forerunner. The sense that 'Barry anticipated us' can shift into the neo-Victorian fantasy that 'Barry needs us': in this configuration Barry is no longer a mere pioneer whose professional reforms heralded and helped bring about modern medical practices and humanitarian thought, but a prophetic figure who in his isolation and under the imperative to protect his identity was instead looking to the future for companionship, desiring to be redeemed by us: 'she seemed almost to court discovery'; 'did James Barry hope [to] … be understood better by a future age?'[16] The neo-Victorian glance in the rear-view mirror in the 'desire to speak with the dead' conjures up an imaginary encounter, a reclamation that, it is implied, enables therapeutic closure for Barry through the recuperation of his story and identity by a community of like-minded individuals: the cathartic release evoked at the close of *Whistling Psyche*.[17] This is why Holmes's biography ends with the invocation of Barry's spirit in the gust of wind stirring and dispersing the pages of her manuscript, bidding it to go forth and prosper.[18]

The oblique allusion to an inverted version of Mary Shelley's lonely and abandoned creature, summoning a salvaged, textualized 'family' bond between Barry and us, the Victorian past and the postmillennial present points to the complex processes of 'worldmaking' in which neo-Victorian life-writing is engaged. Drawing on Nelson Goodman, Caroline Lusin applies this concept to the neo-Victorian construction of the biographee's 'world' from documents brought alive by the imagination, with both biography and biofiction taking inspiration from the tension between 'fact' and 'fiction' in deploying literary plot structures and displaying metafictional awareness of their representational strategies.[19] The 'worldmaking' of Barry biographilia, this book has argued, rests on the dynamic interplay of imagination and documentation, conducted across and between three main forms of life-writing that borrow from and sustain one another. Blurring and intermingling while retaining their broad respective emphases on the reconstruction, reinvention and performative re-enactment of a life, with each making creative use of history and narrative, biography, biofiction and biodrama require a holistic framework of discussion that takes account of the hybridity of their overarching forms.

The scholarly impetus for category paradigms has yielded important models of classification that shed light on the aesthetics and ethics of biographilic world-making. Of these, Max Saunders's auto/biografiction, in this book also adapted to auto/biographiction, constitutes the most organic and significant conceptualization of life-writing as a genre marked by fluidity of form and which offers vital insights into the metaliterary experimentation with life portraiture, mock-authenticity and the counterfeit.[20] That contemporary plays about Barry provide a particularly productive context for investigating the auto/biografictional performance of (trans)gendered selves indicates the broader applicability of Saunders's concept as well as the importance of including biodrama in definitions of neo-Victorian life-writing.

If auto/biografiction focuses attention on the *aesthetics* of life-writing, Marie-Luise Kohlke's differentiation of three modes of biofictional engagement throws into relief the *ethical* conundrum posed by biographilia. Whether it takes the form of an inquisitive prying into the hidden lives of Victorian celebrities, seeks to recuperate marginalized and 'ex-centric' figures for our own purposes, or repurposes real-life Victorians through 'counterfactual fabrication', our neo-Victorian consumption of historical personalities raises probing questions about the ethics of appropriation.[21] Is all life-writing intrinsically predatory? Kohlke's typology affords a fertile understanding of the processes involved in the Victorian to contemporary commodification specifically of 'Othered Subjects' who in their lifetime were subjected to exploitation and abuse.[22] In the remediation of such figures, how can life-writers avoid taking the place of the Victorian showman, and readers that of the freak-show audience? Recalling the case of Saartje Baartman, the 'Hottentot Venus', Kohlke enquires into the politics of recasting Baartman as a curiosity and spectacle possessed by the gaze across the centuries. James Barry, the oddball and loner, of shrill voice and queer body, has equally nourished biofiction's rapacious appetites, as illustrated in Rogers's *A Modern Sphinx,* George Edwin Marvell's 'The Mystery of the Kapok Doctor' and Rutherford's 'Dr. James Barry'. Ultimately, of course, appropriation is an inherent attribute of biographilia and is reflected, in varying degrees of salaciousness or sophistication, in all

Barry life-writing; as Kohlke notes, her categories are prone to overlap.[23] A manifest example is the *ur*-text of Barry life-writing, 'A Mystery Still', which simultaneously excels in the art of biographilic performance and revels in satirizing it, variously celebrates, reclaims and arrogates Barry, and in these acts of appropriation draws so vivid and flamboyant a portrait that it continues to reverberate in Barry biofiction, biodrama and biography today.

Alongside Kohlke's interrogation of the ethics of biofiction, Saunders's conceptualization of auto/biografiction and Ina Schabert's exploration of the overlapping aesthetics of 'factual' and 'fictional' biography, a fourth model that has influenced this book is Ansgar Nünning's meticulous attention to progressive levels of self-reflexivity, revisionism and metatextuality in the postmodernist biographical novel, from 'documentary' and 'realist' approaches, through 'revisionist' fictional biography, to 'biographic metafiction' and 'fictional metabiography'. The strength of this model and particularly of the latter concept is its alertness to postmodernist inter- and hypertextualities. Difficulties, however, arise from erecting boundaries between forms when life-writing is at its most dynamic and alive in breaching them. Like Kohlke, Nünning identifies the 'tendency to cross boundaries and blur genre distinctions' as foundational to biofiction and, by inference, biographilia more generally.[24] The dilemma, then, consists in how to conceptualize discrete typologies in a genre that constitutes itself through intermixing, blending and crossing.

The imposition of strict genre taxonomies, this book contends, not only runs counter to the quintessential fluidity that sustains the biographilic genre; such imposition, I argue, also carries peculiar echoes of the Victorian drive for codification, in particular the project of classifying, and by classifying containing, deviation from regulatory models such as gender binarity. Or, put differently: in its resistance to category injunctions and its substitution of the 'law of genre' for the Derridean 'law of impurity', the 'transgenre' of Victorian and neo-Victorian biographilia retraces the steps of nineteenth-century transgender identity; both are remediated in strikingly similar ways.[25] Just as there is no 'pure' gender, so, this book posits, there is no pure 'genre' of neo-/Victorian life-writing. While my readings distinguish between the broad forms of biography, biofiction and biodrama, their sexual/textual politics and poetics are assessed holistically to enable careful attention to the manner in which these forms draw on and inflect, inspire, play with and 'trans/form' one another.

Existing models of conceptualization, I argue, risk overlooking the fact that biographilic texts across significantly dissimilar time periods, from the Victorian to the contemporary, while differing in form and narrative politics, operate cumulatively and in conjunction in crafting a composite cultural memory of an historical life and identity like James Barry's. Premised on the cultural history of Barry biographilia that this book has undertaken, a key conclusion to be drawn is that, irrespective of considerable variance in levels of literary complexity, aesthetic and ethical choices and likely target markets, Victorian and neo-Victorian forms of life-writing share key motifs and plots in their representation of the biographilic subject. My focus on James Barry has served to explore the predominant textual strategies and narrative structures that all forms of life-writing and types of texts considered (postmodern and popular, self-reflexive and naïve, subtle and sensational) have in common. In re-imagining and remediating prior cultural constructions of the biographilic subject, all texts draw on what, in adaptation of the '"body-part" stories' that Hermione Lee identifies as integral to biography, and Jay Prosser and Rogers Brubaker to transgender life-writing, I discussed as body plots in Chapter 3.[26] Such body stories frequently find further remediation in visual format, in the form of periodical press caricatures or paratextual materials such as book covers: a version of the 'iconisation' which Nünning defines as one of the 'processes of compression' that are key to narrative worldmaking.[27] In the case of an historical transgender personality like James Barry, this book has illustrated, narratives of memorial construction revolve around three central moments and loci of subject constitution, self-affirmation and closure through either revelation or subversion. If the looking glass constitutes a site of external transformation from female to male as signified by change of costume, the duel marks an experience of internal transitioning in the course of the performance of a masculine ritual that enables the expression of queer sensibilities even as it threatens discovery. The bedroom/deathbed scene represents the culmination point of the narrative in which the trope of exposure may turn into an assertion of difference that allows transgender to come into view. The precise nature of such 'body narratives' will be subject to the biographical and historical contexts of the persona in question.

One of the questions that arises here is whether such body stories might be a feature of Victorian and neo-Victorian 'trans'-fictions more broadly, or of nineteenth-century 'trans' representations that are not or only partially biographilic in nature? To probe the wider applicability of this narrative paradigm for Victorian and nineteenth-century studies, it is worth considering two examples related to but different from James Barry's story: Julia Ward Howe's fictional autobiography *The Hermaphrodite* and the intersex memoir of Herculine Barbin.

Begun in 1846–47 but not published until 2004, *The Hermaphrodite* carries semi-autobiographical undertones (about Howe's marriage and internal sense of dislocation) and might thus be placed at the borderline of autobiografiction.[28] An unfinished manuscript novel, it is fragmented in content and heterogeneous in form (a picaresque *Bildungsroman* cum sensation novel with elements of the parable) and thus shares key aspects of Barry biographilia. The titular 'hermaphrodite' Laurence, while self-identifying as a man, is variously perceived by his contemporaries as male, female, neither and both; attracting the passions of both sexes, he resists all advances and painfully suppresses his own desire.[29] The three 'body plots' that shape Barry life-writing are in evidence here, too, though in reverse order. Where Barry biofiction moves from transformation to duel and bedroom discovery (or recovery) scenes, *The Hermaphrodite* inverts and doubles the sequence, so that the first and most momentous crisis in the text is prompted by a bedroom encounter that leads to double exposure and the internalization of abjection. When Laurence rebuffs the advances of a young widow who intrudes into his chamber to seduce him, 'She saw the bearded lip and earnest brow, but she saw also the falling shoulders, slender neck, and rounded bosom – then with a look like that of the Medusa, and a hoarse utterance, she murmured: "monster!"'[30] Though Laurence counters that he is 'as God made me', it is Emma's indictment, replicating as it does his father's rejection, that consolidates his conviction of his inherent monstrosity, inducing him to stifle all emotion and chastise his body's impulses. Even at the close of the novel a fantasized re-union with and embrace by his friend Roland ends with a profound 'consciousness of shame' and a reaffirmation of his state of abjection.[31]

When in the earlier scene Laurence carries the fainted and senseless Emma back to her room, he is discovered and obliged to defend her honour in a duel. In Barry biographilia, the duel threatens disclosure of the protagonist's secret; here it spells spiritual self-annulment as Laurence, though the victor, is compelled to reveal his dispossession: 'I am no man, no woman, nothing.'[32] The bedroom-duel plot replays in reverse order in Laurence's subsequent friendship with Roland, a young aristocrat who saves him from self-starvation. Jealous of his attentions to another man and enraged by the imputation of Laurence's womanhood, Roland initiates a duel with his assumed rival and then launches himself on to his friend, who is able to avert rape only with a hastily drugged drink. The double rerun of these narrative components is followed by two transformation scenes that visualize and then effect release from the 'bondage' of womanhood. In contradistinction to Barry biographilia, the protagonist is disempowered by crossing the gender/dress binary; 'the true meaning of the term "petticoat government"', Laurence learns, is 'that the petticoat governs her who wears it'.[33] In his attempt to slip on female garments, he promptly 'pricked myself with the pins, and strangled myself with the ribbons.'[34] The role of the mirror is here performed by a friend, Berto, who offers a running commentary on the physical and mental stranglehold of femininity.[35] Small wonder, then, if Laurence's return to masculinity is likened to an act of exorcism:

> It was now ... time that I should be released from the ignominious bondage of petticoats, that my legs should be disencumbered of a mass of articles utterly foreign to their use and purpose, and that my diaphragm should be allowed to expand in freedom broader than the lacings of a woman's bodice ... I stripped off the odious disguise, shook the curls back from my brow, and assumed my wonted attire. This being accomplished, Berto and I had a savage carnival over the deposed garments – we danced and shouted around them, we tore and trampled them, we sang them their death song, and then, without pity, consigned them to the flames.[36]

Ironically, however, it is precisely because of the insights he gained from living as a 'woman' and interacting with other women that Laurence learns to unlock his repressed feelings and to grow spiritually into 'one undivided, integral soul'.[37] Womanhood, ultimately, serves to set Laurence free to be himself. As in Barry life-writing, the three body plots thus orchestrate a narrative of *trans/*formation.

The autobiographical narrative of the French intersexual subject Herculine (Abel) Barbin (1838–68) furnishes a considerably less cathartic example of the plot structures of historical accounts of trans experience. Brought up as a girl, christened Adélaïde Herculine and called Alexina, Barbin attended a convent school, subsequently trained as a teacher and attained the position of headmistress in a provincial school before seeking medical advice on her/his condition.[38] Declared 'a man, hermaphrodite, no doubt, but with an obvious predominance of masculine sexual characteristics', Herculine had his civil status changed to Abel Barbin in 1860.[39] After his suicide in 1868 his body attracted medical and periodical press scrutiny. Because Barbin's life story and (inter/sexual) self-representation are significantly dissimilar from Barry's, his papers, printed in extract in 1874 by the physician Ambroise Tardieu under the title *Mes souvenirs*, and reproduced by Foucault in 1978 (first English-language edition 1980) in extended, but still incomplete form alongside a 'Dossier' offer an opportunity to probe the narrative paradigms this study has established for Barry life-writing from an alternative angle.[40]

In stark contrast to Barry, who concealed himself behind his professional accolades and achievements in his 1859 'Memorandum of the Services of Dr James Barry Inspector General of Hospitals', Barbin scripted his trans identity into textual existence, explicitly addressing posterity (both medical/scientific and general) to whom he bequeathed his manuscript: 'O princes of science, enlightened chemists', he wrote, 'I appeal here to the judgement of my readers in time to come'; posthumously, he hoped, he 'shall at last find a homeland, brothers, friends'.[41] By invoking and reaching out to a more enlightened community ('brothers' here echoing the political principle of fraternity, not masculinity *per se*), Barbin claimed agency for himself even at moments of intense anguish: suicide, it is implied, stilled the suffering of the body and mind with the promise of a spiritual afterlife. In contradistinction to Barbin's autobiographical focus on the language of emotion, Barry's strictly career-focused, fact-based self-testimonial, his reserve and indeed the very paucity of extant correspondence and other documents that would throw light on his *inner* experience speak to his determination to curtail posterity's access to his life.

Barbin's memoir ultimately points to his loss of control over his narrative: in title (*Mes souvenirs* being subsumed into *Herculine Barbin dite Alexina B.*) and, more significantly, in gender: Abel's story became Herculine's and Alexina's, as if, Eric Fassin notes, his change of civil status had never taken place, suicide having returned him to a redoubled femininity.[42] Indeed, even though his memoir is divided into two differently gendered parts, with Barbin being addressed as 'Mademoiselle' until his change of civil status and as a male thereafter,[43] Foucault refers to 'Alexina' throughout in the female pronoun:

> It is not a man who is speaking, trying to recall his sensations and his life as they were at the time when he was not yet 'himself.' When Alexina composed her memoirs, she was not far from her suicide; for herself, she was still without a definitive sex.[44]

In actual fact, Barbin's memoir ends with a reassertion of (generic) manhood: 'Perhaps it was that thirst for the unknown, which is so natural to man.'[45] Far from commemorating Barbin's pleasure in occupying an indeterminate (gender) position and revelling in his Otherness ('Elle se plaisisait … à être "autre" sans avoir jamais à être "de l'autre sexe"'), the final part of the memoir records his acute distress about being so absolutely set apart from others in his acquired manhood that he was no longer able to secure a stable livelihood for himself.[46]

Foucault's misrepresentation accentuates Barbin's third loss of control: that over the textual integrity of his narrative.[47] Published in expurgated form, the post-transition account (that Foucault added to Tardieu's edition), covering eight years, is considerably contracted; the original manuscript was never discovered, possibly having been destroyed by Tardieu. What we get to read therefore is Tardieu's version re-presented in expanded, yet nonetheless fragmented format by Foucault – a doubly mediated voice; an echo chamber in which Barbin's address to the afterworld offers up an invitation to the editor (and reader) to indulge in the fantasy of speaking for the past that contemporary Barry life-writing (by Sebastian Barry and Rachel Holmes) invokes for Barry; hence Foucault's overreading of the text in his desire to recognize what Rogers Brubaker defines as a contemporary 'trans of beyond', agender position in Barbin's reminiscences of his erstwhile 'happy limbo of a non-identity'.[48]

The ruptured remains of Barbin's text are self-consciously fashioned as a narrative: a tragic picaresque, a sexual *Bildungsroman* in which the conventions of romance shift into melodrama and sentimental disaster from the moment of the androgynously named 'Camille's' transition to masculinity.[49] Auto/biofiction or auto/biographiction rather than autobiography, in its narrative self-consciousness Barbin's memoir bears resemblance to Barry biofiction, as does the instability of the stories and names (the self-selected Abel and 'Camille' versus Adélaïde Herculine/Alexina; James Barry versus Margaret Bulkley and the biographilic 'James Miranda Barry'). Such interconnections are also reflected in the plot structures of the texts.

As in Howe's *Hermaphrodite*, the autobiographical nineteenth-century trans narrative starts with bedroom revelation scenes: in Barbin's case, an account of the awakening of his sensuality following his romantic crush on a fellow schoolgirl, an affection that resonates literarily with Jane Eyre's worship of Helen Temple. The dawning recognition and then joyful exploration of his sexual desire is recapitulated through a series of night-time encounters, beginning with his literally thunder-struck embrace (in the nude) of his adored Mother Superior during a storm and the '*incredible sensation*' that in that moment takes possession of him.[50] In a second stage he delights in petting Sara, the daughter of his employer (the proprietor of the school in which he is teaching), undressing her at bed-time, kissing her good night and watching over her while asleep. The third iteration of the scene sees the culmination of his passion in their secret sexual union.

Similarly to Barry biographilia and Howe's *Hermaphrodite*, the bedroom constitutes a site of conflicted sentiments: born from confusion, desire co-exists with anxiety and fear of exposure. Exposure, when it does come, is not materialized in a duel that the hero cannot avert or actively seeks out, but takes the shape of penitent self-disclosure: in Barbin's story the physical contest of a duel is replaced by the psychological trial of the confessional and succeeded by externally imposed medical consultation and directive. Confession, as Jay Prosser has noted, is a constitutive element of twentieth-century transsexual autobiography; here, then, Barbin's memoirs anticipate later developments and diverge from the narrative script of Barry biographilia.[51] The three increasingly intensifying bedroom scenes that awaken Barbin's desire and turn him into a sexual agent are followed by three confessions and two medical examinations that cumulatively strip him of the agency he had attained. Condemned and demonized by his first confessor and pathologized by a lewd, 'extraordinarily excit[ed]' provincial doctor, he is, at his second attempt, advised to suppress his impulses and withdraw to contemplative life in of all places a nunnery. Only with the third confessor does he find sympathy and spiritual, medical and legal guidance.[52] That medical acknowledgement is obtained at the prize of the violation of the body can be inferred from the grisly examination and especially autopsy reports included in Foucault's 'Dossier'.[53]

While Barbin takes active steps to change his life and is assisted in his drive for formal recognition of his difference, there is little indication that he follows an overriding inner desire in abandoning the lover with whom he had found happiness and whom he had desired to marry; his internalization of guilt and self-punishment compel him to break with all those who had previously formed the nucleus of his inner life. In contradistinction to Howe's Laurence, who comes into his own during his life as a woman, becoming a man, for Barbin, means not only to strip himself of his womanhood but to forsake women altogether. Paradoxically, as

Fassin observes, in discovering himself a man, Barbin must embrace asexuality.[54] More than that, his change of sex comes at the cost of 'perpetual isolation'.[55]

It is no coincidence, therefore, that the transformation scene – in Barry biographilia an experience of self-empowerment through self-reflection – is here related in the passive voice, as a moment of dispossession in the mirror gaze of heteronormativity: 'On me vit un bon matin assister à la messe en costume d'homme aux côtés de madame de R.., … fille de M. de Sainte-M.' ['I was seen attending mass one fine morning dressed as a man in the company of … the daughter of Monsieur de Saint-M.']. The passage continues: 'Only one or two people had recognized me; that was quite enough. Soon, the whole town was talking about it.'[56] Barbin presents himself 'in the *costume* of' a man; the phrasing implies that his newfound masculinity is a performance that does not represent the inner person any more than the female vestments did. A pair of trousers therefore does not make the man: rather, his manhood must be legitimized, externally and internally, by being placed in juxtaposition to a 'woman' whose sex and gender are irrefutable since she herself stands in relative position to a male authority figure: Abel Barbin thus constitutes himself as the reverse mirror image of Madame R., who herself serves as a mirror to her father, reflecting, in Virginia Woolf's memorable phrase, 'the figure of man at twice its natural size.'[57]

Ironically, the very support that enables Barbin to express his difference and assume a male identity publicly at the same time returns him to the patriarchal family with its binary structures. As a man rather than a relative figure mirroring the authority of another man, he must remove himself from his professional, familial and sexual environment: he deserts Sara and the school (source of a stable income and rising status), leaves his mother, the convent superior and his home province behind and moves to Paris. There, however, without the mirror of a woman who would reflect and stabilize his masculinity, he is unable to establish himself in an occupation that would provide a secure livelihood or new friendships. Trans/formation and transition, here, bring about self-annihilation. In Barbin's narrative, the transformation scene thus has the same fatal connotations as the deathbed discovery and exposure scene of Barry biographilia.

That, for all their differences, Barbin's memoir and Howe's fictional autobiography share key structuring devices with Barry biographilia is significant for the conceptual model this book has developed. Like and unlike contemporary trans life-writing, Victorian and neo-Victorian explorations of historical gender crossing draw on a discrete set of body plots to relay experiences of self-reflection, crisis, transformation and revelation, scripting protagonists' journeys of self-fashioning within narrative forms that perform their own acts of crossing generically. This study has sought to scrutinize this journey through Victorian gender and neo-Victorian genre by tracing the cultural history of James Barry from 1865 to today. The complex inflections of biographilic works on James Barry demonstrably offer an investigative paradigm for examining cultural constructions of nineteenth-century trans/gender identity while enabling a comprehensive conceptualization of the composite genre of neo-Victorian life-writing. If we take closer account of these body narratives, I contend, we will gain significantly new conceptual insights into neo-Victorian biographilia and, more broadly, into the way in which cultural memory is constructed and remediated in life-writing. This, ultimately, is the cultural 'secret' that, to borrow the words of Patricia Duncker and Katriona Gilmore, the textual body of 'Doctor James' *will* impart to us.[58]

Appendices

Appendix 1

Mary Anne Bulkley to James Barry, written in the hand of Margaret Bulkley, 11 April 1804, Wellcome Library, London, RAMC 1264, reproduced courtesy of the Museum of Military Medicine

A. Heilmann, *Neo-/Victorian Biographilia and James Miranda Barry*, https://doi.org/10.1007/978-3-319-71386-1

My Dear brother

I have been always very unwilling to trouble you, knowing the multiplicity of your avocations, or you should have often heard from me, while things were going on prosperously with me. I thought it sufficient if you heard of me & mine, thro my much esteemed friend Mr. Penrose, who I know corresponded with you; I must say he has been ever kind & attentive to me & mine; but I must now trouble you, to inform you, that my Son whom we strained every point to forward in the World, after giving him the best Education this place afforded, we gave a large Apprentice fee to an Eminent Attorney in Dublin, he had served near two years of his Time; When last year a Miss Ward of the City of Dublin, a young Lady of genteel connexions (sister to the late General Ward who was Guilotined in France in Robespeers time) fell in love with him, her friends would not consent till my poor husband, ever anxious to advance his Children, was tempted to settle on him a Farm, for which he paid a Fine & Agents fees, Three hundred pounds Stg. And laid out in building an excellent Dwelling-house, & Offices Manuring &ca more than Twelve hundred pounds (a Lease of Lives renewable for Ever & taken Eleven years ago) and other Interests he had in this Town, and they have been Married. We had embarked some time before this in the Grocery business, and had a well furnished Shop, many Articles for which we were oblidged to lay in on Credit. & our Creditors hearing that my Husband had made over his property on his Son, immediately became importunate, so that we were oblidged to stop payment, this stroke, & the loss of my Husbands employments in the Weigh-houses, in consequence of Party running so high And an Orange faction. Col. Longfield having got at the head of the Weigh-houses, who would not employ him on Account of his Religion

Religion. . These have clouded all our prospects, my Husband
has offered to give up to his Creditors more than would pay them
all, if sold for a fair Value, which things never bring when sold
in this manner. The entire of his debts amount to about Seven
Hundred pounds ~~Stg~~. He was ever partial to John (as being an
only Son) and wished to make him as Respectable as possible,
I fear very much he will not act up to the tenor of his or my ex-
-pectations, as the property settled upon him was intention-
-ally for the purpose of assisting me, and my two Daughters
if Ocasion required his doing so, I received a letter from him, from
Dublin a few days ago which gave me great pain, and which I
imputed to his youth and want of experience. I also fear he
is badly advised, I cannot immediately form any opinion Respecting
himself or his letter, as my Husband is in the Country untill he
he comes home. If he cannot bring his Creditors to a settlement
and give him time to pay them: He purposes going to the West
Indies Untill something Can be done (a very great fall indeed in
the space of about three years from a comfortable situation) &
Remit ~~to~~ us his earning. With the greatest deference I remain

P.S. Most truly & sincerely your

Sir, Most Affectionate ~~Ha Ha~~ Sister

Mary Anne Bulkley

My Mother is not able to write legible on account
of a tremour in her hand, desired me to write for her, My in-
-experience and so much unaccustomed to letter Writing I hope
will be accepted by you as an Apology the length, the many
faults & Errors in this letter. by Sir

by Yours Most Affection

Ha Ha Ha ~~Aunt~~

Merchants Quay

Cork 14th April 1804—

Margaret Anne Bulkley

I am concerned for not being able to
ascertain your address with exactness.—

Transcript[1]

My Dear brother,

I have been always very unwilling to trouble you, knowing the multiplicity of your avocations, or you should have often heard from me, while things were going on prosperously with me. I thought it sufficient if you heard of me & mine, through my much esteemed friend Mr. Penrose, who I know corresponded with you, I must say he has been ever kind & attentive to me and mine, but I must now trouble you, to inform you, that my Son whom we strained every point to forward in the World, after giving him the best Education this place afforded, we gave a large Apprentice fee to an Eminent Attorney in Dublin, he had served near two years of his Time; when last year a Miss Ward of the City of Dublin, a young Lady of genteel connexions (sister to the late General Ward who was Guilotined in France in Robespier's time) fell in love with him, her friends would not consent till my poor husband, ever anxious to advance his Children, was tempted to settle on him a Farm, for which he paid a Fine & Agents fees, Three hundred pounds [letters crossed out] And laid out in building an excellent Dwelling-house, & Offices [illegible] etc. more than Twelve hundred pounds (a Lease of Lives renewable for ever & taken Eleven years ago) and other Interests he had in this Town, and they have been Married. We had embarked some time before this in the Grocery business, and had a well furnished Shop, many Articles for which we were obliged to lay in on Credit. & our Creditors hearing that my Husband had made over his property to his Son, immediately became importunate, so that we were obliged to stop payment, this stroke, & the loss of my Husband's employments in the Weigh-houses, in consequence of Party [running?] so high And an Orange faction. Col. Longfield having got at the head of the Weigh-houses, who would not employ him on account of his Religion. These have clouded all our prospects, my Husband has offered to give up to his Creditors more than would pay them all, if sold for a fair Value which things never bring when sold in this man^{n}er. The entire of his debts amount to about Seven Hundred pounds [letter crossed out]. He was ever partial to John (as being an only Son) and wished to make him as respectable as possible, I fear very much he will not act up to the tenor of his, or my expectations, as the property settled upon him was intentionally for the purpose of assisting me, and my two Daughters if Ocasion required his doing so. I received a letter from him, from Dublin a few days ago, which gave me great pain, and which I imputed to his youth and want of experience, I also fear he is badly advised, I cannot immediately form any opinion respecting himself or his letter, as my Husband is in the Country until he he comes home. If he cannot bring his Creditors to a settlement and give him time to pay them. He purposes going to the West Indies Untill something can be done (a very great fall indeed in the space of about three years from a comfortable situation). & remit ~~to~~ us his earning. With the greatest deference I remain

Most truly & sincerely your most Affectionate etc etc Sister
Mary Anne Bulkley

P.S.
Sir,
My Mother is not able to write legible on account of a tremour in her hand, desired me to write for her, My inexperience and so much unaccustomed to letter writing I hope will be accepted by you as an Apology the length, the many faults & Errors in this letter, by Sir

Merchants Quay — By Yours Most Affectionate etc etc etc
Cork 11 April 1804 — Margaret Anne Bulkley

I am concerned for not being able to ascertain your address with exactness

Appendix 2

James Barry to Sir James McGrigor, St Helena, 23 October 1836, Wellcome Library, London, RAMC 1264, reproduced courtesy of the Museum of Military Medicine

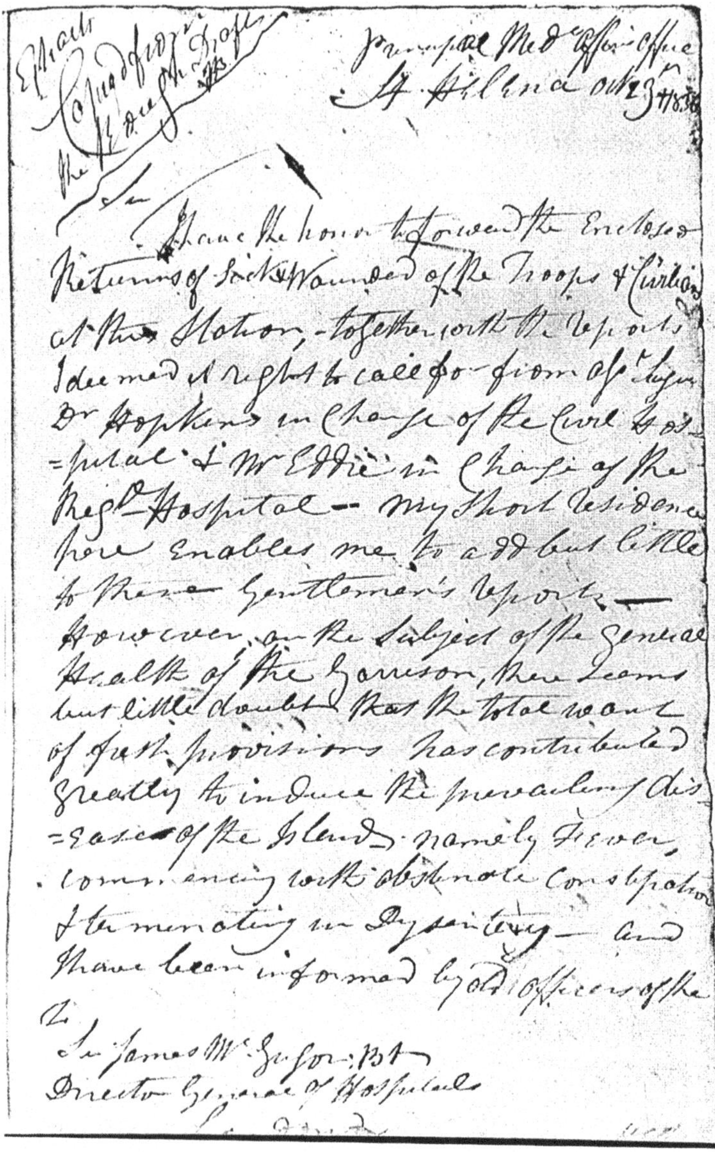

Extracts Correspondence the Rough Drafts

Principal Medl Officer's Office
St Helena Oct 23/1836

Sir

I have the honor to forward the Enclosed Returns of Sick & Wounded of the Troops & Civilians at this Station, — together with the reports I deemed it right to call for from Asst Surgn Dr Hopkins in Charge of the Civil Hos=pital & Mr Eddie in Charge of the Regtl Hospital — my short residence here enables me to add but little to these Gentlemen's reports —

However, on the subject of the general Health of the Garrison, there seems but little doubt that the total want of fresh provisions has contributed greatly to induce the prevailing dis=eases of the Island — namely Fever, commencing with obstinate Constipation & terminating in Dysentery — and I have been informed by old Officers of the

To

Sir James McGrigor Bt
Director General of Hospitals

H E I Company at St Helena; the Other force was
so formidable with them, if not early treated —
that if it were discovered that a Soldier did
not report himself soon after the first Sympt-
(constipation) made its appearance a penalty om
was annexed — Scorbutic affections
also have been evidently induced,
more particularly in persons of a
Scrophulous Diathesis — and I am
of Opinion that the Ration pint of
Cape Wine, has been of Eminent utility
in counteracting this malady, having
almost the effect of an antiscorbutic —
The proceedings of the Medl Board on
Fresh Provisions & Mr Asst Surgeons
Eddie & McLaren's letters — will give ample
information on this Subject —
In regard to the Civil Department; on
my arrival I found a want of arrange-
-ment, more particularly in the disgusting
circumstance of Male attendants on the
female patients — Syphilitic & other
Diseases — and of course the greatest
irregularities — I immediately hired
a respectable woman of Color as Matron
& requested the Milty Chaplain to visit
the Civil side of the Hospital, as well

the Military — I also lost no time in
representing ~~the~~ these matters to the
M. Genl Middlemore, who authorised
me to select a Govt Building close
to the Hospital — & has directed the Ord-
-nance Dept to fit up — one por-
-tion for the reception of females,
& the other for Maniacs — who are
at present in an awfully neglected
State —— Dr Hopkins Asst Staff
Surgeon & P.M.O. in my absence having
a great deal of duty — & every thing
being strange — together with his having
been unaccustomed to these Matters
thought it better to delay any
positive arrangements 'till my
arrival —— I shall conclude
by stating that as Mr Asst Surgeon Oddie
in Charge of the ~~sick~~ 91st Regt was the
only individual here accustomed
to Forms & Returns — thought it right
to call upon him to assist me in
making up the Expenditure, & other
Returns — until my Clerk becomes

becomes accustomed to them.
I enclose the Bill of Mortality for St Helena of 1835 — I am sure it will give you pleasure to hear that to the Zeal, ability & attention of Dr Eddie may be attributed the few deaths of the Patients under his Charge — His Hospital is always clean & well arranged

I have the Honor
to be Sir
Your Most Obedient
Humble Servant
James Barry MD
Surgeon to the Forces
PMO

Copied
A true Copy from my rough Draft made at St Helena
J Barry

Antigua July 10th 1839

Transcript[2]
[Extract] Copied from the Rough Draft JB
Principal Med Affairs Office
St Helena Oct 23 1836
To Sir James McGrigor, Bt
Director General of Hospitals

Sir
I have the honour to forward the enclosed Returns of Sick & Wounded of the Troops & Civilians at this Station, together with the reports I deemed it right to call for from As[sistan]t Surgeon Dr. Hopkins in Charge of the Civil Hospital & Mr. Eddie in Charge of the Reg[u]l[ar] Hospital – My short residence has enabled me to add but little to these Gentlemen's reports. – However, on the subject of the General Health of the Garrison, there seems but little doubt that the total want of fresh provisions has contributed greatly to induce the prevailing disease of the glands namely fever, commencing with obstinate constipation & terminating in Dysentery – and I have been informed by old officers of the HEI [Honourable East India] Company of St Helena that this fever was so formidable with them, if not early treated that if it were discovered that a soldier did not report himself soon after the first symptom (constipation) made its appearance a penalty was arranged – Scorbutic affections also have been evidently induced more particularly in persons of a Scrophulous Diathesis – and I am of opinion that the '[?]Pint' of Cape Wine has been of Eminent utility in counteracting this malady, having almost the effect of an antiscorbutic. The proceedings of the Med^cl^ Board on Fresh Provisions & Mr. Ast Surgeons Eddie & McLaren's letters will give ample information on this Subject –

In regard to the Civil Department; on my arrival I found a want of arrangement, more particularly in the disgusting circumstance of male attendants on the female patients, Syphilitic & other Diseases – and of course the greatest irregularities. – I immediately hired a respectable Woman of Color as Matron & requested the [Military] Chaplain to visit the Civil Side of the Hospital, as well as the military – I also lost no time in representing ~~t~~ these matters to H.E. M. Genl Middlemore, who authorised me to select a Govt Building close to the Hospital & has directed the Ordinance Dept to fill it up: one portion for the reception of females, & the other for Maniacs – who are at present in an awfully neglected State. – Dr. Hopkins Ast Staff Surgeon & P.M.O. [Principal Medical Officer] in my absence having a great deal of duty & every thing being strange, together with his having been unaccustomed to these matters thought it better to delay any possible arrangements 'till my arrival. – I shall conclude by stating that as Mr. Ast Surgeon Eddie, in charge of the [word crossed out] 91st Regt was the only individual here accustomed to Forms & Returns – I thought it right to call upon him to assist me in the making of the Expenditure, & other Returns until my Clerk becomes accustomed to them. –

I enclose the Bill of Mortality for St Helena of 1835 – I am sure it will give you pleasure to hear that to the Zeal, ability & attention of Mr. Eddie may be attributed the fewer deaths of the Patients under his Charge – His Hospital is always clean & well arranged.

I have the Honor
To be Sir
Your most Obedient
Humble Servant
James Barry M.D.
Surgeon to the Forces

Certified
A true Copy from my Rough Draft made at St Helena
Antigua July 18th 1839

Appendix 3

Transcript: James Barry, 'The humble memorial of Dr James Barry, Inspector General of Hospitals', undated draft [1859], Wellcome Library, London, RAMC 373, courtesy of the Museum of Military Medicine.[3]

Therewith that your Memorialist entered the Army as a Medical Officer under the age of fourteen: that he has continuously served to the present time at the Cape of Good Hope, Mauritius, Jamaica, [and had charge of the Windward and Leeward Islands and for twelve months, during the temporary absence of the Inspector General and was thanked in General Orders by Sir (Lord) W[h]ittingham], Trinidad, St Helena, Barbados, Antigua, Malta, Corfu, the Crimea and Canada.

- that your Memorialist when at Malta in 185[1] was promoted to be Deputy Inspector General [word crossed out], and was transferred to Corfu, when he at once volunteered for service in the Crimea; but there being no vacancy at the time for an officer of his rank he, in the meantime, endeavoured to [word crossed out] make himself as useful as possible to the Army before Sebastopol by obtaining permission for 500 sick & wounded men being sent to Corfu, of whom he sent back fit for active Service nearly 400 –

– that during that period the 97th Regt having been ordered from Malta to the Pireus, your Memorialist received a letter from the Officer Com[mandin]g the Reg[imen]t (now M[ajor] Gen[era]l Lockyer) to the effect that his Regt [word crossed out] was unprovided with medical comforts or medicines; ~~and~~ that that he had no means of procuring them, and consequently felt considerable [words crossed out] anxiety and distress, the cholera having broken out, and 92 Men having been already taken ill –

– that in two hours after the receipt of Col Lockyer's letter your Memorialist had embarked a supply of comforts & medicines for the use of the Regt and Hospital, and continued to forward further supplies once a week, there being no other possible means by which such supplies could have been procured –

– that for his conduct on that occasion your Memorialist was thanked by the Medical Board –

– that your Memorialist was also subsequently [word crossed out] thanked by Lord Lyons for discovering the cause of the malignant fever on board HM Ship 'Modeste' (Captain Butler RN) and for his success in remedying the same, and in treating the Sick –

– your Memorialist also received a diamond ring and the thanks, through the British Government of the Arch Duke Charles for services to one of His Imperial 'Highness's[']' men –

– your Memorialist also received the thanks of the late Duke of Wellington for his services during the cholera at Malta in the year –

– your Memorialist might relate many other occasions in which he has proved himself more than ordinarily zealous and useful during a long career in Her Majesty's Service, but he trusts that he has sufficiently shown that he has a claim to some consideration not to say indulgence, from the authorities under whom he is placed –

– your Memorialist has now only to state that having had the influenza in Canada he was ordered Home [words crossed out] to be examined by a Medical Board; that three days after his arrival in England [He arrived 26 May 1859] he attended before the Board, consisting of three Junior Medical Officers, who pronounced your Memorialist to be unfit for further service, the result of which opinion has been that he has been placed on Half Pay [on the 19 July 1859]

Without impinging the desire of the young officers who examined your Memorialist to perform their duty impartially and honestly, he has to observe that not one of them had ever seen your Memorialist before, that your Memorialist owing to his late illness in Canada, and to the effects of a Sea Voyage, from which he suffers greatly, looked unusually delicate and meagre, and that consequently the Board not unnaturally somewhat hastily jumped to the conclusion that your Memorialist was in a bad state of health; whereas the fact is that he feels and believes himself to be stronger & in better health than he has been for the last two or three years, and fully capable of effectively performing the duties of his rank.

Your Memorialist therefore prays that he may be restored to full pay, and ordered back to Canada until he has completed his full [word crossed out] period of Service, of which he requires nearly twenty months; by which means your Memorialist will be saved from great pecuniary loss, and for the grant of which [word crossed out] request your Memorialist will ever pray.

To the Right Hon
The Secretary of State for War

Appendix 4

James Barry, 'Memorandum of the Services of Dr. James Barry Inspector General of Hospitals', stamped 30 January 1859, Wellcome Library, London, RAMC 373, reproduced courtesy of the Museum of Military Medicine

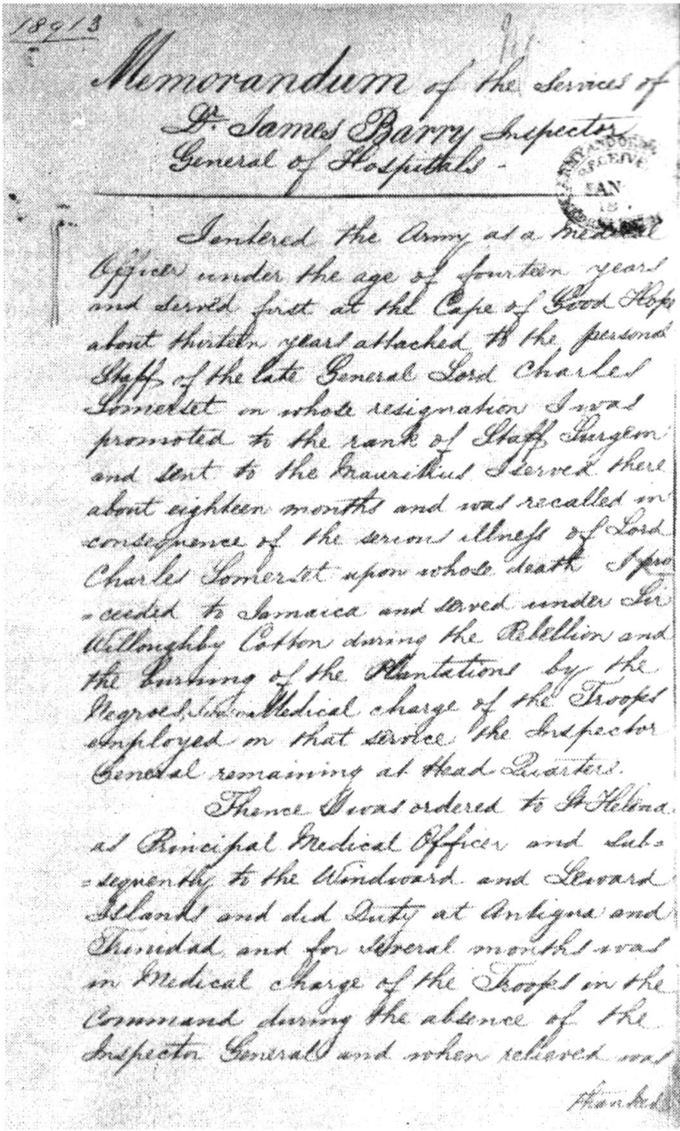

18913

Memorandum of the Services of
Dr James Barry Inspector
General of Hospitals -

I entered the Army as a Medical
Officer under the age of fourteen years
and served first at the Cape of Good Hope
about thirteen years attached to the personal
Staff of the late General Lord Charles
Somerset on whose resignation I was
promoted to the rank of Staff Surgeon
and sent to the Mauritius I served there
about eighteen months and was recalled in
consequence of the serious illness of Lord
Charles Somerset upon whose death I pro-
-ceeded to Jamaica and served under Sir
Willoughby Cotton during the Rebellion and
the burning of the Plantations by the
Negroes in Medical charge of the Troops
employed on that service the Inspector
General remaining at Head Quarters.

Thence I was ordered to St Helena
as Principal Medical Officer and Sub-
-sequently to the Windward and Leeward
Islands and did Duty at Antigua and
Trinidad and for several months was
in Medical Charge of the Troops in the
Command during the absence of the
Inspector General and when relieved was

thanked

thanked in General Order by General
Sir J Whittingham.

Having returned to this Country
on sick leave after a severe attack of
Yellow Fever contracted at Trinidad I was
on my recovery sent to Malta as Principal
Medical Officer and served under General
Sir Patrick Stewart and General Ellice
to both of whom I gave satisfaction
as recorded in the Public Documents at
the Medical Board and I also had the thanks
of the Duke of Wellington for my services
during the period that Island was
visited by the cholera.

I was shortly after promoted
to the rank of Deputy Inspector General
in the Ionian Islands. During the
period of my service there War was declared
against Russia and at my suggestions to
Lord Raglan and Inspector General Sir J
Hall 400 of the sick and wounded from
the Crimea were sent and placed under
my charge at Corfu upwards of 400 of
them returned fit for active service
having been restored to health in an
unusually short period and I myself
proceeded on leave to the Crimea where
I remained about three months with
the 4th Division before Sebastopol and
made myself useful as opportunities
offered which can be testified by Sir
John Hall and the Colonel and Officers
of

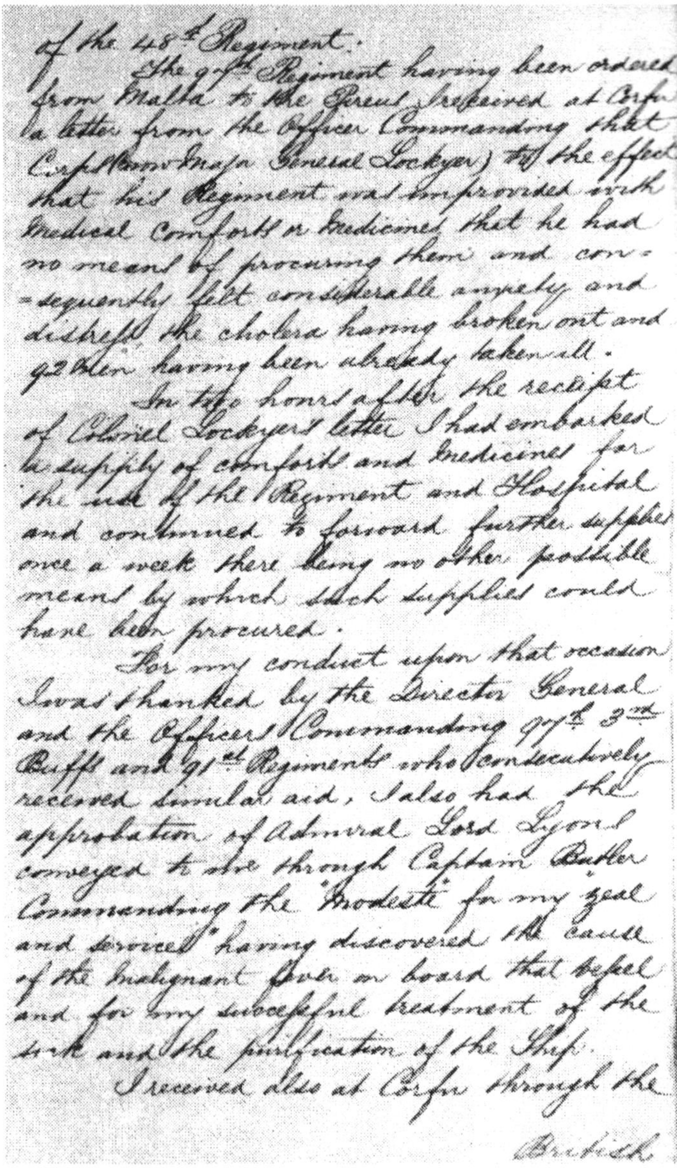

of the 48th Regiment.

The 97th Regiment having been ordered from Malta to the Piraeus I received at Corfu a letter from the Officer Commanding that Corps (Now Major General Lockyer) to the effect that his Regiment was unprovided with Medical Comforts or Medicines that he had no means of procuring them and consequently felt considerable anxiety and distress, the cholera having broken out and 92 men having been already taken ill.

In two hours after the receipt of Colonel Lockyer's letter I had embarked a supply of comforts and medicines for the use of the Regiment and Hospital and continued to forward further supplies once a week there being no other possible means by which such supplies could have been procured.

For my conduct upon that occasion I was thanked by the Director General and the Officers Commanding 97th, 3rd Buffs and 91st Regiments who consecutively received similar aid, I also had the approbation of Admiral Lord Lyons conveyed to me through Captain Butler Commanding the "Modeste" for my zeal and services* having discovered the cause of the malignant fever on board that vessel and for my successful treatment of the sick and the purification of the Ship.

I received also at Corfu through the

British

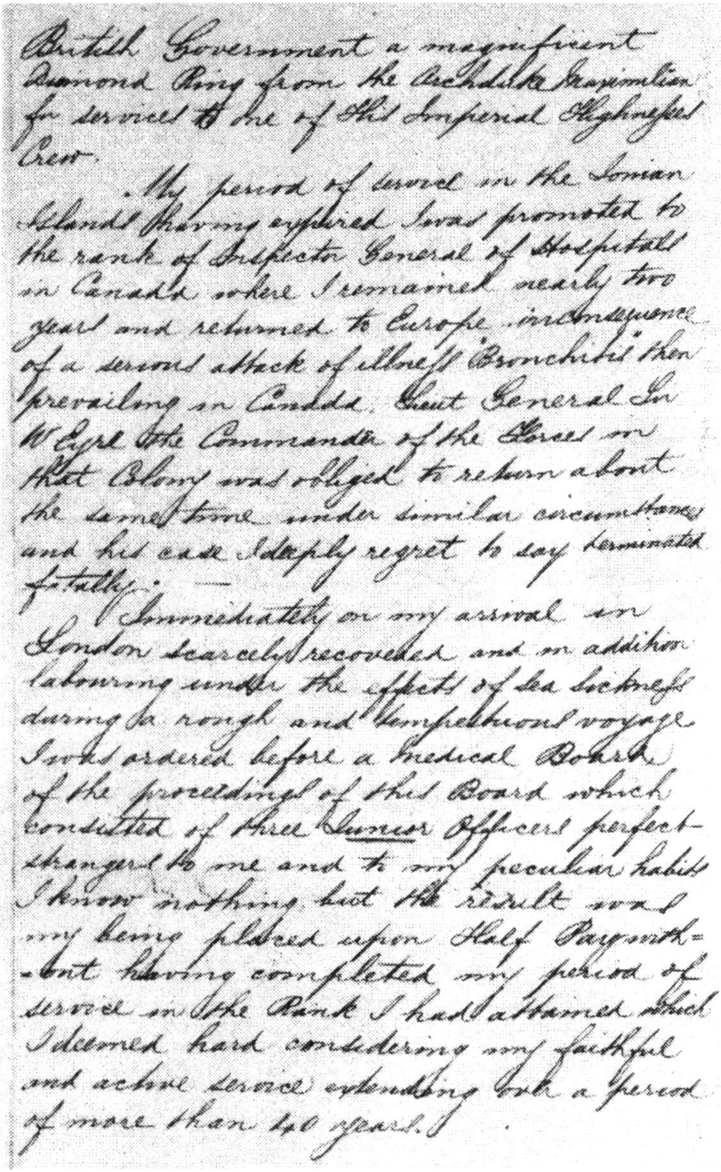

British Government a magnificent Diamond Ring from the Archduke Maximilian for services to one of His Imperial Highness's Crew.

My period of service in the Ionian Islands having expired I was promoted to the rank of Inspector General of Hospitals in Canada where I remained nearly two years and returned to Europe in consequence of a serious attack of illness "Bronchitis" then prevailing in Canada. Lieut General Sir W Eyre the Commander of the Forces in that Colony was obliged to return about the same time under similar circumstances and his case I deeply regret to say terminated fatally. —

Immediately on my arrival in London scarcely recovered and in addition labouring under the effects of sea sickness during a rough and tempestuous voyage I was ordered before a Medical Board of the proceedings of this Board which consisted of three <u>Junior</u> Officers perfect-strangers to me and to my peculiar habits I know nothing but the result was my being placed upon Half Pay with-out having completed my period of service in the Rank I had attained which I deemed hard considering my faithful and active service extending over a period of more than 40 years.

I may add that during this lengthened period of my service I obtained leave of absence on private affairs on only one occasion and then only when I conceived my prospects in the service were seriously compromised for want of a personal appeal at Head Quarters.

On each change of Station I was put to an immense personal outlay the Climates of each being of such different temperatures.

Each move entailed a sacrifice of property then in my possession and an outlay to provide that required for the service in prospect.

I am now prepared to serve Her Majesty in any quarter of the Globe to which I may be sent and am loath to close a career which impartially may be deemed to have been a useful and faithful one without some Special mark of Her Majesty's gracious fa[illegible]

James Barry M.D.

Inspector General

Transcript[4]

Memorandum of the Services of Dr. James Barry Inspector General of Hospitals

I entered the Army as a Medical Officer under the age of fourteen years and served first at the Cape of Good Hope about thirteen years attached to the personal Staff of the late General Lord Charles Somerset on whose resignation I was promoted to the rank of Staff Surgeon and sent to the Mauritius, I served there about eighteen months and was recalled in consequence of the serious illness of Lord Charles Somerset upon whose death I proceeded to Jamaica and served under Sir Willoughby Cotton during the Rebellion and the burning of the Plantations by the Negroes, I was in Medical charge of the Troops employed in that service, the Inspector General remaining at Head Quarters.

Thence I was ordered to St Helena as Principal Medical Officer and subsequently to the Windward and Leward Islands and did Duty at Antigua and Trinidad and for several months was in Medical charge of the Troops in the Command during the absence of the Inspector General and when relieved was thanked in General Orders by General Sir J Whit[t]ingham.

Having returned to this Country on sick leave after a serious attack of Yellow fever contracted at Trinidad I was on my recovery sent to Malta as Principal Medical Officer and served under General Sir Patrick Stewart and General Ellice to both of whom I gave satisfaction as recorded in the Public Document & at the Medical Board and I also had the thanks of the Duke of Wellington for my services during the period that Island was visited by the cholera.

I was shortly after promoted to the rank of Deputy Inspector General in the Ionian Islands. During the period of my service there War was declared against Russia and at my suggestions to Lord Raglan and Inspector General Sir J Hall 500 of the sick and wounded from the Crimea were sent and placed under my charge at Corfu, upwards of 400 of them returned fit for active service, having been restored to health in an unusually short period and I myself proceeded on leave to the Crimea where I remained about three months with the 4th Division before Sebastopol and made myself useful as opportunities offered which can be testified by Sir John Hall and the Colonel and Officers of the 48th Regiment.

The 97th Regiment having been ordered from Malta to the Pireus I received at Corfu a letter from the Officer Commanding that Corp[ora]l (now Major General Lockyer) to the effect that his Regiment was unprovided with Medical Comforts or Medicines, that he had no means of procuring them and consequently felt considerable anxiety and distress, the cholera having broken out and 92 men having been already taken ill.

In two hours after the receipt of Colonel Lockyer's letter I had embarked a supply of comforts and Medicines for the use of the Regiment and Hospital and continued to forward further supplies once a week there being no other possible means by which such supplies could have been procured.

For my conduct upon that occasion I was thanked by the Director General and the Officers Commanding 97th 3rd Buffs and 91st Regiments who consecutively received similar aid, I also had the approbation of Admiral Lord Lyons conveyed to me through Captain Butler Commanding the 'Modeste' for my 'zeal and services' having discovered the cause of the malignant fever on board that vessel and for my successful treatment of the sick and the purification of the Ship.

I received also at Corfu through the British Government a magnificent Diamond Ring from the Archduke Maximilian for services to one of His Imperial Highnesses Crew.

My period of service in the Ionian Islands having expired I was promoted to the rank of Inspector General of Hospitals in Canada where I remained nearly two years and returned to Europe in consequence of a serious attack of illness 'Bronchitis' then prevailing in Canada. Lieut General Sir W Eyre the commander of the Forces in that Colony was obliged to return about the same time under similar circumstances and his case I deeply regret to say terminated fatally. –

Immediately on my arrival in London I scarcely recovered and in addition labouring under the effects of Sea Sickness during a rough and tempestuous voyage I was ordered before a Medical Board, of the proceedings of this Board which consisted of three Junior Officers perfect strangers to me and to my peculiar habits I know nothing, but the result was my being placed upon Half Pay without having completed my period of service in the Rank I had attained which I deemed hard considering my faithful and active service extending over a period of more than forty years.

I may add that during this lengthened period of my service I obtained leave of absence on private affairs on only one occasion and then only when I conceived my prospects in the service were seriously compromised for want of a personal appeal at Head Quarters.

On each change of Station I was put to an immense personal outlay the climates of each being of such different temperatures.

Each move entailed a sacrifice of property then in my possession and an outlay to procure that required for the service in prospect.

I am now prepared to serve Her Majesty in any quarter of the Globe to which I may be sent and am loath to close a career which impartially may be deemed to have been a useful and faithful one without some special mark of her Majesty's gracious favour.

James Barry MD
Inspector General

Notes

1. Transcript mine.
2. Transcript by Mark Llewellyn.
3. Reproduced (with corrections) from a typed transcript included in War Office file RAMC 373 (Wellcome Library), courtesy of the Museum of Military Medicine.
4. Reproduced (with corrections) from a typed transcript included in War Office file RAMC 373 (Wellcome Library), courtesy of the Museum of Military Medicine.

Notes

List of Figures

1. The original press is now under the remit of Pearson UK, and the publisher 'has no objection in principle' to granting permission to reproduce this image, but 'because of the age of this title, the contractual details are no longer available' and the publisher holds 'no record of this title'. The designer of the image is not referenced in the book. Correspondence from the Rights and Permissions Team, Pearson UK, Cape Town, 25 April 2017.
2. This image, entitled 'Murray Miniature' in the Wellcome Library file of the holdings of the Museum of Military Medicine, RAMC 801.6.5.3, is referenced as a 'watercolour painting of Dr James Barry executed at the Cape some time before 1828' in Percival R. Kirby's 'Dr James Barry, Controversial South African Medical Figure: A Recent Evaluation of His Life and Sex', *South African Medical Journal*, 25 April 1970, p. 511, Wellcome Library, RAMC 658.

Chapter 1

1. James Barry's final speech at his court-martial in November/December 1836, as quoted in June Rose, *The Perfect Gentleman: The remarkable life of Dr. James Miranda Barry, the woman who served as an officer in the British Army from 1813 to 1859* (London: Hutchinson, 1977), p. 112. See also Rachel Holmes, *Scanty Particulars: The Mysterious, Astonishing and Remarkable Life of*

A. Heilmann, *Neo-/Victorian Biographilia and James Miranda Barry*, https://doi.org/10.1007/978-3-319-71386-1

Victorian Surgeon James Barry (London: Penguin, 2002), p. 220; hereafter Holmes, *Scanty Particulars* (1). Neither biographer fully references the speech, but both place it in the context of the military trial. Rose refers to the Proceedings of the Court Martial at St. Helena in her bibliographical 'Postscript', p. 154. The US and second UK editions of Holmes's biography reference quotations from the court-martial to file CO 247/52, Public Records Office, London; see Holmes, *Scanty Particulars: The Scandalous Life and Astonishing Secret of Queen Victoria's Most Eminent Military Doctor* (New York: Random House, 2002), p. 207, pp. 336–7, n.204, hereafter Holmes, *Scanty Particulars* (2); and Holmes, *The Secret Life of Dr. James Barry: Victorian England's Most Eminent Surgeon* (Stroud: Tempus, 2007), p. 312, hereafter Holmes, *Secret Life*. I have been unable to trace this document in the James Barry files CO 247/52, CO 247/49 and PRO 30/46/18 held in the National Archives, Kew, Richmond. The probable location of the documents is in the St Helena Archives, Jamestown, St Helena, listed in Michael du Preez and Jeremy Dronfield's most recent biography, *Dr. James Barry: A Woman Ahead of Her Time* (London: Oneworld Publications, 2016), p. 452.

2. Letter dated 24 August 1865, Wellcome Library, London, RAMC 373; see also Rose, *Perfect Gentleman*, p. 13; Isobel Rae, *The Strange Story of Dr. James Barry: Army Surgeon, Inspector-General of Hospitals, Discovered on Death to be a Woman* (London: Longmans, Green and Co, 1958), pp. 115–16. For more detailed discussion see Holmes, *Scanty Particulars* (1), pp. 258–62.
3. Rogers Brubaker, *trans: Gender and Race in an Age of Unsettled Identities* (Princeton: Princeton University Press, 2016), p. 73.
4. Ansgar Nünning, 'Fictional Metabiographies and Metaautobiographies: Towards a Definition, Typology and Analysis of Self-Reflexive Hybrid Metagenres', in *Self-Reflexivity in Literature*, ed. Werner Huber, Martin Middeke and Hubert Zapf (Würzburg: Königshausen & Neumann, 2005), p. 198. Nünning's essay is reprinted in Michael Lackey (ed.), *Biographical Fiction: A Reader* (New York: Bloomsbury, 2016), pp. 363–79.
5. Linda Hutcheon prominently argued in *A Poetics of Postmodernism: History, Theory, Fiction* (1988; London: Routledge, 1996) that it is the 'ex-centric[s]', the 'formerly excluded (women – but also the working class, gays, ethnic and racial minorities …)' that are the

focus of historiographic metafiction, i.e. the postmodern historical novel (p. 95). Arguably, as Christian Gutleben reminds us, the one-time outsider in our own time represents the mainstream, at least in academic study, so that the 'subversion at play' in adopting the voice of the Other 'appears anachronistic'; see his *Nostalgic Postmodernism: The Victorian Tradition and the Contemporary British Novel* (Amsterdam: Rodopi, 2001), p. 175. This notion of neo-Victorianism's retrospective mirror glance is also discussed in Simon Joyce's 'The Victorians in the Rearview Mirror', in *Functions of Victorian Culture at the Present Time*, ed. Christine L. Krueger (Athens: Ohio University Press, 2002), pp. 3–17.

6. Only the office of Director General outranked the Inspector General; see du Preez and Dronfield, *Dr. James Barry*, p. 352.
7. See epigraph 2. The charwoman sought to obtain remuneration she claimed had been promised, and then withheld, by Barry's landlady. That the layer-out had kept quiet about her discovery up until this point and expected to be paid for her silence casts doubt on her testimony; on the other hand, as Rachel Holmes observes, she would have been unlikely to make such a claim without being convinced 'that what she had seen was a woman's body' (*Scanty Particulars* [1], p. 321). After her revelations were made public, several of Barry's earlier acquaintances alleged that they had always suspected him to be a woman; that these testimonies followed in the wake of sensational newspaper reporting weakens their credibility. Details of McKinnon's full name and his friendship with Barry are sourced from du Preez and Dronfield, *Dr. James Barry*, p. 369.
8. In *The Perfect Gentleman* biographer June Rose laid the groundwork for tracing James Barry's origins to one of the daughters of Mary Anne Bulkley, sister of the Irish-born history painter James Barry; William L. Pressly was the first scholar to discover correspondence with the Bulkleys' family solicitor David Reardon that established James Barry's identity as that of the elder Bulkley sister, Margaret, and to reproduce handwriting samples of Margaret Bulkley and James Barry in his 'Portrait of a Cork Family: The Two James Barrys', *Cork Historical and Archaeological Society*, vol. 90 (1985), pp. 137–49. Holmes's *Scanty Particulars* and Michael du Preez provided further documentary evidence. See H. M. du Preez, 'Dr James Barry: the early years revealed', *South African Medical Journal*, vol. 98 (2008), pp. 52–58, and 'Dr James Barry

(1789–1865): the Edinburgh years', *Journal of the Royal College of Physicians of Edinburgh*, vol.42: 3 (2012), pp. 258–65. Du Preez's essays will hereafter be referenced as 'The early years' and 'The Edinburgh years'. See also du Preez and Dronfield, *Dr. James Barry*.

9. For radio broadcasts see June Rose, *Quest for Dr. James Barry*, prod. Madeau Stewart (BBC radio broadcast, 27 June 1973), Wellcome Library, London, RAMC 1089; also Jean Binnie, 'Dr Barry', radio play broadcast by the BBC in the *Who Sings the Hero?* series on 19 August 1992; for details see 'BBC Afternoon Plays, 1984–2002', http://www.suttonelms.org.uk/lost10.html [accessed 29 November 2015]. For TV productions see 'An Experiment', *A Skirt through History*, dir. Philippa Lowthorpe (BBC, 1994), http://explore.bfi.org.uk/4ce2b7d7be08e [accessed 17 April 2017].
10. The biopic currently under development is *Dr. James Barry,* with Rachel Weisz in the lead role (and co-produced by her); screenplay by Nick Yarborough. Another biopic, *Heaven and Earth*, directed by Marleen Gorliss and with Natascha McElhone in the lead role, appears to have stalled. Andrew Pulver, 'Rachel Weisz to play real-life gender-fluid Victorian doctor', *Guardian,* 13 December 2016, https://www.theguardian.com/film/2016/dec/13/rachel-weisz-stars-james-barry-film-gender-fluid-victorian-doctor [accessed 12 December 2016]. For *Heaven and Earth* see *Movie Insider* (entry dated 5 February 2009), http://www.movieinsider.com/m2261/barry#plot [accessed 15 December 2016]. Mystery and enigma are often referenced in titles, both primary and critical; for the latter see, for example, Alice Wilson, 'The Enigma of Dr. James Barry', *Health, Law & Ethics*, downloaded from *LJSM*, vol.1, 30 April 2010, pp. 243–45. http://issuu.com/lsjm/docs/hle [accessed 2 November 2015]; Mary Hammond, 'The Enigma of James Barry' [review of Patricia Duncker's *James Miranda Barry*], *Women: A Cultural Review*, vol. 13:1 (2010), pp. 104–106; also Van Hunks, 'The Mysterious Doctor James Barry: Dr. James "Miranda" Barry in South Africa', http://www.vanhunks.com/cape1/barry1.html [accessed 8 November 2015].
11. For 'author fiction' see Laura E. Savu's study of postmodernist metafiction that takes authors as their subject in *Postmortem Postmodernists: The Afterlife of the Author in Recent Narrative* (Madison: Fairleigh Dickinson University Press, 2009), p. 9.
12. See Jan Morris's autobiography, now a classic of the transgender canon, *Conundrum* (London: Faber and Faber, 1974).

13. See the first chapter, 'Trans*', of Jack Halberstam, *Trans: A Quick and Quirky Account of Gender Variability* (Oakland, CA: University of California Press, 2018), p. 4. For a brief discussion of the use of the asterisk see also Jack Halberstam, 'Trans* – Gender Transitivity and New Configurations of Body, History, Memory and Kinship', *Parallax*, vol. 22:3 (2016), p. 368.
14. See the essays collected in Robyn Warhol and Susan S. Lanser (eds), *Narrative Theory Unbound: Queer and Feminist Interventions* (Columbus: Ohio State University Press, 2015). Intersectionality is discussed in Lanser's position piece, 'Toward (a Queerer and) More (Feminist) Narratology' (pp. 23–42) as well as by a number of other contributors.
15. Monique Rooney, 'Grave endings: the representation of passing', *Australian Humanities Review*, vol. 23 (Sept. 2001), http://australianhumanitiesreview.org/2001/09/01/grave-endings-the-representation-of-passing/ [accessed 22 December 2016].
16. For a recent example of the tensions between two of these positions see Historic England's decision to include Barry's grave in its listing of the nation's LGTBQ landmarks and the instant rejoinder see Mark Brown, 'Secret transgender Victorian surgeon feted by Historic England,' *Guardian* online, 25 July 2017, https://www.theguardian.com/society/2017/jul/25/secret-transgender-victorian-surgeon-feted-by-heritage-england and response by Louise Perry, 'Dr James Barry had no choice but to pretend to be a man', *Guardian* online, 25 July 2017, https://www.theguardian.com/world/2017/jul/25/dr-james-barry-had-no-choice-but-to-pretend-to-be-a-man [both accessed 26 July 2017].
17. Marjorie Garber, *Vested Interests: Cross-Dressing and Cultural Anxiety* (1992; London: Penguin, 1993), p. 166.
18. The date of death was 25 not 15 July 1865 as inscribed on the gravestone. Rose, *Perfect Gentleman*, p. 16, and Holmes, *Scanty Particulars* (1), p. 153.
19. The appellation 'Doctor James' derives from the first biofiction, 'A Mystery Still' in Charles Dickens's *All the Year Round*, vol. XVII (1866–67), 18 May 1867, pp. 492–95. This form of address has since been adapted in popular culture; see Katriona Gilmore, Gilmore & Roberts, 'Doctor James', *The Innocent Left*, released by Navigator Records, 2012, https://soundcloud.com/gilmoreroberts/doctor-james [accessed 5 November 2015].

20. Olga Racster and Jessica Grove, 'Preface' to *The Journal of Dr. James Barry* (London: Lane, 1932), n.p.; Olga Racster, *Curtain Up! The Story of Cape Theatre* (Cape Town: Juta and Co, 1951), p. 101. Barry's spectre is also summoned in George Edwin Marvell's story 'The Mystery of the Kapok Doctor', *Cape Times Christmas Annual*, December 1904, p. 13; here Barry is said to be invoked as a warning to naughty children. The story's reference to Barry's ghost also appears in Rae's *Strange Story*, p. 58.
21. Holmes, *Scanty Particulars* (1), p. 326.
22. See Terry Castle's argument, in *The Apparitional Lesbian: Female Homosexuality and Modern Culture* (New York: Columbia University Press, 1993), that the figure of the lesbian haunts Western culture.
23. Judith Halberstam, *In a Queer Time and Place: Transgender Bodies, Subcultural Lives* (New York: New York University Press, 2005), p. 78. While Halberstam's first books appeared under his original first name Judith, the author has since published under the name Jack, and subsequent discussion will therefore refer to Jack while referencing works where applicable to Judith Halberstam.
24. See Rachel Carroll's introductory chapter to *Transgender and the Literary Imagination: Changing Gender in Twentieth Century Writing* (Edinburgh: Edinburgh University Press, 2018); see also Halberstam, *Trans*, p. 8, and *In a Queer Time and Place*, p. 49; also Stephen Whittle, 'Foreword', and Susan Stryker, '(De)Subjugated Knowledges: An Introduction to Transgender Studies', in *The Transgender Studies Reader*, ed. Susan Stryker and Stephen Whittle (London: Routledge, 2006), p. xi, p. 3; Brubaker, *trans*, p. xii p. 17. See also Jacqueline Rose, 'Who do you think you are', *London Review of Books*, vol. 38: 9, 5 May 2016, http://www.lrb.co.uk/v38/n09/jacqueline-rose/who-do-you-think-you-are [accessed 16 December 2016]; and Danielle Audet, 'The "T" in LGBT: What CASAs Need to Know', http://nc.casaforchildren.org/files/public/site/conference/HO2015/E%20-%20The%20T%20in%20GLBT.pdf [accessed 18 September 2016].
25. As Stryker notes in her introduction to the *Transgender Studies Reader*, '(De)Subjugated Knowledges' (p. 4), the term 'transgender' was first used in the 1980s but its contemporary meaning can be traced to Leslie Feinberg's *Transgender Liberation: A Movement Whose Time Has Come* (New York: World View Forum, 1992); the pamphlet is reproduced in the anthology. For transgender mainstreaming see Brubaker, *trans*, p. 43. For international examples and

the legal implementation of a 'third' or ambiguous'/undisclosed sex option on documents see Brubaker, pp. 43–46.

26. See the 'Becoming Christine' exhibition at the Galway Arts Centre, Ireland, in June 2017, http://www.galwayartscentre.ie/exhibitions/123-becoming-christine; see 'Transgender woman's selfies document transition', *BBC News*, 18 June 2017, http://www.bbc.co.uk/news/av/world-europe-40290864/transgender-woman-s-selfies-document-transition [both sources accessed 18 June 2017]. See also the *Transvengers* site for young trans people, Wellcome Library, London, https://wellcomecollection.org/transvengers [accessed 8 July 2016], and the 'Transgender Hirstory in 99 Objects' exhibition organized by Chris E. Vargas's Museum of Transgender Hirstory & Art, or MOTHA, ONE National Gay & Lesbian Archives, Los Angeles, 21 March to 11 July 2015, http://www.sfmotha.org/post/113084736715/one and website, http://www.sfmotha.org/; see Sabine Heinlein, 'The transgender body in art: finding visibility "in difficult times like these"', *Guardian* online, 18 November 2016, https://www.theguardian.com/artanddesign/2016/nov/18/transgender-art-trans-hirstory-in-99-objects [both sources accessed 19 November 2016]. The 'Studying transgender and transvestism archive' opened at the Wellcome Library, London, in December 2014, http://blog.wellcomelibrary.org/2014/12/studying-transgender-and-transvestism-a-new-archive/ [accessed 15 July 2015]. For symposia see the BSA Postgraduate Forum on 'Moving Beyond the Binaries of Sex and Gender: Non-Binary Identities, Bodies and Discourses' hosted in the School of Sociology and Social Policy at the University of Leeds on 22 March 2016, http://tumblr.genderedintelligence.co.uk/post/137551961199/bsa-conference-on-non-binary-identities [accessed 16 September 2016].
27. Jane Fay, 'Anti-trans campaigners are determined to say new gender identity legislation will change everything – it won't', *Independent*, 25 July 2017, http://www.independent.co.uk/voices/gender-identity-law-legislation-trans-transgender-rights-lgbt-legal-confirmation-a7859376.html [accessed 25 July 2017]; Jon Stone, 'People to be allowed to pick their own gender without doctor's diagnosis, under Government plans', *Independent*, 23 July 2017, http://www.independent.co.uk/news/uk/politics/transgender-rules-reform-gender-dysphoria-changes-2004-gender-recognition-self-identify-a7855381.html [accessed 23 July 2017]; May Bulman, 'Mr, Ms., or Mx? HSBC bank offers trans customers gender-neutral titles',

Independent, 31 March 2017, http://www.independent.co.uk/news/uk/home-news/hsbc-bank-transgender-customers-neutral-titles-mx-ind-mre-a7659686.html [accessed 1 April 2017]; Rebecca Flood, 'Judge grants person the right to be genderless in landmark ruling', *Independent*, 26 March 2017, http://www.independent.co.uk/news/world/americas/judge-gender-genderless-legal-patch-us-landmark-ruling-a7651036.html [accessed on 26 March 2017]; 'Maria Miller and Kellie Maloney on "de-gendering" passports', *BBC News*, 14 January 2016, http://www.bbc.co.uk/news/uk-politics-35311636 [accessed 17 January 2016]. See also Avinash Chak, 'Beyond "he" and "she": The rise of non-binary pronouns', *BBC News Magazine*, 7 December 2015, http://www.bbc.co.uk/news/magazine-34901704; 'The Growing Use of Mx as a Gender-inclusive Title in the UK', http://polyinpictures.com/wp-content/uploads/mxevidencelowres.pdf; 'Transgender Americans seek birth certificate rule change', *BBC News Magazine*, 5 January 2012, http://www.bbc.co.uk/news/magazine-16420819; [last two sources accessed 7 December 2015]; Rozina Sini, '"We don't care" – the new sign for gender-neutral toilets', *BBC News*, 25 August 2016, http://www.bbc.co.uk/news/world-us-canada-37187370 [accessed 25 August 2016].

28. Gender Recognition Act 2004, http://www.legislation.gov.uk/ukpga/2004/7/contents [accessed 20 January 2016].
29. House of Commons, Woman and Equalities Committee, 'Transgender Equality: First Report of Session 2015–16', 14 January 2016, http://www.publications.parliament.uk/pa/cm201516/cmselect/cmwomeq/390/390.pdf; see also 'Transgender Equality Enquiry' and its findings of 3 November 2015, Women and Equalities Committee, http://www.parliament.uk/business/committees/committees-a-z/commons-select/women-and-equalities-committee/inquiries/parliament-2015/transgender-equality/ [both accessed 20 January 2016].
30. See Halberstam, *Trans*, p. 19.
31. See the 'Transgender' collection of the *Independent*, http://www.independent.co.uk/topic/transgender and the 2012–2015 news items available under 'Transgender: A collection of programmes and clips looking at Transgender issues', *BBC Player Radio* (2016), http://www.bbc.co.uk/programmes/p02dt14s – for a selection of subsequent news items see Deirdre Finnerty, 'The transgender Republican trying to change her party', *BBC World Service*, 28

September 2016, http://www.bbc.co.uk/news/magazine-37256151. See also Ben Kentish, 'Second World War veteran aged 90 is transitioning to a woman', *Independent*, 30 March 2017, http://www.independent.co.uk/news/uk/home-news/econd-world-war-veteran-patricia-davies-leicestershire-transition-woman-aged-90-years-old-a7658736.html and Rachel Hosie, 'Trans artist helps break down period stigma with bold post', *Independent*, 23 July 2017, http://www.independent.co.uk/life-style/transgender-cass-clemmer-periods-women-photo-poem-menstruation-gender-non-binary-a7855521.html [all sources last accessed 25 July 2017].

32. See Juliet Jacques' *Trans: A Memoir* (London: Verso, 2012), a collection of her 'Transgender Journeys' article series in the *Guardian*, 2010–12, https://www.theguardian.com/lifeandstyle/series/transgender-journey [accessed 4 August 2016]. *The Danish Girl*, dir. Tom Hooper (Working Title Films, Pretty Pictures, ReVision Pictures, 2015), was adapted from David Ebershoff's bionovel of 2000 on the early twentieth-century pioneering transgender artist Einar Wegener/Lili Elbe, *The Danish Girl* (London: Weidenfeld & Nicolson, 2000). For Lili Elbe's mediated memoirs, see Niels Hoyer (ed.), *Man into Woman: The First Sex Change. A Portrait of Lili Elbe*, trans. H.J. Stenning (1933; London: Blue Boat, 2004), discussed alongside the novel and film in Carroll, *Transgender and the Literary Imagination*, chapters 4 and 6. See also concern in the transgender community about casting decisions made for transgender films: Maisie Smith-Walters, 'Hollywood trans roles under fire – again', *BBC News Magazine*, 15 September 2016, http://www.bbc.co.uk/news/magazine-37312338 [accessed 16 September 2016].
33. See Chantal da Silva, 'Jennifer Lopez lauded for use of gender-neutral pronouns', *Independent*, 24 July 2017, http://www.independent.co.uk/arts-entertainment/music/news/jennifer-lopez-gender-neutral-pronouns-they-nibling-the-fosters-a7856941.html [accessed 25 July 2017]. For media debates in 2015 about *Glamour* Woman of the Year Caitlyn Jenner, formerly Olympian athlete Bruce Jenner, see 'GLAAD responds to Vanity Fair cover featuring Caitlyn Jenner, releases updated top sheets for journalists', GLAAD, 1 June 2015, http://www.glaad.org/blog/glaad-responds-vanity-fair-cover-featuring-caitlyn-jenner-releases-updated-tip-sheet [accessed 16 November 2015]; 'Protesters gather against Caitlyn Jenner outside Chicago House', *AXS Entertainment*, 14 November 2015, http://www.examiner.com/article/protesters-gather-against-caitlyn-jenner-outside-chicago-house

[accessed 16 November 2015]. For an in-depth discussion of transgender debates around Jenner in the context of related debates about Rachel Dolezal's transracial self-identification see Brubaker, *trans*, especially the Preface, Introduction and chapter 1; also Zeba Blay, 'What it Really Means to be Transracial and Black', *Huffington Post*, 1 February 2016, http://www.huffingtonpost.com/2015/07/08/what-it-means-to-be-transracial-and-black_n_7666088.html?utm_hp_ref=rachel-dolezal and Lucy Pasha-Robinson, 'Rachel Dolezal: White woman who identifies as black calls for "racial fluidity" to be accepted', *Independent*, 28 March 2017, http://www.independent.co.uk/news/people/rachel-dolezal-white-woman-black-racial-fluidity-accepted-transracial-naacp-a7653131.html [both journal sources accessed 29 March 2017].

34. Rachel Hosie, 'Hanne Gaby Odiele: Top intersex model on how doctors tried to change her gender as a child', *Independent*, 24 April 2017, http://www.independent.co.uk/life-style/health-and-families/hanne-gaby-odiele-intersex-model-doctors-gender-change-child-belgian-fashion-lifestyle-a7698796.html [accessed 24 April 2017]. See also Nicola Gill, 'We are Intersex', *Times Magazine Supplement*, 12 December 2015, pp. 28–36; Olivia Blair, 'Vogue model Hanne Gaby Odiele comes out as intersex', *Independent*, 24 January 2017, http://www.independent.co.uk/life-style/health-and-families/vogue-model-hanne-gaby-odiele-intersex-comes-out-gender-belgian-sex-x-y-chromosome-chanel-prada-a7542851.html [accessed 25 January 2017].
35. Shehab Khan, 'Transgender man gives birth to baby boy in Oregon', *Independent*, 31 July 2017, http://www.independent.co.uk/news/world/americas/transgender-man-birth-baby-boy-oregon-portland-leo-trystan-reese-biff-chaplow-lgbt-a7868301.html [accessed 31 July 2017]; Kashmira Gander, 'British trans man claims he is the first man to have a baby in the UK', *Independent*, 9 July 2017, http://www.independent.co.uk/life-style/health-and-families/trans-man-pregnancy-birth-labour-eggs-donor-uk-british-hayden-cross-scott-parker-gloucester-brighton-a7831571.html, and Chris Baynes, 'Britain's first pregnant man gives birth to girl', *Independent*, 8 July 2017, http://www.independent.co.uk/news/uk/home-news/britains-first-pregnant-man-gives-birth-to-girl-hayden-cross-a7830346.html [last two sources both accessed 9 July 2017]; Sarah Young, 'Transgender dad and partner announce they are

expecting first biological child', *Independent*, 1 June 2017, http://www.independent.co.uk/life-style/transgender-dad-gay-partner-first-biological-child-trystan-reese-biff-chaplow-oregon-a7767271.html [accessed 1 June 2017]; Olivia Crellin, 'The transgender family where the father gave birth', *BBC Magazine* online, 23 September 2016, http://www.bbc.co.uk/news/magazine-37408298 [accessed 24 September 2016]; 'Watching my son become my daughter', *BBC Magazine*, 1 June 2017, http://www.bbc.co.uk/news/av/magazine-40111723/watching-my-son-become-my-daughter [accessed 1 June 2017]; 'BBCtrending: Meet my transgender kid', *BBC News Magazine*, 7 March 2015, http://www.bbc.co.uk/news/magazine-31697046 [accessed 7 December 2015]; Regan Morris, 'Transgender 13-year-old Zoey having therapy', *BBC News* online, Los Angeles, 12 January 2015, http://www.bbc.co.uk/news/world-us-canada-30783983 [accessed 15 January 2016]; Victoria Derbyshire, 'The story of two transgender children', *BBC News Magazine* online, 7 April 2015, http://www.bbc.co.uk/news/magazine-32037397 [accessed 15 January 2016]; Stefanie Hirst, 'My son wants to be a girl', *BBC News*, 16 January 2016, http://www.bbc.co.uk/news/uk-35323211 [accessed 17 January 2016]; 'I'm a non-binary ten-year-old', *BBC News Magazine*, 18 September 2016, http://www.bbc.co.uk/news/magazine-37383914 [accessed 18 September 2016]; 'Modern family will feature a transgender child actor in a forthcoming episode', *BBC Newsbeat*, 27 September 2016, http://www.bbc.co.uk/newsbeat/article/37481561/modern-family-will-feature-a-transgender-child-actor-in-a-forthcoming-episode [accessed 27 September 2016]; Mario Cacciottolo and Monica Soriano, 'Transgender child: The boy putting his female puberty on hold', *BBC News* online, 1 December 2016, http://www.bbc.co.uk/news/health-38132301 [accessed 1 December 2016]; Ashraf Padanna, 'India opens first school for transgender pupils', *BBC News* online, 30 December 2016, http://www.bbc.co.uk/news/world-asia-india-38470192 [accessed 31 December 2016]; Sally Weale, 'Book explaining gender diversity to primary school children sparks furore', *Guardian* online, 2 January 2017, https://www.theguardian.com/society/2017/jan/02/book-explaining-gender-diversity-to-primary-school-children-sparks-furore [accessed 2 January 2017]; Hannah Ellis-Petersen, 'BBC film on child transgender issues worries activists',

Independent, 11 January 2017, https://www.theguardian.com/society/2017/jan/11/bbc-film-on-child-transgender-issues-worries-activists [accessed 11 January 2017]; Miles Dilworth, 'Single sex schools "failing in their legal duties to accommodate transgender pupils"', *Independent*, 9 April 2017, http://www.independent.co.uk/news/education/education-news/single-sex-schools-failing-legal-duties-accommodate-transgender-pupils-stonewall-women-equalities-a7674896.html [accessed 10 April 2017].

36. See Lucy Pasha-Robinson, 'Trans woman receives police payout after being forced to strip naked and being sprayed with mace', *Independent*, 20 June 2017, http://www.independent.co.uk/news/uk/home-news/trans-woman-police-payout-stripped-naked-mace-spray-avon-somerset-constabulary-a7799166.html [accessed on 20 June 2017]; 'Transgender pension case to be examined by EU judges', *BBC News* online, 10 August 2016, http://www.bbc.co.uk/news/uk-37033868 [accessed 10 August 2016]. See also 'US judge rules against Virginia transgender toilet ban', *BBC News*, 19 April 2016, http://www.bbc.co.uk/news/world-us-canada-36087908, and 'US Supreme Court blocks transgender ruling', *BBC News*, 4 August 2016, http://www.bbc.co.uk/news/world-us-canada-36971310 [both accessed 4 August 2016]; Charlotte England, 'US Supreme Court throws out transgender bathroom case after Donald Trump retracts anti-discrimination law', *Independent*, 7 March 2017, http://www.independent.co.uk/news/world/americas/us-supreme-court-transgender-bathroom-case-donald-trump-anti-discrimination-law-barack-obama-a7615236.html [accessed 7 March 2017]. See also 'Caitlin Jenner on Donald Trump's failure to protect trans people: "This is a disaster"', *Independent*, 24 February 2017, http://www.independent.co.uk/news/world/americas/caitlyn-jenner-donald-trump-transgender-bathroom-row-twitter-video-lgbt-rights-a7596816.html [accessed on 24 February 2017].

37. See concern about trans policies in schools, in the workplace and in prisons. For schools see: May Bulman, 'Almost half of all trans pupils have tried to take own lives, study finds', *Independent*, 28 June 2017, http://www.independent.co.uk/news/uk/home-news/trans-pupils-attempt-suicide-take-own-lives-lgbt-education-schools-study-stonewall-cambridge-a7809841.html [accessed 29 June 2017]; Rachel Pells, 'Transgender policies in schools "a waste of time and

money", claims leading academic', *Independent*, 23 June 2017, http://www.independent.co.uk/news/education/education-news/transgender-policies-school-gender-identity-neutral-toilets-waste-of-time-money-dr-joanna-williams-a7805511.html [accessed 23 June 2017]. For the workplace see: Jeremy B. White, 'Transgender "curriculum" launched to help tech firms with diversity problems', *Independent*, 2 August 2017, http://www.independent.co.uk/news/world/americas/transgender-curriculum-tech-firms-diversity-silicon-valley-diversity-problem-slack-a7874066.html [accessed 2 August 2017]; 'Changing the rules: Breaking transgender taboos at work', a news item on new developments in international business cultures, *BBC News* online, 6 May 2016, http://www.bbc.co.uk/news/business-36194759 [accessed 31 December 2016]; 'Transgender-friendly toilets planned for 2020 Olympics in Tokyo', *Guardian* online, 2 March 2017, https://www.theguardian.com/sport/2017/mar/01/tokyo-2020-olympics-transgender-friendly-toilets [accessed 2 March 2017]. For prisons see Sarah Baker, *Transgender Behind Prison Walls* (Hook, Hampshire: Waterside Press, 2017), reviewed by Mia Harris, 'An insider guide to being transgender in prison', *The Conversation*, 17 May 2017, http://theconversation.com/an-insiders-guide-to-being-transgender-in-prison-74970 [accessed 23 July 2017]; 'Transgender woman Tara Hudson moved to female prison', *BBC News* online, 30 October 2015, http://www.bbc.co.uk/news/uk-34683418; 'Tara Hudson: "I didn't choose to be this way"', *BBC News* online, 30 October 2015, http://www.bbc.co.uk/news/uk-34683418; 'Transgender Prisoner: I was absolutely terrified', *BBC News* online, 7 December 2015, http://www.bbc.co.uk/news/uk-35029928; 'Transgender prisoner Tara Hudson "feared being raped"', *BBC News* online, 7 December 2015, http://www.bbc.co.uk/news/uk-england-somerset-35030241; 'Transgender woman Vikki Thompson found dead at Armley jail', *BBC News* online, 19 November 2015, http://www.bbc.co.uk/news/uk-england-leeds-34869620; Sally Chidzoy, 'Transgender inmate found dead in Woodhill prison cell', *BBC News* online, 1 December 2015, http://www.bbc.co.uk/news/uk-england-beds-bucks-herts-3497222 [last six sources accessed 7 December 2015]; 'Transgender woman found dead in cell at HMP Doncaster', *BBC News* online, 5 January 2017, http://www.bbc.co.uk/news/uk-england-south-yorkshire-38518833 [accessed 6 January 2017].

38. See Clark Mindock, 'Second US federal court blocks Trump's transgender military ban', *Independent*, 23 December 2017, http://www.independent.co.uk/news/world/americas/us-politics/donald-trump-transgender-military-ban-latest-second-court-blocks-washington-a8126811.html; Mythili Sampathkumar, 'The seven words Trump "banned" a health agency from using were projected onto his hotel', *Independent*, 21 December 2017, http://www.independent.co.uk/news/world/americas/us-politics/donald-trump-hotel-cdc-banned-words-lgbt-fetus-science-evidence-a8121311.html; Hannah Lawrence, 'LGTB group criticizes proposals by Trump administration officials to ban the word "transgender"', *Independent*, 17 December 2017, http://www.independent.co.uk/news/world/americas/trump-centre-disease-control-and-prevention-lgbt-criticism-transgender-latest-department-of-health-a8115246.html; Lolita C. Baldor, 'Pentagon says transgender troops will be able to enlist in military next month despite Trump's opposition', *Independent*, 11 December 2017, http://www.independent.co.uk/news/world/americas/us-politics/transgender-troops-enlist-trump-ban-pentagon-go-ahead-latest-a8104481.html [all previous sources accessed 23 December 2017]; Mythili Sampathkumar, 'Transgender members of US military speak out against Trump's ban', *Independent*, 26 August 2017, http://www.independent.co.uk/news/transgender-us-military-donald-trump-ban-james-mattis-a7914746.html; Robert Burns, 'Trump officially directs Pentagon to ban transgender recruits', *Independent*, 25 August 2017, http://www.independent.co.uk/news/world/americas/us-politics/trump-transgender-ban-trans-troops-medical-treatment-latest-a7913686.html and Clark Mindock, 'Senator who lost both legs in Iraq war blasts Trump on transgender military ban', *Independent*, 24 August 2017, http://www.independent.co.uk/news/world/americas/us-politics/trump-transgender-ban-tammy-duckworth-statement-response-us-senator-criticism-a7911526.html [last three items accessed 26 August 2017]; Andrew Buncombe, 'Donald Trump's transgender ban criticised by 56 former generals and admirals', *Independent*, 1 August 2017, http://www.independent.co.uk/news/world/americas/us-politics/donald-trump-transgender-ban-us-military-56-generals-admirals-criticise-palm-center-a7871641.html [accessed 1 August 2017]; Emily Shugerman, '"This is discrimination, plain and simple": Trump's ban on transgender

military service deemed a "vile attack" on LGTBQ Americans', *Independent*, 26 July 2017, https://www.independent.co.uk/news/world/americas/us-politics/trump-transgender-ban-us-military-nancy-pelosi-lgbt-rights-americans-vile-congress-democrats-a7861611.html [accessed 26 July 2017]; Clark Mindock, 'Donald Trump bans transgender people from serving in US military due to "disruption" they would cause', *Independent*, 26 July 2017, http://www.independent.co.uk/news/world/americas/us-politics/donald-trump-bans-transgender-people-us-military-army-chelsea-manning-lgbt-rights-gay-president-a7861196.html [accessed 26 July 2017].

39. Stephen Whittle, *The Transgender Debate: The Crisis Surrounding Gender Identity* (Reading: South Street Press, 2000), p. 1; see also Whittle's 'Forward' to *The Transgender Reader*, pp. xi–xii.
40. A search for 'transgender' on Google Image and Flickr, for example, almost exclusively brings up images of transwomen [accessed March 2017].
41. Second-wave and radical feminism's difficult relationship with transgender, from Janice G. Raymond's *The Transsexual Empire: The Making of the She-Male* (1979; New York: Teacher's College Press, 1994) to ongoing debate about whether transwomen should have access to women-only spaces, has raised questions about feminist transphobia and the validity of TERF ('trans-exclusionary radical feminist') identities (Rose, 'Who do you think you are'). For a discussion of feminism's complex response to transgender see Carroll's introductory chapter to *Transgender and the Literary Imagination.* For examples of debates see criticism of Chimamanda Ngozi Adichie and the outcry over *Woman's Hour* presenter Jenni Murray and Germaine Greer's refusal to acknowledge trans-women as 'real' women: Maya Oppenheim, 'Author Chimamanda Ngozi Adichie faces backlash for suggesting transgender women are not real women', *Independent*, 12 March 2017, http://www.independent.co.uk/arts-entertainment/books/news/chimamanda-ngozi-adichie-transgender-women-channel-four-a7625481.html [accessed 12 March 2017]; Sarah Ditum, 'I'm not surprised that the BBC chastised Jenni Murray over her transgender comments – this is what institutional sexism looks like', *Independent*, 7 March 2017, http://www.independent.co.uk/voices/jenni-murray-sunday-times-transgender-india-willoughby-a7616151.html [accessed 7 March 2017]. For protest

against Cardiff University's hosting of Greer for the 2015 Haydn Ellis Lecture on 18 November 2015 see 'Germaine Greer: Transgender women are "not women"', *BBC News* online, 24 October 2015, http://www.bbc.co.uk/news/uk-34625512 [accessed 5 November 2015]; Kate Lyons, 'I think Germaine Greer is wrong on trans issues – but banning her isn't the answer', *Guardian* online, 27 October 2015, http://www.theguardian.com/commentisfree/2015/oct/27/germaine-greer-transphobia-cardiff-feminism-inclusive [accessed 5 November 2015]; Helen Lewis, 'What the row over banning Germaine Greer is really about', *New Statesman* online, 27 October 2015, http://www.newstatesman.com/politics/feminism/2015/10/what-row-over-banning-germaine-greer-really-about [accessed 5 November 2015]; Yanan Wang, 'Feminist Germaine Greer still pummelled for "misogynistic views toward transwomen"', *Washington Post* online, 3 November 2015, https://www.washingtonpost.com/news/morning-mix/wp/2015/11/03/feminist-germaine-greer-still-being-pummelled-for-misogynistic-views-toward-transwomen/ [accessed 5 November 2015]; 'Germaine Greer gives university lecture despite campaign to silence her', *Guardian* online, 18 November 2015, http://www.theguardian.com/books/2015/nov/18/transgender-activists-protest-germaine-greer-lecture-cardiff-university [accessed 19 November 2015]; Colin Riordon, 'Germaine Greer: Having her speak at Cardiff University was the right thing to do', *Times Higher Education*, 3 December 2015, https://www.timeshighereducation.com/comment/germaine-greer-having-her-speak-at-cardiff-university-was-the-right-thing-to-do [accessed 4 December 2015].

42. Brubaker, *trans*, p. 79. See also Halberstam, who in *Trans* notes that transwomen (particularly of colour) face the highest incidence of violence and social ostracism in the trans community (p. 18).
43. Katrina Roen, '"Either/Or" and "Both/Neither": Discursive Tensions in Transgender Politics', *Signs*, vol. 27: 2 (Winter 2002), pp. 501–22. Roen offers an excellent explication of the juxtaposition of contemporary passing/transsexual and crossing/transgender politics. For a discussion of conflictual positions within the transgender community, see also Rose, 'Who do you think you are?'. Jay Prosser distinguishes between transgender's positioning 'in an interstitial space between sexes' and transsexuality's 'invest[ment] in the sexed body as home'; *Second Skins: The Body Narratives of Transsexuality* (New York: Columbia University Press, 1998), p. 201.

44. Kate Bornstein, *Gender Outlaw: On Men, Women, and the Rest of Us* (New York: Random House, Vintage, 1995), p. 72. For Barry's wish to be buried in his clothes see Edward Bradford, 'The Reputed Female Army Surgeon: Letter from Deputy-Inspector Bradford', *Medical Times and Gazette*, vol. 2, 9 September 1865, p. 293, http://babel.hathitrust.org/cgi/pt?id=mdp.39015021328169;view=1up;seq=299 [accessed 2 December 2015]; also Wellcome Library, London, RAMC 373. See also my discussion of Ebenezer Rogers's use of Bradford's account in Chapter 3.
45. The Chevalier d'Éon, who identified and dressed as both 'male' and 'female', was forced, at the risk of expatriation, to commit her/himself to living in one gender only: femininity. See Garber, *Vested Interests*, pp. 259–66, and my discussion in Chapter 2.
46. Brubaker, *trans*, p. 10.
47. Bradford, 'The Reputed Female Army Surgeon', p. 293. Bornstein, *Gender Outlaw*, pp. 72–74. For the contradictions and problematic politics of Bornstein's conceptualization see Roen's '"Either/Or" and "Both/Neither"', pp. 506–509.
48. Brubaker, *trans*, pp. 10–11.
49. As Brubaker notes, 'transgender' encompasses a double position of both '*changing* gender .... and *challenging* gender' (*trans*, p. 17).
50. Halberstam, *In a Queer Time and Place*, p. 18.
51. Virginia Goldner, 'Trans: Gender in Free Fall', in 'Transgender Subjectivities: Theories and Practices', ed. Virginia Goldner, special issue of *Psychoanalytic Dialogues*, vol. 21:2 (2011), p. 165 (emphases in original).
52. See chapter 2 of Cora Kaplan's *Victoriana: Histories, Fictions, Criticism* (Edinburgh: Edinburgh University Press, 2007), pp. 37–84.
53. Hermione Lee, *Body Parts: Essays on Life-Writing* (London: Chatto & Windus, 2005), p. 100.
54. Beth Palmer and Benjamin Poore, 'Introduction: Performing the Neo-Victorian', special issue of *Neo-Victorian Studies*, vol. 9: 1 (2016), p. 4.
55. Ibid., p. 4.
56. Benjamin Poore, *Heritage, Nostalgia and Modern British Theatre: Staging the Victorians* (Basingstoke: Palgrave Macmillan, 2012), p. 97.
57. See the title of chapter 4 ('Staging Life Stories') in Poore's *Heritage, Nostalgia and Modern British Theatre*, p. 97.

58. See epigraph 3; Brubaker, *trans*, p. 73.
59. Prosser, *Second Skins*, p. 191.
60. Ibid., p. 101.
61. Ibid., p. 103.
62. Garber, *Vested Interests*, p. 71 (emphases in original).
63. Ibid., *Vested Interests*, p. 353.
64. Robert J. C. Young, *Colonial Desire: Hybridity in Theory, Culture and Race* (London: Routledge, 1995), p. 26.
65. See Rae, *Strange Story*, pp. 2–7.
66. Ibid., p. 6. Similarly, du Preez and Dronfield see the elderly Inspector General coming 'full circle, back to the origin of James Barry, having grown into the same irascible, eccentric old man his uncle had been' (*Dr James Barry*, p. 370).
67. See Stephen W. Baskerville, 'Barry, James, fourth earl of Barrymore (1667–1748)', *Oxford Dictionary of National Biography* (Oxford: Oxford University Press, 2004), online edn, http://www.oxforddnb.com/view/article/65188 [accessed 1 December 2015].
68. For myths about 'Hellgate' Barrymore having fathered Barry, see June Rose, *Perfect Gentleman*, p. 17. Ironically, Rose later herself conjectures about Barry's noble family connections (see Chapter 3). For Barrymore as a spouse see Olga Racster and Jessica Grove's unpublished play, *Dr. James Barry: A romantic play founded on South African history* (Lord Chamberlain's Office, British Library, LCP 1919/17 I No.2338) and their subsequent novel, *The Journal of Dr. James Barry* (London: Lane, 1932). In both drama and novel Barrymore is Barry's abusive husband and the cause of her flight into manhood. Speculation about Barry's aristocratic father sometimes led to confusion between 'Barrymore' and 'Buchan' (David Steuart Erskine, 11th Earl of Buchan). See Ebenezer Rogers's letter to the editor, 'A Female Member of the Army Medical Staff', *Lancet*, vol. 3792, 2 May 1896, p. 264.
69. '[O]b curam paternam', dedication to Miranda, p. 2 of Barry's M.D. dissertation, 'Disputatio Medica Inaugralis, de Merocele, vel Hernia Crurali' (June 1812), Edinburgh Research Archive, https://www.era.lib.ed.ac.uk/handle/1842/417 [accessed 8 November 2015]. The name on the title page is rendered in Latin, 'Jacobus Barry'. For Barry's signature on extant letters see Pressly, 'Portrait of a Cork Family', p. 141; du Preez, 'The early years', p. 55. See also Barry's letters in the Wellcome Library, London, held in various RAMC files, and Appendices 2 and 4 in this volume.

70. Elizabeth Longford, 'James Barry', *Eminent Victorian Women* (1981; Stroud: History Press, 2008), p. 213.
71. James Barry, 'Memorandum of the Services of Dr. James Barry Inspector General of Hospitals', stamped 30 Jan 1859, Wellcome Library, London, RAMC 373; see Appendix 4.
72. For example, Barry's year of birth is dated to 'c.1799' in Sydney Brandon's 'Barry, James' entry in the *Oxford Dictionary of National Biography* (Oxford: Oxford University Press, 2004), online edn, http://www.oxforddnb.com/view/article/1563 [accessed 1 December 2015]. Interestingly, twentieth-century transgender autobiography also at times constructs transition as an experience of rejuvenation; see Morris's *Conundrum*: 'All this helped to make me younger. It was not merely a matter of *seeming* younger; except in the matter of plain chronology, it was actually true' (p. 93, emphasis in original). This might offer a measure of insight into Barry the student's experience, once he had become confident of his act and new identity; it may also provide a context for Barry's exuberance during his early years at the Cape.
73. See Rae, *Strange Story*, p. 2. This date also appears in Reginald Hargreaves, 'Dr James Barry (1795–1865)', *Women-at-Arms: Their Famous Exploits Throughout the Ages* (London: Hutchinson, [1930]), pp. 175–90, and his later brief reference in 'Women-at-Arms', *Journal of the Royal United Service Institution*, vol. 101:601 (February 1956), p. 8. For later examples see J. L. Reyner, 'Visible Difference', *The Stage and Television Today*, vol. 5613, 10 November 1988, p. 16, and Charles G. Roland, 'Barry, James', in *Dictionary of Canadian Biography*, vol. 9 (University of Toronto / Université Laval, 2003), http://www.biographi.ca/en/bio/barry_james_9E.html [accessed 8 November 2015].
74. Given Mary Anne Bulkley's reference to her daughter Margaret's age in her letter to her brother James Barry RA of 14 January 1805 (Wellcome Library, London, RAMC 1264), Barry was almost certainly born in 1789; see also du Preez and Dronfield, *Dr. James Barry*, p. 394 n.6. For further discussion see the biographical section in the next chapter.
75. Du Preez cites 'Wednesday 29 or Thursday 30 November 1809' as the crucial date; see 'The Edinburgh years', p. 259 (emphasis added).
76. Magnus Hirschfeld's *Transvestites* (originally published in 1910) and an article (authored by G.E.C.) entitled 'An Amazing Male Impersonation: The Strange Story of Dr. James Barry, Esq. M.D.' in

the *Illustrated London News* of 16 March 1929 refer to India as a posting (p. 148); Hirschfeld, *Transvestites: The Erotic Drive to Cross-Dress*, trans. Michael A. Lombardi-Nash (New York: Prometheus, 1991), p. 411. India is also referenced in Jenni Murray's *Votes for Women! The Pioneers and Heroines of Female Suffrage* (London: Oneworld Publications, 2018), p. 28.

77. [Major-General] G[eorge] Middlemore, document entitled 'General Orders, 7 December 1836', Wellcome Library, London, RAMC 1264. See also Holmes, *Scanty Particulars* (1), p. 218. Barry was court-martialed for displaying contempt for the military establishment at St Helena. When his complaint about lack of supplies for the civil branch of the military hospital for which he was responsible was ignored, he took the case straight to the Secretary of War (letters dated 14 and 15 November 1836, Wellcome Library, London, RAMC 1264; see also CO 247/52, National Archives, Kew, London). Following his acquittal, the Commissariat was ordered to make precisely those provisions Barry had demanded; see Barry's triumphant cover note to the verdict, Wellcome Library, RAMC 1264; also CO 247/52, National Archives. For further details see Holmes, *Scanty Particulars* (1), pp. 213–21.
78. Holmes, *Scanty Particulars* (1), p. 220.
79. Garber, *Vested Interests*, p. 204 (emphasis in original).
80. Judith Butler, *Gender Trouble: Feminism and the Subversion of Identity* (London: Routledge, 1990), p. 33.
81. See discussions of Barry in Julie Wheelwright, *Amazons and Military Maids: Women Who Dressed as Men in Pursuit of Life, Liberty and Happiness* (London: Pandora, 1989), pp. 69–70; Garber, *Vested Interests,* pp. 203–205; Alison Moulds, 'Groundbreakers: James Miranda Barry', FWSA blog, 27 November 2013, http://fwsablog.org.uk/2013/11/27/james-miranda-barry/ [accessed 18 April 2015]. For transgender readings see E. E. Ottoman, 'Dr. James Barry and the specter of trans and queer history', GLBT History, 24 November 2014, https://acosmistmachine.com/2015/11/24/dr-james-barry-and-the-specter-of-trans-and-queer-history/ [accessed 12 August 2017]; Jess Rota, 'James Barry, unsung hero', *Unsung LGTB Heroes*, repr. From *We Are Family Magazine*, vol. 6 (Summer 2014), https://wearefamilymagazine.co.uk/unsung-lgbt-heroes-james-barry/ [accessed 10 August 2017]; Hamish Copley, 'Dr. James Miranda Barry', *The Drummer's Revenge: LGTB*

history and politics in Canada, posted 2 December 2007, https://thedrummersrevenge.wordpress.com/2007/12/02/dr-james-miranda-barry/ [accessed 29 October 2015]; 'Dr. James Miranda Barry (1789–1865): Transgender British Surgeon', *The Legacy Project*, http://www.legacyprojectchicago.org/James_Miranda_Barry/imag000.jpg [accessed 12 August 2017]; and Juliet Jacques's 'Five trans role models you should know about', *Guardian* online, 8 June 2012, http://www.theguardian.com/commentisfree/2012/jun/08/five-trans-role-models [accessed 3 November 2015], where Barry is discussed alongside the Chevalier d'Éon, Sylvia Rivera, Jayne Counti, Leslie Feinberg and Vladimir Luxuria. See also 'Dr James Barry', *The Secret Histories Project* blog, 12 December 2012, http://secrethistoriesproject.tumblr.com/post/37785045159/17-dr-james-barry-when-dr-james-barry-died-in [accessed 1 December 2015]; and 'James Miranda Stuart Barry (1795–1865) Military Surgeon', *A Gender Variance Who's Who*, 16 January 2008, http://zagria.blogspot.co.uk/2008/01/james-miranda-stuart-barry-1795-1865.html#.Vl5Chr_ziNN [accessed 1 December 2015].

82. See Pressly, 'Portrait of a Cork Family'; Susan Neuhaus and Sharon Masall-Dare, 'Before Federation: women in military medicine', chapter 1 of *Not for Glory: A Century of Service by Medical Women to the Australian Army and its Allies* (Salisbury, Qld: Boolarong Press, 2014), pp. 1–6.
83. See Percival R. Kirby, 'The Centenary of the Death of James Barry, M.D., Inspector-General of Hospitals (1795–1865): A Re-examination of the Facts relating to his Physical Condition', Read at the Annual General Meeting of the South African Museums Association held at King William's Town on Wednesday, 24 March 1965, *Africana Notes and News*, vol. 16: 6 (June 1965), pp. 223–227, Wellcome Library, RAMC 455; James Ross MacMahon, M.D., C.M. IV, 'Dr James Barry: A Study in Deception', *McGill Medical Journal*, vol. 37:1 (February 1968), pp. 25–32; copy held in June Rose collection of papers re James Barry, Wellcome Library, London, RAMC 1264/6; Mr. A. Dickson Wright, 'Caesarian Section', *St Mary's Hospital Gazette*, vol. 74 (January to February 1968), pp. 22–23, Wellcome Library, RAMC 748; Prof. Percival R. Kirby, [posthumous] 'Dr James Barry, Controversial South African Medical Figure: A Recent Evaluation of his Life and Sex', *South African*

Medical Journal, 25 April 1970, pp. 506–16, Wellcome Library, RAMC 658; Kathleen M. Smith, 'Dr. James Barry: Military man – or woman?', *Canadian Medical Association Journal*, vol. 126, 1 April 1982, pp. 854–57; Earl F. Nation, M.D., 'James Barry, M.D., Inspector General of Hospitals: Man or Woman?', *Urology*, vol. 31:2 (February 1988), pp. 184–88; Brian Hurwitz and Ruth Richardson, 'Inspector General James Barry MD: Putting the Woman in her Place', *British Medical Journal*, vol.298: 6669, 4 February 1989, pp. 299–305; A. K. Kubba, 'The Life, Work and Gender of Dr. James Barry MD (1795–1865)', *Proceedings of the Royal College of Physicians of Edinburgh*, vol.31 (2001), pp. 352–56; Robert Leitch, 'The Barry Room: The Tale of a Pioneering Military Surgeon', *U.S. Medicine*, July 2001, http://web.archive.org/web/20070928030206/, http://www.usmedicine.com/column.cfm?columnID=53&issueID=28 [accessed 1 December 2015]; du Preez's 2008 and 2012 articles, 'The early years' and 'The Edinburgh years'; Wilson, 'The Enigma of Dr. James Barry'.

84. James Bannerman, 'The Double Life of Dr. James Barry', *Maclean's Magazine*, 1 December 1950, pp. 49–55, Wellcome Library, London, RAMC238; Van Hunks, 'The Mysterious Doctor James Barry'; Nic Fleming, 'Revealed: Army surgeon actually a woman', *Telegraph* online, 5 March 2008, http://www.telegraph.co.uk/news/science/science-news/3334909/Revealed-Army-surgeon-actually-a-woman.html [accessed 7 December 2015]; Angela *[sic]*, 'Margaret Ann Bulkley: The extraordinary Doctor James Barry', *A Silver Voice from Ireland* blog, 17 July 2011, https://thesilvervoice.wordpress.com/2011/07/17/the-most-hardened-creaturedoctor-james-barry/ [accessed 14 August 2016]. See also the 2009 National Lottery list of 50 'unsung heroes'; Barry features in the select few showcased by Tom Geoghegan, 'Five British heroes overlooked by history', *BBC News Magazine*, 15 November 2009, http://news.bbc.co.uk/1/hi/magazine/8364465.stm [accessed 10 August 2017]. Barry is also featured on Facebook: OGM Facts, 14 March 2017, https://www.facebook.com/omgfactsofficial [accessed 21 March 2017].

85. See June Rose's radio broadcast *Quest for Dr. James Barry* (produced by Madeau Stewart), transmitted on 27 June 1973, and her related article 'James Barry, the First Woman Doctor', *Listener*, vol. 90: 2321, 20 September 1973, pp. 369–70; both at the Wellcome

Library, London, RAMC 1089. For a synopsis of the radio programme see http://genome.ch.bbc.co.uk/067c12ad2b544f0398e4ea0e806418bc [accessed 10 August 2017]. Rose was interviewed in part two (on Barry) of 'An Experiment' of the BBC's *A Skirt through History*, directed by Philippa Lowthorpe in 1994 (and featuring Anna Massey as Barry and Rosalie Crutchley as Florence Nightingale), http://explore.bfi.org.uk/4ce2b7d7be08e [accessed 28 October 2015]. *BBC News Magazine* includes 'Margaret Ann Bulkley' in a list of 'The heroes Britain accidentally forgot', last updated 17 November 2009, http://news.bbc.co.uk/1/hi/magazine/8364465.stm#margaret [accessed 8 November 2015]. For reference to a *Heritage Television* episode on Barry's Canadian posting, 'produced by then-independent superchannel CHCH in Hamilton, and hosted by Canadian historian Pierre Berton', see 'James Miranda Barry', Project Gutenberg Self-Publishing Press, http://self.gutenberg.org/articles/james_miranda_barry [accessed 1 December 2015].

86. For Sebastian Barry see Christina Hunt Mahony's collection *Out of History: Essays on the Writings of Sebastian Barry* (Dublin: Carysfort Press, 2006). For Patricia Duncker see Hammond, 'The Enigma of James Barry' [review of *James Miranda Barry*], pp. 104–6; Christian Gutleben, 'An aesthetic of performativity: Patricia Duncker's art of simulation in *James Miranda Barry*', *Études Anglaises: revue du monde Anglophone*, vol. 60:2 (2007), pp. 212–25; Jana Funke, 'Obscurity and Gender Resistance in Patricia Duncker's *James Miranda Barry*', *European Journal of English Studies*, vol. 16:3 (2012), pp. 15–25; Georges Letissier, 'Nomadic Transgender Identity: Patricia Duncker's *James Miranda Barry* and Wesley Stace's *Misfortune*', *Neo-Victorian Studies*, vol. 9: 2 (2017), pp. 15–40; Carroll, chapter 3 of *Transgender and the Literary Imagination*.
87. Jacques Derrida and Avital Ronell, 'The Law of Genre', *Critical Inquiry* ('On Narrative'), vol. 7:1 (1980), p. 59.
88. Derrida and Ronell, 'The Law of Genre', p. 57.
89. Hayden White, 'Anomalies of Genre: The Utility of Theory and History for the Study of Literary Genres', *New Literary Theory*, vol. 34:3 (Summer 2003), p. 602.
90. See Nadine Boehm-Schnitker and Susanne Gruss's introduction to their edited essay collection, 'Fashioning the Neo-Victorian – Neo-Victorian Fashions', *Neo-Victorian Literature and Culture:*

Immersions and Revisitations (London: Routledge, 2014), p. 1. See also their special issue 'Spectacles and Things: Visual and Material Culture and/in Neo-Victorianism', *Neo-Victorian Studies*, vol. 4:2 (2011), and Rachel A. Bowser and Brian Croxall's special issue on 'Steampunk, Science, and (Neo)Victorian Technologies', *Neo-Victorian Studies*, vol. 3:1 (2010). For an example of neo-Victorian exhibition aesthetics, see Sonia Solicari (ed.), *Victoriana: A Miscellany* (London: Guildhall Art Gallery, 2013).

91. Linda Hutcheon's definition of postmodern historical fiction has been widely adopted as a framework for neo-Victorian studies; see 'Historiographic Metafiction: "The Pastime of Past Time"', *A Poetics of Postmodernism: History, Theory, Fiction* (1988; London: Routledge, 1996), pp. 105–23. For a study of metafiction and post-millennial neo-Victorianism see Ann Heilmann and Mark Llewellyn, *Neo-Victorianism: The Victorians in the Twenty-First Century* (Basingstoke: Palgrave Macmillan, 2010). For further discussion of historiography see Alan Robinson's *Narrating the Past; Historiography, Memory and the Contemporary Novel* (Basingstoke: Palgrave Macmillan, 2011).
92. For nostalgia see Gutleben, *Nostalgic Postmodernism*; Simon Joyce, *The Victorians in the Rearview Mirror* (Athens: Ohio University Press, 2007). For cultural memory see Kaplan, *Victoriana*, and Kate Mitchell, *History and Cultural Memory in Neo-Victorian Fiction: Victorian Afterimages* (Basingstoke: Palgrave Macmillan, 2010). For adaptation see Sarah Cardwell, *Adaptation revisited: Television and the classic novel* (Manchester: Manchester University Press, 2002); Dianne F. Sadoff, *Victorian Vogue: British Novels on Screen* (Minneapolis: University of Minnesota Press, 2010); Linda Hutcheon, with Siobhan O'Flynn, *A Theory of Adaptation*, second edition (London: Routledge, 2013), and, most recently, Antonija Primorac, *Neo-Victorianism on Screen: Postfeminism and Contemporary Adaptations of Victorian Women* (Basingstoke: Palgrave Macmillan, 2018). For trauma see Marie-Luise Kohlke and Christian Gutleben (eds), *Neo-Victorian Tropes of Trauma: The Politics of Bearing After-Witness to Nineteenth-Century Suffering* (Amsterdam: Rodopi, 2010).
93. See Kirsten Shepherd-Barr, *Science on Stage: From Doctor Faustus to Copenhagen* (Princeton, NJ: Princeton University Press, 2006), in particular chapter 5 on 'Evolution in Performance: The Natural

Sciences on Stage', pp. 111–27; John Glendening, *Science and Religion in Neo-Victorian Novels: Eye of the Ichthyosaur* (London: Routledge, 2013); Eckart Voigts, Barbara Schaff and Monika Pietrzak-Franger (eds), *Reflecting on Darwin* (Farnham: Ashgate, 2014).

94. Rosario Arias and Patricia Pulham (eds), *Haunting and Spectrality in Neo-Victorian Fiction: Possessing the Past* (Basingstoke: Palgrave Macmillan, 2010); Helen Davies, *Gender and Ventriloquism in Victorian and Neo-Victorian Fiction: Passionate Puppets* (Basingstoke: Palgrave Macmillan, 2012).
95. Jeannette King, *The Victorian Woman Question in Contemporary Feminist Fiction* (Basingstoke: Palgrave Macmillan, 2005); Mariadele Boccardi, *The Contemporary British Historical Novel: Representation, Nation, Empire* (Basingstoke: Palgrave Macmillan, 2009); Elizabeth Ho, *Neo-Victorianism and the Memory of Empire* (London: Continuum, 2012).
96. See Antonija Primorac and Monika Pietrzak-Franger's special issue on 'Neo-Victorianism and Globalisation: Transnational Dissemination of Nineteenth-Century Cultural Texts', *Neo-Victorian Studies*, vol. 8:1 (2015). In her 'Introduction' to the inaugural issue of *Neo-Victorian Studies* (vol.1:1 [2008], p. 2) Marie-Luise Kohlke conceptualized neo-Victorianism as 'includ[ing] the whole of the nineteenth century, its cultural discourses and products, and their abiding legacies, not just within British and British colonial contexts and not necessarily coinciding with Queen Victoria's realm; that is, to interpret neo-Victorianism outside of the limiting nationalistic and temporal identifications that "Victorian", in itself or in conjunction with "neo-", conjures up for some critics.' Kohlke reaffirmed this definition in 'Mining the Neo-Victorian Vein: Prospecting for Gold, Buried Treasure and Uncertain Material', in *Neo-Victorian Literature and Culture: Immersions and Revisitations*, ed. Nadine Boehm-Schnitker and Susanne Gruss (London: Routledge, 2014), p. 21.
97. Nadine Boehm-Schnitker and Susanne Gruss, 'Introduction: Fashioning the Neo-Victorian – Neo-Victorian Fashions', *Neo-Victorian Literature and Culture: Immersions and Revisitations*, ed. Nadine Boehm-Schnitker and Susanne Gruss (London: Routledge, 2014), p. 2.
98. White, 'Anomalies of Genre', p. 602.

99. Leon Edel, 'Biography: A Manifesto', *Biography*, vol. 1:1 (Winter 1978), p. 1, p. 3.
100. White, 'Anomalies of Genre', p. 602.
101. Joanna Scott, 'On Hoaxes, Humbugs, and Fictional Portraiture', special issue on 'Biofictions', ed. Michael Lackey, *a/b: Auto/Biography Studies*, vol. 31:1 (2016), p. 30. For Scott's bionovel see *Arrogance* (New York: Linden, 1991). The essay is reproduced in Michael Lackey (ed.), *Biographical Fiction: A Reader* (New York: Bloomsbury, 2016), pp. 98–104.
102. Jay Parini, 'Writing Biographical Fiction: Some Personal Reflections', special issue on 'Biofictions', ed. Michael Lackey, *a/b: Auto/Biography Studies*, vol. 31:1 (2016), p. 26.
103. Michael Lackey argues that biofiction has superseded historical fiction; my argument is that the two forms are at their most powerful when interpellated. See Lackey, 'The Rise of the Biographical Novel and the Fall of the Historical Novel', in 'Biofictions', ed. Michael Lackey, special issue of *a/b: Auto/Biography Studies*, vol. 31:1 (2016), p. 34.
104. Kaplan, *Victoriana*, p. 65.
105. See Halberstam, *In a Queer Time and Place*, p. 2. For the 'bi-temporal' aspects of biofiction see Michael Lackey, 'Introduction: A narrative space of its own', in *Biographical Fiction: A Reader*, ed. Michael Lackey (New York: Bloomsbury, 2016), p. 10.
106. For fictional biography see Ina Schabert, 'Fictional Biography, Factual Biography, and their Contamination', *Biography*, vol. 5:1 (Winter 1982), p. 2. For Ansgar Nünning's five types of fictional biography see his 'Fictional Metabiographies and Metaautobiographies: Towards a Definition, Typology and Analysis of Self-Reflexive Hybrid Metagenres', in *Self-Reflexivity in Literature*, ed. Werner Huber, Martin Middeke and Hubert Zapf (Würzburg: Königshausen & Neumann, 2005), pp. 201–202.
107. For 'metabiographical fiction' see Eckart Voigts, 'Bio-Fiction: Neo-Victorian Revisions of Evolution and Genetics', in *Neo-Victorian Literature and Culture: Immersions and Revisitations*, ed. Nadine Boehm-Schnitker and Susanne Gruss (London: Routledge, 2014), p. 82. For 'fictional metabiography' see also Ansgar Nünning, 'An Intertextual Quest for Thomas Chatterton: the Deconstruction of the Romantic Cult of Originality and the Paradoxes of Life-Writing in Peter Ackroyd's Fictional Metabiography *Chatterton*', in *Biofictions: The Rewriting of Romantic Lives in Contemporary Fiction*

and Drama, ed. Martin Middeke and Werner Huber (London: Camden House, 1999), pp. 27–49.

108. Nünning, 'An Intertextual Quest for Thomas Chatterton', p. 29, p. 30, p. 28; Nünning, 'Fictional Metabiographies and Metaautobiographies', p. 199, p. 202, p. 209.
109. Hutcheon, 'Historiographic Metafiction', p. 106.
110. Marie-Luise Kohlke, 'Neo-Victorian Biofiction and the Special/Spectral Case of Barbara Chase-Riboud's *Hottentot Venus*', *Australasian Journal of Victorian Studies*, vol. 18:3 (2013), pp. 4–21.
111. Lucia Boldrini, '"Allowing it to speak out of him": The Heterobiographies of David Malouf, Antonio Tabucchi and Marguerite Yourcenar', in 'Autobiografictions: Comparatist Essays', ed. Lucia Boldrini and Peter Davies, special issue of *Comparative Critical Studies*, vol. 1:3 (2004), p. 252; see also Lucia Boldrini, *Autobiographies of Others: Historical Subjects and Literary Fiction* (London: Routledge, 2012). For autobiofiction see Marie-Luise Kohlke, 'Neo-Victorian Biofiction and the Special/Spectral Case of Barbara Chase-Riboud's *Hottentot Venus*', *Australasian Journal of Victorian Studies*, vol.18:3 (2013), p. 6.
112. For 'autobiografiction' see Max Saunders, *Self-Impression: Life-Writing, Autobiografiction, and the Forms of Modern Literature* (Oxford: Oxford University Press, 2010). For autobiographiction see Faysal Mikdadi's novel *Return* (n.p., Lulu.com, 2008), a fictionalized autobiography that draws on *David Copperfield* for its representation of a twentieth-century Palestinian-Lebanese family (p. 260). In email conversation (15 November 2015) the author explained: 'I did consider using the term "autobiofiction". I decided against using it partly because of the implication of the word "fiction" which would have instantly denied the biographical aspect of the novel. Although the novel is based on my own life, it is only true to the emotional reality of that life – hence its claim to being a "rewrite" of *David Copperfield* since, as a novel, it seeks to reflect the human condition through one particular life. That life obviously has events that may resemble the character David Copperfield's but it does not replicate them. It occurred to me that the coined word "phiction" in "autobiographiction" would include the autobiographic element whilst retaining the fictional element of rearranging a life in order to make sense of it – to take the reader through the protagonist's journey as his character develops into that final entity

whose life now makes some sense. "Biofiction" … is about a fiction pretending to be reality – "that plays with a real life personality". … [U]sing any other term would impede the pen on paper "that is embedded in the 'graphilic' element".'

113. Stephen Reynolds, 'Autobiografiction', *Speaker*, n.s. 16:55 (1906), p. 28, p. 30, accessed from Max Saunders's Homepage, https://blogs.kcl.ac.uk/maxsaunders/autobiografiction/autobiografiction-scan/ [accessed 27 February 2018]. For discussion of Reynolds see chapter 4 of Saunders's *Self-Impression*, pp. 165–207. For 'biografiction' as a derivative of 'autobiografiction' see pp. 216–18. For earlier uses of autobiografiction, as discussed by Saunders, see Peter J. Bailey, '"Why Not Tell the Truth?": The Autobiographies of Three Fiction Writers', *Critique*, vol. 32 (1991), p. 211; Lucia Boldrini and Peter Davies's special issue on 'Autobiografictions: Comparatist Essays', *Comparative Critical Studies*, vol. 1:3 (2004).
114. Saunders, *Self-Impression*, p. 218.
115. The series of titles have been translated into (purple prose-titled) German but no English translation as yet exists: Floortje Zwigtman, *Schijnbwegingen* [*Ich, Adrian Mayfield*] (Baarn: De Fontein, 2005), *Tegenspel* [*Adrian Mayfield: Versuch einer Liebe*] (Baarn: De Fontein, 2007), *Spigeljongen* [*Adrian Mayfield: Auf Leben und Tod*] (Baarn: De Fontein, 2011). For the earlier examples see Peter Ackroyd, *The Last Testament of Oscar Wilde* (London: Penguin, 1993) and Gyles Brandreth's six titles in the John Murray series: *Oscar Wilde and the Candlelight Murders* (2007), *Oscar Wilde and the Ring of Death* (2008), *Oscar Wilde and the Dead Man's Smile* (2009), *Oscar Wilde and the Nest of Vipers* (2010), *Oscar Wilde and the Vatican Murders* (2011), *Oscar Wilde and the Murders at Reading Gaol* (2012). As Susanne Gruss points out, the iconic nature of Wilde's queerness can have an unexpectedly heteronormative effect; the series, she argues, conspicuously circumvents the depiction of Wilde's homosexuality and instead 'uses the genre of historical crime fiction … to create a comparatively tame twenty-first century aestheticist'. See Gruss's 'Wilde Crimes: The Art of Murder and Decadent (Homo) Sexuality in Gyles Brandreth's Oscar Wilde Series', 'Neo-Victorian Masculinities', ed. Ann Heilmann and Mark Llewellyn, special issue of *Victoriographies*, vol. 5:2 (2015), p. 167.
116. See Michael Slater's biography *Dickens and Women* (London: Dent, 1983); Miriam Margolyes' and Sonia Fraser's biofictional play

Dickens's Women (1989), published by London Hesperus Press in 2011; Gaynor Arnold's bionovel on Catherine Dickens, *Girl in a Blue Dress* (Birmingham: Tindal Street Press, 2008) and Lillian Nayder's biography of *The Other Dickens: A Life of Catherine Hogarth* (Ithaca: Cornell University Press, 2011) as well as Claire Tomalin's biographies of Ellen Ternan, *The Invisible Woman* (London: Viking, 1990) and *Charles Dickens: A Life* (London: Penguin, 2012). For an exploration of Ruskin's marital fiasco see Emma Thompson (writer) and Richard Laxton's (director) *Effie Gray* (Sovereign Films, 2014).

117. Kaplan, *Victoriana*, p. 47.
118. Janet Malcolm, *The Silent Woman: Sylvia Plath and Ted Hughes* (London: Papermac, 1995), p. 9.
119. See Steven Marcus's study of Victorian pornography, *The Other Victorians: A Study of Sexuality and Pornography in Mid-Nineteenth-Century England* (London: Weidenfeld and Nicolson, 1964), which influenced John Fowles's *French Lieutenant's Woman* (London: Panther, 1969) and also later novels such as Michel Faber's *The Crimson Petal and the White* (London: Canongate, 2002). Sarah Waters's neo-Victorian trilogy of novels, in particular *Tipping the Velvet* (London: Virago, 1998) and *Fingersmith* (London: Virago, 2003), offer female and lesbian explorations of Victorian pornography. For Henry James see *The Aspern Papers*, in *The Turn of the Screw and The Aspern Papers* (Ware: Wordsworth Editions, 1993), p. 217. James's unnamed protagonist seeks to ingratiate himself with a spinster who lives in Venice with her aunt (modelled on Claire Clairmont) in order to purloin the latter's correspondence with a famous American poet (based on Shelley). The charge of 'publishing scoundrel' is issued by the aunt who, having started up from sleep, surprises her ostensible lodger in her private apartments, fingering her escritoire.
120. Kaplan, *Victoriana*, pp. 58–59; Marie-Luise Kohlke, 'Sexsation and the Neo-Victorian Novel: Orientalising the Nineteenth Century in Contemporary Fiction', in *Negotiating Sexual Idioms: Image, Text, Performance*, ed. Marie-Luise Kohlke and Luisa Orza (Amsterdam: Rodopi, 2008), p. 67. Kohlke argues that in its obsession with the sexual lives of the Victorians, 'neo-Victorianism … has become the new Orientalism, a significant mode of imagining sexuality in our hedonistic, consumerist, sex-surfeited age.'
121. Davies, *Gender and Ventriloquism in Victorian and Neo-Victorian Fiction*, p. 7.

122. Holmes, *Scanty Particulars* (1), p. 323.
123. Brubaker, *trans*, p. 92.
124. Ibid., *trans*, p. 92. The exemplar cited is Morris's *Conundrum*.
125. Lee, *Body Parts*, p. 8.
126. Kit Brennan, *Tiger's Heart* (1996; Vancouver: Scirocco Drama, revised edn 1998), Act II, Scene 26, p. 111.
127. Julia Thomas, *Nineteenth-Century Illustration and the Digital: Studies in Word and Image* (Basingstoke: Palgrave, 2017), p. 3, p. 7. See also her chapter on 'Illustration and the Victorian Novel', in *The Oxford Handbook of Victorian Literary Culture*, ed. Juliet John (Oxford: Oxford University Press, 2016), pp. 617–36.
128. Thomas, *Nineteenth-Century Illustration and the Digital*, p. 10.

Chapter 2

1. 'A Female Medical Combatant', *Medical Times and Gazette*, 26 August 1865, p. 228, http://babel.hathitrust.org/cgi/pt?id=mdp.39015021328169;view=1up;seq=299 [accessed 2 December 2015].
2. Katriona Gilmore, Gilmore & Roberts, 'Doctor James', *The Innocent Left*, released by Navigator Records, 2012, https://soundcloud.com/gilmoreroberts/doctor-james [accessed 5 November 2015]. I am grateful to Katriona Gilmore for permission to quote from the lyric here and elsewhere in this book.
3. Astrid Erll and Ann Rigney, 'Introduction: Cultural Memory and its Dynamics', in *Mediation, Remediation, and the Dynamics of Cultural Memory*, ed. Astrid Erll and Ann Rigney in collaboration with Laura Basu and Paulus Bijl (Berlin: Walter de Gruyter, 2009), p. 4.
4. Colonel N.J.C. Rutherford, 'Dr. James Barry: Inspector-General of the Army Medical Department', *Journal of the Royal Army Medical Corps*, vol. LXIII (July–Dec. 1939), p. 109. The full name is sourced from the index of Michael du Preez and Jeremy Dronfield's *Dr. James Barry: A Woman Ahead of Her Time* (London: Oneworld Publications, 2016), p. 477.
5. Judith Halberstam, *In a Queer Time and Place: Transgender Bodies, Subcultural Lives* (New York: New York University Press, 2005), p. 17, p. 55. As noted in the Notes section to the introductory chapter, I follow Halberstam's preference and most recent publishing practice by referring to Jack while referencing books to the name under which they appeared.

6. Katriona Gilmore's use of 'Doctor James' in Gilmore & Roberts' lyric is borrowed from the first biostory, 'A Mystery Still', where '*Doctor James*' is explained as the name given 'as it stood in the Army List in 1865', *All the Year Round*, XVII (1866–67), 18 May 1867, p. 493 (emphasis in original), *Dickens Journals Online*, http://www.djo.org.uk/all-the-year-round.html [accessed 7 April 2015].
7. Sebastian Barry, *Whistling Psyche*, in *Whistling Psyche. Fred and Jane* (London: Faber and Faber, 2004), p. 14.
8. Isobel Rae discovered the connection to Mary Anne Bulkley; June Rose identified Barry as one of Mary Anne's daughters. William Pressly found proof of Margaret Bulkley's identity as James Barry in the female Bulkleys' correspondence with their solicitor Daniel Reardon and reproduced handwriting samples of a letter Margaret drafted to her brother John, probably in September 1808, and a letter James Barry sent to Reardon in 1809. H.M. du Preez reproduces a full page of the 1809 letter to Reardon, with the sender identified by Reardon as 'Miss Bulkley' on the cover, a copy of which is included in the essay; he also cites a 'professional forensic document analyst' who examined Margaret Bulkley and James Barry's letters of 1808–1809 and declared them to be by the same hand. (A similar forensic examination is recorded in Florida Ann Town's *With a Silent Companion* [1999; Alberta: Red Deer Press, 2000], p. 176). That Margaret was born in 1789 can be inferred from her mother, Mary Anne's, letter of 14 January 1805 to her brother, the painter James Barry, in which she refers to 'Margaret being but 15 years old'. Critics variously refer to 'Mary Anne' or 'Mary Ann' and 'Margaret' or 'Margaret Anne' Bulkley; the signature on the 14 January 1805 letter reads 'Mary Anne Bulkley', and Margaret signed her mother's earlier (11 April 1804) letter to James Barry as 'Margaret Anne Bulkley'. For references see Isobel Rae, *The Strange Story of Dr. James Barry* (London: Longman's 1958), p. 5; June Rose, *The Perfect Gentleman* (London: Hutchinson, 1977), p. 18; Rachel Holmes, *Scanty Particulars: The Mysterious, Astonishing and Remarkable Life of Victorian Surgeon James Barry* (London: Penguin, 2002), pp. 285–93, hereafter *Scanty Particulars* (1); William Pressly, 'Portrait of a Cork Family: The Two James Barrys', *Cork Historical and Archaeological Society*, vol. 90 (1985), pp. 137–49; H.M. du Preez, 'Dr. James Barry: the early years revealed', *South African Medical Journal*, vol. 98 (2008), pp. 52–53, and 'Dr. James Barry (1789–1865): the Edinburgh years', *Journal of*

the Royal College of Physicians of Edinburgh, vol.42: 3 (2012), p. 258, pp. 261–62. For Mary Anne and Margaret's letters to James Barry see Wellcome Library, London, RAMC 1264, and Appendix 1. Holmes dates Barry's birth to 1790 (*Scanty Particulars* [1], p. 295); because of her mother's 14 January 1805 reference, Margaret's birthday would then have to have fallen in the first two weeks of January. 1789 is therefore the birth year identified in du Preez and Dronfield's biography *Dr. James Barry*, p. 393 n.5. Previous biographers cite the years 1795 (Rae, *Strange Story*, p. 2) and 1799 (Rose, *Perfect Gentleman*, p. 17), in which case Barry would have graduated (in 1812) between the ages of 13 and 17 rather than 23.

9. The Bulkleys faced financial ruin after their only son (and eldest child) John had demanded an extravagant settlement to enable his upwardly mobile marriage in 1803. Du Preez refers to Jeremiah Bulkley's subsequent internment in Dublin's Marshalsea prison ('The Edinburgh years', p. 259) and Pressly to Mary Anne 'abandon[ing] her husband' ('Portrait of a Cork Family', p. 137). In her 14 January 1805 letter to her brother, Mary Anne claims, however, that she had been 'thrown out of house & home by a Husband & Son'; Wellcome Library, RAMC 1264. For further details and transcripts of Mary Anne's letters to James Barry see Holmes, *Scanty Particulars* (1), pp. 287–91; for the 1804 letter (written in Margaret's hand) see also Appendix 1.
10. James Barry was elected to the Royal Academy in 1773 on the strength of his *Medea* (1772) and three earlier monumental paintings and in 1779 was the only member to be expelled from the Academy. See William L. Pressly, *The Life and Art of James Barry* (New Haven: Yale University Press, 1981), p. 1, p. 37, pp. 139–41. For a discussion of Barry's mental imbalance see Pressly, 'Portrait of a Cork Family', pp. 130–32. For his response to Mary Anne Bulkley and her appropriation of his estate after his death (by buying out Redmond) see Pressly (ibid., pp. 138–39), Holmes, *Scanty Particulars* (1), p. 20, p. 293, and du Preez and Dronfield, *Dr. James Barry*, pp. 35–36.
11. In 'Portrait of a Cork Family' Pressly records that Margaret Bulkley enquired for a position in a note to the solicitor Daniel Reardon on 19 May 1808 (p. 140); du Preez ('The early years', 54) gives the date of the letter as 19 May 1806. For Margaret's draft letter to her brother, responding to John's begging letter to his mother of 2

September 1808, see Pressley, 'Portrait of a Cork Family', pp. 139–40.

12. See *The Life and Adventures of Mrs. Christian Davies, commonly called Mother Ross* (London: R. Montagu, 1740), and *The Female Soldier or the Surprising Life and Adventures of Hannah Snell* (London: R. Walker, 1750), repr. in *Women Adventurers: The Lives of Madame Velazquez, Hannah Snell, Mary Anne Talbot, and Mrs. Christian Davies*, ed. Ménie Muriel Dowie (London: Fisher Unwin, 1893), pp. 55–119, pp. 197–288. See also Reginald Hargreaves, *Women-at-Arms: Their Famous Exploits Throughout the Ages* (London: Hutchinson, [1930]), pp. 33–63, pp. 89–110; Julie Wheelwright, *Amazons and Military Maids: Women Who Dressed as Men in Pursuit of Life, Liberty and Happiness* (London: Pandora, 1989), passim; Jo Stanley, *Bold in Her Breeches: Women Pirates Across the Ages* (London: Pandora, 1996), passim.
13. Moll Cut-Purse is one of the few women included in James Caulfield's *Portraits, Memoirs and Characters of Remarkable Persons from the Reign of Edward the Third to the Revolution*, 2 vols (London: James Caulfield, 1794); for the quotation see I, p. 106. Given the publication date of this book, it is possible that Margaret Bulkley came across it before making herself over into James Barry. Mary Read and Anne Bonney are prominent figures in Daniel Defoe's *A General History of the Pyrates, from their first Rise and Settlement in the Island of Providence to the present Time. With the remarkable Actions and Adventures of the two Female Pyrates Mary Read and Anne Bonny* (London: T. Warner, 1724), Project Gutenberg ebook, http://www.gutenberg.org/files/40580/40580-h/40580-h.htm [accessed 29 March 2016]. See also Hargreaves, *Women-At-Arms*, pp. 112–27, pp. 64–7.
14. In a letter dated 7 January 1810 Barry thanks General Miranda for giving him access to the 'Treasure' of his 'very extensive and elegant Library', and after Mary Anne Bulkley's departure from Edinburgh Barry spent his holidays in the Earl of Buchan's house or country estate. The 1810 letter is reproduced as a typed transcript in vol. 23 of the *Archivo del General Miranda*, ed. José Nucete Sardi, Antonio Alamo, Jacinto Fombona Pachano and Eduardo Arroyo Lamela, Academia Nacional de la Historia (CARACAS) (Caracas, 1929–50), pp. 265–67, British Library, Reference Collection 9774.h.1. See also Rae, *Strange Story*, p. 5; Holmes, *Scanty Particulars* (1), p. 28, p. 30.

15. Mary Anne Talbot, *The Life and Surprising Adventures of Mary Anne Talbot in the Name of John Taylor* (London: J.G. Barnard, 1809), repr. in Dowie, *Women Adventurers*, pp. 136–96; see also Wheelwright, *Amazons and Military Maids*, p. 97. Talbot's memoirs are also reproduced in Heike Bauer (ed.), *Women and Cross-Dressing 1800–1939*, 3 vols (London: Routledge, 2006), II, pp. 69–130.
16. Rose's *Perfect Gentleman* (p. 21) and the BBC's 'An Experiment' in the *Skirt through History* series posit that the creation of 'James Barry medical student' was entirely the brainchild of three men: Barry senior (who had died in 1806), Lord Buchan and General Miranda, the latter two close friends of the painter; it was these men who 'decided that Mary Anne Bulkley's … daughter … should have an education worthy of her'. Du Preez has suggested that after Mary Anne's letter Barry consulted his friends Dr. Fryer and Miranda, and that they jointly developed a plan of education for Margaret as early as 1805 ('The early years', 54). Given Barry's intestate state, the indignation that speaks from Mary Anne's second (14 January 1805) letter to her brother about his discourteous treatment of Margaret ('What did you give my Child when she was here last June, did you ask her to Dinner, in short did you act as an Uncle or as Christian to a poor unprotected, unprovided for Girl'), and the lack of any evidence that he discovered a sudden interest in his niece (such as letters to this effect kept by Daniel Reardon alongside Mary Anne's), his involvement in such a plan is doubtful. It is more likely that Barry's friends, engaged on editing his works posthumously, were asked for assistance by Mary Anne or Margaret herself. Du Preez and Dronfield note that Margaret was introduced to Miranda by his partner, Sarah Andrews, who had been a close friend of James Barry Senior (*Dr. James Barry*, p. 38).
17. Du Preez, 'The Edinburgh years', p. 259, p. 265 n.14; see also 'The early years', p. 55.
18. Holmes, *Scanty Particulars* (1), p. 11, p. 39; also Rae, *Strange Story*, p. 8. For the importance for Barry's later medical practice of Edinburgh's emphasis on the 'omnicompetent' physician and the 'combination of theory and practice in the medical training' he received see Howard Phillips, 'Home Taught for Abroad: The Training of the Cape Doctor, 1807–1910', in *The Cape Doctor in the Nineteenth Century: A Social History*, ed. Harriet Deacon, Howard Phillips and Elizabeth van Heyningen (Amsterdam: Rodopi, 2004), pp. 114–15.

19. Kathryn Hughes, *Victorians Undone: Tales of the Flesh in the Age of Decorum* (London: 4th Estate, 2017), p. xi; Rosemary Ashton, entry on Thomas Carlyle in *Makers of Nineteenth Century Culture 1800–1914*, ed. Justin Wintle (London: Routledge & Kegan Paul, 1982), pp. 102–4.
20. See Janet Carphin's 'Letter to the Editors' (dated 14 October 1895), 'Notes, Comments, and Answers to Correspondents' section, *Lancet*, vol. 3764, 19 October 1895 (p. 1021), where she comments on her deceased friend Dr. [John] Jobson's recollections of Barry. When taught boxing, Barry 'never would strike out, but kept his arms over his chest to protect it from blows.' While Jobson was introduced to Mrs. Bulkley as Barry's mother, elsewhere Mrs. Bulkley was referenced as his 'Aunt'; see Barry's letter to General Miranda of 7 January 1810, reproduced in vol. 23 of the *Archivo del General Miranda*, pp. 265–67, British Library, Reference Collection 9774.h.1. (See also Rae, *Strange Story*, pp. 4–5; Rose, *Perfect Gentleman*, pp. 24–25; Holmes, *Scanty Particulars* [1], pp. 28–29).
21. Carphin, letter to *Lancet*, 19 October 1895, p. 1021.
22. Holmes, *Scanty Particulars* (1), pp. 38–39.
23. The quotation is taken from the Greek dramatist Menander; Holmes, *Scanty Particulars* (1), p. 39. See title page of Barry's M.D. thesis, 'Disputatio Medica Inauguralis, de Merocele, vel Hernia Crurali' (June 1812), Edinburgh Research Archive, https://www.era.lib.ed.ac.uk/handle/1842/417 [accessed 8 November 2015]. See also du Preez and Dronfield, *Dr. James Barry*, pp. 77–78.
24. 'James Miranda Barry', Commemorative Plaques, University of Edinburgh, 16 October 2015, http://www.ed.ac.uk/about/people/plaques/barry [accessed 5 August 2016]. Another plaque honours female medical pioneer Sophia Jex Blake.
25. Holmes cites Astley Cooper's motto that a surgeon should have 'an eagle's eye, a lady's hand, and a lion's heart' as key to Barry's professional practice; Barry came to be known for his small, delicate and skillful surgeon's hands. James Hamilton, a specialist in midwifery, was in support of the medical education of women and had conducted two (unsuccessful) Caesarian sections. Dr. James Gregory and Dr. Andrew Duncan were both advanced thinkers, and Holmes suggests that Barry's later iconoclasm, love of eccentricity (also in dress style) and humanitarian spirit were influenced by these early role models. See *Scanty Particulars* (1), pp. 13–15, pp. 35–49,

p. 167. For E. Fryer see vol. 1 of *The Works of James Barry, Esq.: Historical Painter*, 2 vols (London: Cadell and Davies, 1809), which contains 'Some Account of the Life and Writings of the Author', including correspondence with William Burke and Joshua Reynolds, pp. 1–338; https://books.google.co.uk/books?id=AZIOAQAAMAAJ&dq=bibliogroup%3A%22The%20Works%20of%20James%20Barry%20...%20Historical%20Painter%22&pg=PA4#v=thumbnail&q&f=false [accessed 10 November 2015]. For the collaboration of Fryer, Buchan and Miranda see Holmes, *Scanty Particulars* (1), p. 23. For Mary Anne Bulkley's involvement in editing her brother's works see Pressly, 'Portrait of a Cork Family', p. 238. For biographical information on Miranda see Robert Harvey, *Liberators: Latin America's Struggle for Independence 1810–1830* (London: John Murray, 2000), p. 19, p. 36.

26. For Buchan's promotion of women's education see David Steuart Erskine, 11th earl of Buchan, *The anonymous and fugitive essays of the earl of Buchan, collected from various periodical works* (Edinburgh: n.p., 1812). For Fryer see Barry's 7 January 1810 letter to Miranda, in which he referred to him as 'my inestimable friend' (vol. 23 of the *Archivo del General Miranda*, p. 265; see also Rae, *Strange Story*, p. 4). Buchan approached Anderson about assisting Barry in 1810. For the influence of these men see Holmes, *Scanty Particulars* (1), pp. 22–33; for details of Buchan and Miranda see pp. 23–33. For Miranda's library see also Rae, *Strange Story*, p. 7. According to du Preez and Dronfield, only Reardon, Fryer and Miranda knew of Barry's new identity in Edinburgh (see *Dr. James Barry*, p. 52, pp. 64–65; see also du Preez's 'The early years', p. 55). Barry's postscript in his January 1810 letter to Miranda asking him and Fryer not to 'mention in any of your correspondence any thing' about 'Mrs. Bulkby's Daughter' *[sic]* certainly indicates their complicity (for the postscript to the letter see vol. 23 of the *Archivo del General Miranda*, pp. 266–67; the misspelling of 'Bulkley' must be a transcription error).

27. For this paragraph's biographical details on Miranda, and his eventual betrayal to the Spanish government by Simón Bolivar, see Harvey, *Liberators,* pp. 1–97; quotations are from p. 20, p. 23, p. 32.

28. A 'Pupil Dresser' was 'above the ordinary pupil and below the surgeon's apprentice'; a 'Hospital Assistant' was a junior medical officer

in the Army Medical Department (Rae, *Strange Story*, p. 15, pp. 18–19).

29. For Barry's treatment of Georgina Somerset's illness, see du Preez and Dronfield, *Dr. James Barry*, pp. 122–23. For his intervention in the case of Lord Charles Somerset see his letter to the Principal Medical Officer of Malta, dated 13 October 1848 (Wellcome Library, London, RAMC 1264): 'when I was young, very young, I took on myself the heavy responsibility of differing in opinion from the Inspector General and three eminent professional men, in the case of the Governor ... [T]hese gentlemen having reported ... that His Excellency had not twenty-four hours to live – at my earnest request the Colonial Secretary stopped the dispatches for forty-eight hours and I was left in sole possession of the case: the event justified this difference of opinion. – His Lordship survived many years.'
30. Holmes, *Scanty Particulars* (1), p. 162; Rose, *Perfect Gentleman*, p. 151; du Preez and Dronfield, *Dr. James Barry*, pp. 213–17. The first successful Caesarian was conducted in Zürich in 1818, but it was not until 1833 that the UK saw the section performed with success (Rae, *Strange Story*, p. 28). Barry's tutor James Hamilton had attempted the operation twice, unsuccessfully (Holmes, ibid., p. 167).
31. In a note of 3 August 1857, Barry wrote that he had been ordered to Canada to 'cool myself after such a long dependence on the tropics and hot countries'; Wellcome Library, London, RAMC 1264/3.
32. For details see the biographies by Rae, Rose, Holmes. Du Preez and Dronfield draw attention to Barry's departure from Canada having been hastened by another altercation, during which he made unfounded allegations of corruption against a fellow officer, a situation which determined the presiding military commander, Lieutenant General Sir William Eyre, to object to a continuation of his services in a letter to the Military Secretary to the Commander in Chief of the Forces: 'the uncontrollable temperament of this officer ... renders him unfit for his high position. ... [T]he utmost allowance has been made by every one for Doctor Barry's peculiar constitution & eccentricities of character but it is clear that there must be a limit to such consideration & and it is most desirable that some arrangement should be made by which this officer may retire from the active duties of his Profession, for which, from age & and natural infirmities, he is now *totally unfit*.' (Quoted in du Preez and Dronfield's *Dr. James Barry*, pp. 361–62, emphases by the authors).

33. While at the Cape, Barry objected to the unregulated sale of drugs and refused to grant an apothecary's licence to the son of a local dignitary because of his lack of a professional qualification (this is often referred to as the 'Liesching affair'). The candidate's father, president of the South African Medical Society, was an equally unqualified apothecary who, however, had practiced for many years, and his son had undergone a lengthy apprenticeship. As Harriet Deacon notes, Barry's actions led to 'tighter regulations on drug sales in the regulations of 1823'. He also exposed the horrendous conditions to which inmates of the (mostly black) leper colony and the civil and convict prisons were subjected, implying that the local authorities were not only criminally negligent in the pursuit of their duties but actively complicit with abuse. See Deacon's 'Medical Gentlemen and the Process of Professionalisation before 1860', in Deacon, Phillips and van Heyningen, *The Cape Doctor*, p. 91, p. 139; Harriet Deacon and Elizabeth van Heyningen, 'Opportunities Outside Private Practice before 1860', in ibid., p. 143; Elizabeth Longford, 'James Barry', *Eminent Victorian Women* (1981; Stroud: History Press, 2008), pp. 221–22; Holmes, *Scanty Particulars* (1), pp. 100–57; and du Preez and Dronfield, *Dr. James Barry*, pp. 165–81, pp. 188–202.
34. The first quotation is referenced to the State Archives, Cape Town, CO 180 and/or Public Records Office (National Archives), London, CO 48/97 (reference not fully identified); the second quotation is sourced to Brink, State Archives, Cape Town, CO 226, both as quoted in Rachel Holmes, *Scanty Particulars: The Scandalous Life and Astonishing Secret of Queen Victoria's Most Eminent Military Doctor* (New York: Random House, 2002), p. 108, p. 90; hereafter *Scanty Particulars* (2).
35. Holmes, *Scanty Particulars* (1), p. 174.
36. In 1825 Barry's post of Colonial Medical Inspector was abolished after his exposure of failing professional standards and institutional abuse had alienated senior officials, including Her Majesty's Fiscal, Daniel Denyssen, and the Colonial Secretary, Sir Richard Plasket. Barry was subsequently cleared of all charges by an official enquiry (Holmes, *Scanty Particulars* [1], pp. 101–57). These events were the culmination of several key interventions Barry made into the medical management of the Cape in the years 1822–1825: he reorganized the Somerset Hospital that had become inoperative; he

remained firm in his refusal to issue apothecary licences to unqualified individuals (see the 'Liesching affair' above); he implemented humanitarian and sanitary guidelines on discovering the extreme neglect and abject insanitary conditions in the newly established leper colony; he drew attention to the inhumane treatment and battery of prisoners, implicating the Fiscal, Denyssen, in colluding with prisoner abuse. While later, in St Helena, Barry would be court-martialed for breaking with protocol and writing to the Secretary of War instead of going through the formal line of command, in this case he fell victim to the Colonial Secretary's own impropriety in passing his report on conditions in the prison straight to the Fiscal. Barry was, however, not without backing: he was supported by Somerset throughout; a medical board Barry set up also found Liesching Junior ineligible for examination (though a later board established by Plasket complied with the Colonial Secretary's wishes), and the Commissioners involved in the Inquiry into Somerset's government at the Cape vindicated his conduct when he was threatened with civil imprisonment following the altercations ensuing from the row over conditions in the Tronk (town prison) and recommended that he be left in charge (Rose, *Perfect Gentleman*, p. 87; Holmes, *Scanty Particulars* [1], pp. 96–127, pp. 146–157; for the commissioners' report see pp. 155–57). Ultimately, this was a stand-off between medical professionalism and humanitarianism on the one hand and civil service autocracy on the other. Barry was not imprisoned, but he lost his civil appointment and a substantial part of his income. To add insult to injury, he was offered a junior, not the leading role on the newly implemented Supreme Medical Committee that replaced his post. For details see also Rae, *Strange Story*, pp. 34–54, Rose, *Perfect Gentleman*, pp. 54–87, and du Preez and Dronfield, *Dr. James Barry*, pp. 166–77. For another account of the various altercations see Michael Gelfand, 'The Somerset Tradition', *S. A. Medical Journal*, 26 June 1965, Wellcome Library, London, RAMC 801/6/5/1, http://wellcomelibrary.org/item/b18495370 [accessed 13 September 2016].

37. Letter to Sir James McGrigor, St Helena, 23 October 1836, Wellcome Library, London, RAMC 1264, repr. in Appendix 2.
38. See Holmes for a discussion of Barry's 'Report upon the Arctopus Echinatus or Plat Doorn of the Cape of Good Hope' (1827), *Scanty Particulars* (1), pp. 172–74.

39. Holmes refers to a 90% reduction in *Scanty Particulars* (1), p. 241.
40. Holmes, *Scanty Particulars* (1), p. 251.
41. See Longford, 'James Barry', p. 225. The first two of the three Contagious Diseases Acts (1864, 1866, 1869) that regulated the forcible examination and registration of women considered to be 'prostitutes' bookend the last year of Barry's life. In 1869 Josephine Butler established the Ladies National Association for the Repeal of the Contagious Diseases Acts. The acts were not repealed until 1886.
42. Barry was court-martialed, shortly after his arrival in St Helena in 1836, for complaining directly to the Secretary of State at the War Office about the island's Assistant Commissary for refusing to supply the civilian alongside the military hospital. Two years after his acquittal, in a scene dramatized in 'A Mystery Still' (p. 493), Barry was arrested on unspecified charges and deported from St Helena, only to be released on his arrival in Britain; Holmes refers to 'an unresolved mystery' since, once the case was referred to James McGrigor and Fitzroy Somerset, 'Barry's arrest was lifted and no charges were pressed' (*Scanty Particulars* [1], p. 225). Isobel Rae, June Rose and Holmes place Barry's arrest in the context of his protest against the allowance for civil duties having been discontinued and for medical officers, including himself, being required to make retrospective repayments (Rae, *Strange Story*, p. 84; Rose, *Perfect Gentleman*, pp. 109–10; Holmes, *Scanty Particulars* [1] pp. 221–30). Du Preez and Dronfield attribute Barry's arrest to Major General Middlemore taking exception to his 'highly insubordinate and insulting' conduct in refusing to examine an officer's health when thus instructed (because he believed he was expected to collude with the desired repatriation of this officer on the grounds of illness); *Dr. James Barry*, p. 280.
43. Edward Bradford [Deputy-Inspector-General of Hospitals], 'The Reputed Female Army Surgeon: Letter from Deputy-Inspector Bradford', *Medical Times and Gazette*, vol. 2, 9 September 1865, p. 293, http://babel.hathitrust.org/cgi/pt?id=mdp.39015021328169;view=1up;seq=299 [accessed 2 December 2015]; also Wellcome Library, London, RAMC 373.
44. Nightingale and Barry famously clashed in Scutari in 1855; see discussion below. For speculation about Nightingale interfering in the award of a knighthood see Dickson Wright, 'Caesarian Section', p. 23, and June Rose in the BBC episode 'An Experiment' of *A Skirt through History*.

45. James Barry, 'Memorandum of the Services of Dr. James Barry Inspector General of Hospitals' and 'The humble memorial of Dr. James Barry, Inspector General of Hospitals' (undated), with transcripts, Wellcome Library, London, RAMC 373, repr. in Appendices 3 and 4. Also see Holmes, *Scanty Particulars* (1), p. 253.
46. Wheelwright, *Amazons and Military Maids*, pp. 69–70. A similar point is made in Sylvie Ouellette's novel *Le Secret du docteur Barry* (2012; Paris: Terres de femmes, De Borée, 2013), p. 253.
47. Count [Emmanuel] de Las Cases, *Mémorial de Sainte Hélène: Journal of the Private Life and Conversations of the Emperor Napoleon at Saint Helena*, 4 vols (London: Henry Colburn & Co, 1823), vol. IV, part 8, p. 96. Barry is discussed in the section headed 'My Residence at the Cape', and this entry is dated January 1817.
48. Sir Henry William Dillon, *A Narrative of My Professional Adventures* (1790–1839), ed. Michael A. Lewis, 2 vols (n.p.: Navy Records Society, 1956), vol. II (1802–1839), p. 408. The reference to Barry appears in a section headed 'September 1816'. Barry was 'considered extremely clever' and, in treating Dillon, expressed his disapproval of the previous medication he had received. *Narrative* was first published in 1856; see Rose, *Perfect Gentleman*, p. 33.
49. Holmes, *Scanty Particulars* (1), p. 279.
50. George Thomas, Earl of Albemarle, *Fifty Years of My Life*, 2 vols (London: Macmillan, 1876), II, p. 100.
51. Albemarle, *Fifty Years of My Life*, II, p. 100.
52. Lord Buchan is explicitly named as progenitor – father rather than grandfather – in Ebenezer Rogers's late-Victorian account of Barry's life in his letter to the reader discussion entitled 'A Female Member of the Army Medical Staff', *Lancet*, vol. 3792, 2 May 1896, p. 264. For further rumours about Barry's high-born origins see discussion in Chapter 3.
53. Albemarle, *Fifty Years of My Life*, II, p. 101.
54. Las Cases, *Mémorial de Sainte Hélène*, vol. IV, part 8, p. 97. A supporter of Napoleon, Las Cases was held at the Cape as a political prisoner and met Barry when the latter attended his son during an illness. Given the conditions of their captivity, Las Cases had wanted Barry to encourage his son, Emanuel, to return home, but Emanuel refused to leave his father and was warmly commended for his loyalty by Barry (p. 109). As Holmes argues, Las Cases may have reminded Barry of Miranda, who had died in captivity the year

before (*Scanty Particulars* [1], pp. 68–69). Barry introduced Emanuel to Somerset's daughters (p. 109). He may have had a hand in the Las Cases being moved from their constrained conditions in prison to the luxurious environment of Somerset's country residence (du Preez and Dronfield, *Dr. James Barry*, p. 127). A more intimate acquaintance, however, was cut short by Barry accompanying Somerset on his tour of the Cape and the Las Cases departing for Britain.

55. After his death, one of Barry's colleagues recalled that he courted the reputation of 'quite a lady-killer' and at society functions would 'tack herself on to the finest and best-looking woman in the room'; Colonel Wilson, quoted in E[benezer] R[ogers], 'A Female Member of the Army Medical Staff', *Lancet*, vol. 3768, 16 November 1895, p. 1269.
56. See Rae, *Strange Story*, pp. 91–94.
57. Holmes, *Scanty Particulars* (1), pp. 128–44; for the wording of the placard see p. 130. See also du Preez and Dronfield, *Dr. James Barry*, pp. 181–87.
58. Holmes, *Scanty Particulars* (1), p. 130, p. 138. The 'placard affair' developed in the context of Dutch settler complaints about Somerset's governorship of the Cape. Somerset stood accused of corruption to fund his extravagant lifestyle and of exerting an authoritarian rule. The man at the heart of the plot, the attorney William Edwards, was already in prison, having been convicted of sending abusive letters to Somerset and his officials; he had a long-standing criminal career as an impostor. Edwards was associated with the Cape's then only independent paper, the *South African Commercial Advertiser*; Somerset shut the press down to pre-empt publication of the libel. This in turn consolidated accusations of press censorship and Somerset's dictatorial rule (Holmes, pp. 128–45).
59. Holmes, *Scanty Particulars* (1), p. 133. The petitioner, Bishop Burnett, held grievances against both the Somerset governance and against Barry, having been the target of the latter's satiric wit (p. 133).
60. [Staff Surgeon Major David Reid] McKinnon to [George Graham, the Registrar General], 24 August 1865, Wellcome Library, London, RAMC 373.
61. Rose, *Perfect Gentleman*, p. 14; Holmes, *Scanty Particulars* (1), pp. 260–69.

62. See letter by George Graham, General Registrar, of 23 August, and reply by McKinnon on 24 August 1865, Wellcome Library, London, RAMC 373.
63. *Saunders's News-Letter*, 14 August 1865, repr. in Kirby, 'The Centenary of the Death', pp. 230–31, Wellcome Library, RAMC 455; the original article was reprinted with a commentary in 'A Female Medical Combatant', *Medical Times and Gazette*, 26 August 1865, pp. 227–28, http://babel.hathitrust.org/cgi/pt?id=mdp.39015021328169;view=1up;seq=299 [accessed 2 December 2015]. For the charwoman's separate identity from Sophia Bishop see du Preez and Dronfield, Appendix B, 'Who Discovered Dr. Barry's Secret?', *Dr. James Barry*, pp. 390–91.
64. 'A Strange Story', *Manchester Guardian*, 21 August 1865; 'A Female Medical Combatant', *Medical Times and Gazette*, 26 August 1865, p. 228. This latter article was reprinted in full in *Timaru Herald*, vol. 2:80, 25 November 1865, p. 7, National Library of New Zealand, http://paperspast.natlib.govt.nz/cgi-bin/paperspast?a=d&d=THD18651125.2.19&dliv=&e=-------10--1----0-- [accessed 1 December 2015]. Holmes references a further report in *Whitehaven News*, 24 August 1865 (*Scanty Particulars* [1], p. 265). The *Medical Times and Gazette* report is reproduced, in French translation, with a lengthy commentary by René Arnold, as 'A Female Medical Combatant – Le médecin militaire femelle', alongside Edward Bradford's letter to the *Medical Times* of 6 September 1865; see extended note in the *Revue Étrangère*, vol. and date unknown, pp. 97–112, in Longmore Pamphlet Collection, vol.4 (1863–1882), Wellcome Library, London, RAMC 423/4. Another typed-up copy, with English translation, can be found in RAMC 801/6/5/1, http://wellcomelibrary.org/item/b18495370 [accessed 13 September 2016].
65. 'A Female Medical Combatant', p. 228.
66. Ibid., p. 228.
67. Holmes, *Scanty Particulars* (1), pp. 264–74. For later examples see the *Lancet* correspondence on 'A Female Member of the Army Medical Staff', *Lancet*, vol. 3764, 19 October 1895, p. 1021; vol. 3765, 26 October 1895, p. 1086; vol. 3768, 16 November 1895, p. 1269; vol. 3792, 2 May 1896, p. 264.
68. McKinnon cited by Ebenezer Rogers, 'A Female Member of the Army Medical Staff', *Lancet*, vol. 3765, 26 October 1895, p. 1086.
69. Many stories abound about multiple duels, but as Barry biographers note, only one of these was substantiated by Barry's fellow-duelist

Abraham Josias Cloete (Cleote in contemporary and earlier twentieth-century accounts). For further discussion see Chapter 3. For other references see Bradford, 'The Reputed Female Army Surgeon', p. 293.

70. Bradford, 'The Reputed Female Army Surgeon', p. 293.
71. Ibid.
72. 'Pourquoi n'aurait-il pas eu affaire à l'un de ces êtres semblables aux fabuleux fils d'Hermès et d'Aphrodite, participant des deux sexes, sans en posséder aucun?', René Arnold, 'A Female Medical Combatant – Le médecin militaire femelle', *Revue Étrangère*, vol. and date unknown, p. 112, in Longmore Pamphlet Collection, vol. 4 (1863–1882), Wellcome Library, London, RAMC 423/4 (translation mine).
73. See E. Gujon's autopsy report of Abel (Herculine) Barbin, 'Étude d'un cas d'hermaphrodisme imparfait chez l'homme', *Journal de l'anatomie et de la physiology de l'homme* (1869), pp. 609–39, repr. in *Michel Foucault présente Herculine Barbin dite Alexina B. suivi de Un scandal au couvent d'Oscar Panizza* ([Paris]: Gallimard, 2014), p. 160; English-language edition: Michel Foucault [ed.], *Herculine Barbin: Being the Recently Discovered Memoirs of a Nineteenth-Century French Hermaphrodite*, trans Richard McDougall (New York: Vintage, 2010), p. 140. Hereafter references to the two editions will appear as 'Gallimard' or 'Vintage' editions. – For intersexuality being linked to 'disorders of sex development', see Vernon A. Rosario, 'The History of Aphallia and the Intersexual Challenge to Sex/Gender', in *A Companion to Lesbian, Gay, Bisexual, Transgender, and Queer Studies*, ed. George E. Haggerty and Molly McGarry (Blackwell Publishing, 2007), p. 92, Blackwell Reference Online, http://www.blackwellreference.com/subscriber/tocnode.html?id=g9781405113298_chunk_g978140511329814 [accessed 16 December 2016].
74. Katharine Park and Robert A. Nye, 'Destiny is Anatomy – Making Sex: Body and Gender from the Greeks to Freud by Thomas Laqueur', *New Republic*, 18 February 1991, p. 56.
75. Thomas Laqueur, *Making Sex: Body and Gender from the Greeks to Freud* (Cambridge, Massachusetts: Harvard University Press, 1990), pp. 61–62.
76. Michel Foucault refers to 'simplisme réducteur' in his 'Préface: Le vrai sexe', *Michel Foucault présente Herculine Barbin dite Alexina B*

suivi de Un scandal au couvent d'Oscar Panizza (1978; [Paris]: Gallimard, 2014), pp. 11–12; for the English translation see Foucault, 'Introduction' to *Herculine Barbin: Being the Recently Discovered Memoirs of a Nineteenth-Century French Hermaphrodite*, [ed.] Michel Foucault, trans. Richard McDougall (1980; New York: Vintage, 2010), pp.viii–ix.

77. As Park and Nye point out, Aristotle embraced a two-sex model and nineteenth-century medicine maintained Galenic ideas alongside theories of hermaphroditism ('Destiny is Anatomy', p. 56).
78. Gujon's 1869 report refers to 'masculine hermaphroditism' (Vintage edition, p. 129; Gallimard edition, p. 152).
79. See also Eveline Kilian, *GeschlechtSverkehrt: Theoretische und literarische Perspektiven des gender-bending* (Königstein: Ulrike Helmer Verlag, 2004), p. 59. This logic discounts the possibility of impeded *female* development (p. 63). Vernon Rosario notes that nineteenth-century medicine generally classified as male 'individuals with testicular issue and feminine genitalia', while 'individuals with ovarian tissue, no matter how masculine their external appearance, were designated female pseudohermaphrodites'; see 'The History of Aphallia and the Intersexual Challenge to Sex/Gender', p. 95.
80. Prof. Percival R. Kirby, [posthumous] 'Dr. James Barry, Controversial South African Medical Figure: A Recent Evaluation of his Life and Sex', *South African Medical Journal*, 25 April 1970, p. 515. For Klinefelter's as an intersexual condition, see Intersex Society of North America, http://www.isna.org/faq/conditions [accessed 2 December 2015].
81. Holmes, *Scanty Particulars* (1), pp. 263–69.
82. Elizabeth Crawford, 'Women and the First World War: The Work of Women Doctors', originally published in *Ancestors* (July 2006), repr. on Crawford's website 'Woman and Her Sphere', http://womanandhersphere.com/2014/05/06/women-and-the-first-world-war-the-work-of-women-doctors/ [accessed 18 April 2015].
83. For Blackwell see Catriona Blake, *The Charge of the Parasols: Women's Entry to the Medical Profession* (London: Women's Press, 1990), p. 43. From 1860, physicians who had gained their degrees abroad could be excluded from the Register. Garrett, after four years of medical studies in St Andrews, Edinburgh and London, obtained the License of the Society of Apothecaries in 1865 and was entered on the medical register in 1866, but did not qualify as an M.D.

(Paris) until 1870 (ibid., pp. 216–17). See also Rose, *Perfect Gentleman*, p. 12.

84. Geertje Mak, *Doubting Sex: Inscriptions, bodies and selves in nineteenth-century hermaphrodite case histories* (Manchester: Manchester University Press, 2012), p. 2.
85. See Las Cases's *Mémorial de Sainte Hélène*, vol. IV, part 8 (1823) and Dillon's *Narrative of My Professional Adventures*, vol. II, p. 408, as discussed above.
86. As Mak argues (*Doubting Sex*, p. 57), sex was closely tied to location: geographical, social, economic and legal: 'Rather than rooted in an interior sense of self, sex appears to be a location: a literal location (at home or in the fields, with men or women in church), a social location (the people you work, play or sleep with), an economic location (within the context of a gendered division of labour), a sexual location (whom you desire and have sex with) and, finally, a legal position (a civil status which also defines whom you can marry).'
87. The 'Dedication' of Ebenezer Rogers's sensation novel assures readers that 'the incidents … will be recognized as *founded on facts*', the latter passage being explicitly emphasized. Other than that the character of the crabby and idiosyncratic Doctor Fitzjames is loosely based on Barry, the incidents are entirely fictive. The text is set in British Guiana (where Rogers himself had served). See Major E. Rogers, *A Modern Sphinx*, 3 vols (London: John and Robert Maxwell, 1881), British Library Historical Print editions. For examples of the incorporation of fictional sequences into biographies see Chapter 4.
88. George Edwin Marvell, 'The Mystery of the Kapok Doctor', section on 'Romances of the Cape', *Cape Times Christmas Annual*, December 1904, p. 13, National Library of South Africa, Cape Town, General Reference Collection 1876–1910.
89. Olga Racster and Jessica Grove, 'Appendix' to *The Journal of Dr. James Barry* (London: Lane, 1932), p. 180. This edition is reproduced in *Fictions and Lives* (Part 2), vol. III of Heike Bauer's anthology set *Women and Cross-Dressing 1800–1939* (London: Routledge, 2006), pp. 100–363.
90. Racster and Grove, *The Journal of Dr. James Barry*, n.p.
91. Ibid., n.p.
92. Racster and Grove, 'Preface', ibid., n.p. and 'Appendix', p. 180.
93. Racster and Grove, 'Appendix', ibid., p. 180. For 'shameful failure' see p. 13.

94. The 'Appendix' seeks to substantiate the historical facts that inspired the novel by citing and referencing a range of source materials.
95. For 'chameleon figure' see Holmes, *Scanty Particulars* (1), p. 19.
96. Olga Racster and Jessica Grove's *Dr. James Barry: Her Secret Story* (London: Gerald Howe, 1932) contains five illustrations, including of Barry (a version of the portrait reproduced in Fig. 3.5), Charles Somerset, Barry's gravestone and death certificate. Apart from some minor alteration in the dates of journal entries, the text is identical.
97. Janet Carphin, 'Letter to the Editors', *Lancet*, vol. 3764, 19 October 1895, p. 1021.
98. Holmes, *Scanty Particulars: The Mysterious, Astonishing and Remarkable Life of Victorian Surgeon James Barry* (Penguin); *Scanty Particulars: The Scandalous Life and Astonishing Secret of Queen Victoria's Most Eminent Military Doctor* (Random House).
99. Rachel Holmes (*Scanty Particulars* [1], p. 83) suggests that Barry's choice of a name for the dog served as a coded reference to a secret relationship with Somerset. For Mary Tighe's *Psyche, or, The Legend of Love*, published privately in 1805 and posthumously in 1811, see Simon Avery's entry in *The Cambridge Guide to Women's Writing in English*, ed. Lorna Sage (Cambridge: Cambridge University Press, 1999), p. 625. I am grateful to Jane Moore for drawing my attention to this connection.
100. See the second title of Racster and Grove's novel (*Dr. James Barry: Her Secret Story*) and Anne and Ivan Kronenfeld's *The Secret Life of Dr. James Barry* (2000) discussed below. A more recent example of the titular trope is Sylvie Ouelette's *Le Secret du docteur Barry* (2012), also discussed below. There are very slight differences mainly consisting of adjustments to the formatting of notes between Holmes's *Secret Life* and the earlier US edition of *Scanty Particulars.*
101. The representation of this Barry's undercover femininity may reflect a 'cover trend' of depicting women in headless positions. See Sayantani DasGupta, 'Downcast, Decapitated and Dead: Why Don't Women in Book Covers and Ads Stare Back?', *Adios Barbie: the body image site for everybody*, 22 March 2012, http://www.adiosbarbie.com/2012/05/downcast-decapitated-and-dead/ [accessed 18 April 2017]. Notably, the withheld face conceals more than one secret, most prominently that this is not 'the' James Barry who is the subject of the book. For details see my Preamble.

102. Intersexuality and transgender identity are sometimes aligned in contemporary criticism, with scholars pointing out that what Rogers Brubaker calls narratives of 'transmigration' may invoke biology to account for an inherent and essential sense of identity at odds with the sex the individual in question was assigned at birth. Gender reassignment surgery can be termed gender confirmation surgery to draw attention to the way in which surgery 'corrects' the body's deviation from self-identification. This correlates with intersexuality in that Rosario records that, irrespective of upbringing and surgical interventions early on, intersexual children as young as three can insist on an immutable sense of their gender identity. Brubaker's other two transgender positions of 'trans of between' and 'trans of beyond', however, are identities that embrace ambiguity and fluid both/neither ontologies and that are thus significantly different from intersexuality. Rogers Brubaker, ***trans**: Gender and Race in an Age of Unsettled Identities* (Princeton: Princeton University Press, 2016), p. 7, pp. 10–11; Rosario, 'The History of Aphallia and the Intersexual Challenge to Sex/Gender', pp. 103–104.
103. E. Rogers, Lieutenant-Colonel (late Staff Officer of Pensioners and formerly Captain 3rd West India Regiment), 'A Female Member of the Army Medical Staff', 'Notes, Comments, and Answers to Correspondents' section, *Lancet*, vol. 3764, 19 October 1895, p. 1021. According to British Library records, Rogers was born in 1835, so would have been 22 at the time of meeting Barry – if they did meet in the way reported. As an unsigned and undated note headed 'Unreliable', filed in papers collected in RAMC 801/5/1, Wellcome Library, London, indicates, 'Barry could not have been aboard the steamer with Rogers in 1857. … In August, 1857, Barry was at Corfu; on September 18 he, or she, arrived at Portsmouth en route to a new appointment at Montreal. It is unlikely that the journey from England to Canada would have taken in several thousand miles to the Windward Islands.' See http://wellcomelibrary.org/item/b18495370 [accessed 13 September 2016]. Du Preez and Dronfield date the encounter to 1860/61 when, after his retirement, Barry visited friends in Jamaica (*Dr. James Barry*, pp. 366–69).
104. Henry James, Preface to *The Tragic Muse*, volume 7 of the New York Edition (1908), http://www.henryjames.org.uk/prefaces/page_inframe.htm?page=text07 [accessed 5 November 2015].

105. Rogers, *A Modern Sphinx*; Major E. Rogers, *Madeline's Mystery*, edited by the author of Lady Audley's Secret (London: J. and R. Maxwell, [1882]), Harry Ransom Center, The University of Texas at Austin, WOLFF 752.
106. Lieut.-Colonel E. Rogers, *A Modern Sphinx: A novel.* Edition de luxe, with seven illustrations. In one volume (London: n.p. [1896]), British Library General Reference Collection C.194.a.672. Rogers's 'Introduction' is dated 18 November 1895 (p.xvi). In his final letter submitted to the *Lancet* (vol. 3792, p. 264) under the heading 'A Female Member of the Army Medical Staff', dated 2 May 1896, Rogers refers to the recent republication of his novel.
107. 'A Mystery Still', *All the Year Round*, vol. XVII (1866–67), 18 May 1867, pp. 492–95.
108. The flamboyancy and wit of Barry's portrait carries Dickensian echoes; other passages have a different texture. For further discussion see Chapter 3. I am grateful to Holly Furneaux for advising on Dickens's authorial/editorial role. *Dickens Journals Online* has no author attribution for this article: http://www.djo.org.uk/indexes/articles/a-mystery-still.html [accessed 31 December 2016]. Barry biographilia typically references Dickens as the editor of *All the Year Round* in which the story was published, and thus as the publisher of the text, thereby inadvertently blurring the question of authorship. An example can be found in Rachel Holmes's 'Preface': 'Charles Dickens publicized a heavily embellished version of the life of the "Inspector General" in his best-selling magazine *All the Year Round*' (*Scanty Particulars* [1]), p. 5. A later reference to the 'author of the article on Barry's life published by Dickens' disambiguates the two roles (p. 224). Similarly, du Preez and Dronfield's *Dr. James Barry* lists Dickens as the editor of the story in the bibliography but credits him with its authorship in the text: 'as Charles Dickens later related it' (p. 231).
109. Halberstam, *In a Queer Time and Place*, p. 35.
110. Silas Lesnick, 'Rachel Weisz to Headline Dr. James Barry Biopic', *Movie News*, 12 December 2016; the other producers listed are Celine Rattray and Trudy Styler, http://www.comingsoon.net/movies/news/794263-james-barry-biopic [accessed 15 December 2016]. Preparations for an earlier biopic, *Heaven and Earth*, dir. Marleen Gorris, produced by Focus Films, lead roles to be played by Natascha McElhone and Pierce Brosnan, appear to have stalled; see

Movie Insider (entry dated 5 February 2009), http://www.moviein-sider.com/m2261/barry#plot [accessed 15 December 2016].

111. O. Racster and J. Grove, *Dr. James Barry: A romantic play founded on South African history*, Lord Chamberlain's Office, British Library, LCP 1919/17 I No.2338. Sybil Thorndike played the lead role; Racster and Grove's subsequent novel is dedicated to her. For the comment about the implausible plot see the letter approving the play for licence, Lord Chamberlain's Office, 1 July 1919, British Library, LCP 1919/17 I No.2338.
112. Réné Juta, *Cape Currey* (1920; Memphis: General Books, 2010).
113. Max Saunders, *Self-Impression: Life-Writing, Autobiografiction, and the Forms of Modern Literature* (Oxford: Oxford University Press, 2010), p. 9.
114. Racster and Grove, *The Journal of Dr. James Barry*, p. 168, p. 105.
115. Journalist, novelist and playwright Olga Racster, Baroness de Wagstaffe, was Russian born and moved to South Africa after working as a journalist in London; as 'Treble Violl' she acted as drama and music critic for the *Cape Times*; see online *Encyclopaedia of South African Theatre, Film, Media and Performance* (ESAT), http://esat.sun.ac.za/index.php/Olga_Racster. Beyond her having co-authored Barry biographilia and a number of plays and novels with Racster, little is known of Jessica Grove, and even less of George Edwin Marvell. For Grove see http://esat.sun.ac.za/index.php/Jessica_Grove [both sources accessed 28 March 2016].
116. James Barry Munnik Hertzog, Prime Minister of the first Africaner government of South Africa from 1926, took his name from his godfather, who himself was the grandson of James Barry Munnik, the child Barry had delivered a century earlier, in 1826. Barry waived his fee but asked that the child be named after him, starting a tradition in the Munnik family of the first-born son being given his name. See Rae, *Strange Story*, p. 28, and Holmes, *Scanty Particulars* (1), pp. 162–70.
117. Racster and Grove, *Dr. James Barry*, Act II, p. 54. For Barry's freeing of a slave and/or an indentured black boy see Holmes, *Scanty Particulars* (1), p. 163, p. 202, and du Preez and Dronfield, *Dr. James Barry*, pp. 160–61.
118. 'The humble memorial of Dr. James Barry, Inspector General of Hospitals' is an undated draft, revised as 'Memorandum of the

Services of Dr. James Barry Inspector General of Hospitals', in which Barry outlines his career and services to the Crown in order to appeal against the retirement imposed in 1859. See Wellcome Library, London, RAMC 373, and Appendices 3 and 4. For further context see Holmes, *Scanty Particulars* (1), p. 252.

119. While other biographies trace Barry's mother, Mary Anne Bulkley, no further than 1812, du Preez and Dronfield uncovered details of her and the other Bulkleys' later lives. Having committed an unspecified crime, Jeremiah was deported to New South Wales in 1823. Mary Anne, at age seventy, was so destitute that she faced admittance to the workhouse in Cork in 1835. Her kinship with James Barry the painter appears to have saved her; she subsequently moved in with her son John and continued to live with his wife, Elizabeth, after John's death. Du Preez and Dronfield suggest that Barry would have become aware of his mother's plight (reported in the *Times* and elsewhere) and that his absence from service in this particular year may suggest that he came to her rescue: 'No trace survives of James having been in touch [with his mother] since he joined the Army in 1813, nor any record of them establishing contact now. All that is known for certain is that at this point, in the middle of 1835, for the only time in his long career … Dr. James Barry vanishes from the record. He continued to be in the Army and on full pay; but other than a note that he was "At Home" for a year and two months – without apparent duties and not sick – he goes missing, during a change in postings that should not have involved his visiting England at all. … If she [Margaret] helped her mother, it would have been in strict secrecy … After a year in mysterious obscurity, on 19 April 1836 Dr. Barry emerged again into the light, when he and his manservant John took ship at last for their long-delayed voyage to St Helena. What happened to Mrs. Bulkley is not clear, but she eventually found her way back to England and joined her son John's family.' (*Dr. James Barry*, pp. 255–57, p. 350).

120. Du Preez and Dronfield, Appendix B, 'Who Discovered Dr. Barry's Secret?', *Dr. James Barry*, pp. 390–91. In her altercation with McKinnon, the layer-out claimed to have discovered stretch marks, which she said she had identified because, as 'a married woman and the mother of nine children', she 'ought to know' (McKinnon's letter to the Registrar General, 24 August 1865, Wellcome Library, London, RAMC 373). Sophia Bishop, then around 30, was unmar-

ried 'with no sign of children'; see England censuses of 1851, 1861, 1871 and 1881 as noted in *Dr. James Barry*, p. 291, p. 449 n.7 and 8.

121. Intersex is generally defined as an atypical sexual anatomy that may involve a discrepancy between external and internal organs. See Intersex Society of America, 'What is intersex?', http://www.isna.org/faq/what_is_intersex [accessed 29 October 2015].
122. Holmes, *Scanty Particulars* (1), p. 300. For historical diagnoses of intersex discovered as the result of hernia treatment, see Alice Domurat Dreger, *Hermaphrodites and the Medical Invention of Sex* (Cambridge: Harvard University Press, 1998), p. 50, p. 94.
123. Marjorie Garber, *Vested Interests: Cross-Dressing and Cultural Anxiety* (1992; London: Penguin, 1993), p. 69.
124. Hamish Copley, 'Dr. James Miranda Barry', *The Drummer's Revenge: LGTB history and politics in Canada*, posted 2 December 2007, https://thedrummersrevenge.wordpress.com/2007/12/02/dr-james-miranda-barry/ [accessed 29 October 2015].
125. Du Preez and Dronfield, *Dr. James Barry*, p. 63; see also their stereotypical depiction of Barry's 'mothering urge' towards children and specifically 'little girls', p. 367.
126. Ibid., p. 62, p. 153.
127. Ibid., p. 63.
128. Ibid., p. 79.
129. Ibid., p. 422, n.10. Du Preez and Dronfield's conceptualization of transvestism pays scant attention to the fact that, historically, at a time of women's educational, professional, social and political disenfranchisement, ambition and the material benefits of masculinity would have been substantial contributory factors in underpinning a 'male' sense of identity.
130. Ibid., p. 351.
131. Jean Binnie's *Colours: Jean Barry Esq* was premiered by the Abbey Theatre, Dublin on 3 October 1988 and saw twenty-two performances in that month. (The subtitle is reproduced as on the Abbey Theatre website, but this is likely to be an error as Barry's first name on the cast list is given as Jane, and that is also the name used in the script held in the Bristol Theatre Collection). See the listing of Binnie's play on http://www.doollee.com/PlaywrightsB/binnie-jean.html [accessed 5 August 2017]. The play was directed by Jude Kelly, with Veronica Quilligan as Jane and Kevin Flood as James Barry. The extensive cast list can be downloaded from the Abbey

Theatre Archive, https://www.abbeytheatre.ie/archives/production_detail/702/ [accessed 5 August 2017]. For the Leeds Playhouse production of *Colours*, premiered on 13 October 1988 and directed by John Harrison, with Hetta Charnley as Barry, see Robin Thornber, 'Double firsts', *Guardian*, 30 September 1989, p. 31, and J.R.L. Reyner, 'Visible Difference', *The Stage and Television Today*, vol. 5613, 10 November 1988, p. 16. For play scripts see *Colours* (1988), British Library, London, MPS3993, and *Colours: James Barry – Her Story* (1989), Bristol Theatre Collection, Bristol, WTC/PS/000047. I am grateful to Angela V. John for drawing my attention to this play, to Bronwen Blatchford for alerting me to the play text being held at Bristol Theatre Collection, and to Jill Sullivan for granting me access at short notice at a time the collection was closed for refurbishment. Binnie later wrote a radio play, 'Dr. Barry', broadcast by the BBC in the *Who Sings the Hero?* series on 19 August 1992; for details see 'BBC Afternoon Plays, 1984–2002', http://www.suttonelms.org.uk/lost10.html [accessed 29 November 2015]. Binnie refers to being commissioned to write a play in 'First among women', [letter to] *British Medical Journal*, vol. 304, 25 January 1992, p. 257.

132. 'I so want teenage girls to see this and say "This is our story" as well as having a very, very good time'; Thornber, 'Double firsts', p. 31. The men's ages are discussed in the play: Erskine is 60 and Miranda 51; Arthur Wellesley, though younger, is still some twenty years (the under-aged) Jane's senior.
133. The later Duke of Wellington was an Irish compatriot. In 'The humble memorial of Dr. James Barry, Inspector General of Hospitals' (undated, 1859) Barry recorded that he was formally thanked by Wellington 'for his services during the cholera at Malta'; Wellcome Library, London, RAC 373; see Appendix 3.
134. Binnie, *Colours*, Act I:7, p. 30; Act I:8, p. 36; Act II:1, p. 49 (Bristol Theatre Collection).
135. Frederic Mohr, *Barry: Personal Statements, Five Solo Plays* (Edinburgh: [David McKail], [1994]), pp. 43–76; see also 1984 play script, National Library of Scotland, Edinburgh, Traverse Theatre Inventory, Acc. 9285/8 and Scottish Theatre Archive, Glasgow, STA Mn 63/7. The original handwritten manuscript and (slightly longer) typescript are also held at the Scottish Theatre Archive, STA Mn 57/2.

136. The play was first performed in the US, in 1983, under the direction of Allan Harari, by Aspect Theatre, Paramus, New Jersey, with Jane Sharp in the title role. Its first British premiere was in 1984, at the Traverse Theatre Club, Edinburgh, with Gerda Stevenson as Barry and Stephen Unwin as director. This was followed, also in 1984, by a second British production at the Traverse Festival Fringe, and accompanied by two radio broadcasts, in 1983. More recently, Mohr's play was adapted for a 25th anniversary production in the US in 2008 by Rowan Tree Theatre, Glasgow, with Isabella Jarrett in the lead role and under the direction of John Carnegie; in personal email correspondence (14 May 2015) McKail dissociated himself from this version. For the production history see 'Frederic Mohr's Radio Plays', http://www.suttonelms.org.uk/david-mckail.html; see also 'BBC Afternoon Plays, 1984–2002', http://www.suttonelms.org.uk/lost10.html [both accessed 29 November 2015]. Also Mohr, *Barry: Personal Statements, Five Solo Plays*, p. 44. For the 2008 production see 'Barry', https://www.list.co.uk/article/6107-barry/ [accessed 17 April 2015] and 'Recent Reviews', Rowan Tree Theatre Company, http://www.rowantreetheatrecompany.co.uk/article_57.shtml [accessed 17 April 2015]. For the Traverse Theatre script and cuts to the original see National Library of Scotland, Edinburgh, Traverse Theatre Inventory, Acc. 9285/8. TV dramatization: in 1985 David McKail started to adapt the play for television, framing Barry's memories of his life with an opening that begins with his last day and death, contextualizing the charwoman's anger at being denied the (rather trivial) household objects he promised her. After his death a gold-coroneted carriage with liveried footmen collects Barry's possessions (p. 7). The text dramatizes the layer-out's discovery and its communication to the landlady and the authorities (McKinnon and MacGregor). Barry has left a lengthy autobiographical manuscript, which MacGregor begins to read. This then blends into Barry's flashback on his life. The text breaks off with Barry's recognition of his loneliness during his student days in Edinburgh. The manuscript of the TV script is held in the Scottish Theatre Archive, Glasgow, STA Mn 57/1.

137. In an undated, handwritten manuscript filed with correspondence on and reviews of the 1984 production, David McKail states that Barry is 'about discrimination' and 'also to some extent a comment on the feminist movement' in that it reflects, through the figure of

Barry, contemporary pressure on women to deploy 'masculine techniques' in male-dominated careers; as such the play articulates anxieties about whether, in order to succeed, 'women must become more like men'. National Library of Scotland, Edinburgh, Traverse Theatre Inventory Acc. 9285/8.

138. Mohr, *Barry*, 1984 play script, p. 37; *Five Solo Plays*, p. 76.
139. Mohr, *Barry*, 1984 play script p. 37; *Five Solo Plays*, p. 76.
140. See Claire Gleitman, '"In the dank margins of things": *Whistling Psyche* and the Illness of Empire', in *Out of History: Essays on the Writings of Sebastian Barry*, ed. Christina Hunt Mahony (Dublin: Carysfort Press, 2004), p. 209.
141. Sebastian Barry, *Whistling Psyche*, p. 48. Premiered in May 2004 at the Almeida Theatre, London, the play was directed by Robert Delamere and starred Kathryn Hunter as Barry and Claire Bloom as Nightingale; see *Whistling Psyche*, p. 1, and Andrea Lopaz's review on *Curtain Up*, http://www.curtainup.com/whistlingpsyche.html [accessed 28 October 2015]. For the February 2014 staging of the play, at the Alliance Theatre Black Box in Atlanta, directed by Rebecca Frank, with Kathleen McManus as Barry and Joanna Daniel as Nightingale, see 'Whistling Psyche by Sebastian Barry', Indiegogo, https://www.indiegogo.com/projects/whistling-psyche-by-sebastian-barry#/ [accessed 29 October 2015].
142. Sebastian Barry, *Whistling Psyche*, p. 51.
143. Kit Brennan, *Tiger's Heart* (1996; Vancouver: Scirocco Drama, revised edn 1998), back cover. The notes on the 'Production History' (n.p.) cite three Canadian performances: in 1995 by the Great Canadian Theatre Company, Ottowa, directed by Colin Tylor; in 1996 as part of the *1996 Women in View Festival* at the Frederick Wood Theatre, University of British Columbia, directed by Jan Selman; and in 1998 at the Ship's Company theatre, in Parrsboro, Nova Scotia, directed by R. H. Thomas. For details of the cast see also 'Casting Requirements' (n.p.), which indicates that the play is conceived for a cast of between five to twelve actors.
144. Dantzen/Danzer was in Barry's employ from 1818; in 1827 Barry applied for a permit for him for Mauritius. Holmes speculates that this may have been the black man photographed with the elderly Barry in Kingston (Fig. 2.4; see *Scanty Particulars* [1], p. 82, p. 178). In pictorial and other representations Dantzen's ethnicity is usually referenced as Malay; du Preez and Dronfield note his

Khoikhoi or San origins and cite the Cape Town Register of Shipping as evidence of 'Danzer' leaving Barry's employ on their return from Mauritius in 1829. Drawing on the fictionalized account in 'A Mystery Still', they speculate that Barry replaced Danzer with a black soldier named 'John' in Jamaica (*Dr. James Barry*, p. 229, p. 433 n.1; p. 252, 435 n.18).

145. Roy Foster, '"Something of us will remain": Sebastian Barry and Irish History', in *Out of History: Essays on the Writings of Sebastian Barry*, ed. Christina Hunt Mahony (Dublin: Carysfort Press, 2004), p. 184.
146. The quotation is from Brennan, *Tiger's Heart*, Act I, Scene 10, p. 51; see also Sebastian Barry, *Whistling Psyche*, p. 11.
147. Brennan, 'Casting Requirements', ibid., n.p.
148. Brennan, 'Pronunciations' and 'Casting Requirements', ibid., n.p.
149. Brennan, ibid., Act I, Scene 16, p. 79.
150. Patricia Duncker, 'James Miranda Barry 1795–1865' (1989), *Monsieur Shoushana's Lemon Trees* (London: Serpent's Tail, 1997), pp. 37–42. Patricia Duncker, *James Miranda Barry* (London: Serpent's Tail, 1999).
151. Duncker, *James Miranda Barry*, p. 35.
152. Virginia Goldner, 'Transgender Subjectivities: Introduction to Papers by Goldner, Suchet, Saketopoulou, Hansbury, Salamon & Corbett, and Harris', editorial to 'Transgender Subjectivities: Theories and Practices', ed. Virginia Goldner, special issue of *Psychoanalytic Dialogues*, vol. 21: 2 (2011), p. 153.
153. Anne and Ivan Kronenfeld, *The Secret Life of Dr. James Miranda Barry* (2000; Cambridge, MD: Write Words, ebooksonthenet, 2004), p. 233.
154. For a biographical framework, earlier scholarship either appears to have been overlooked or remains unreferenced. The text comes to very similar conclusions to June Rose's 1977 biography but presents them as original new insights, and draws on biographical detail provided at length in Pressly's 'Portrait of a Cork Family', but neither source is acknowledged; see my discussion of biographiction in Chapter 4. For novelistic shortfalls see reader comments about the 'dull[ness]' of the narration and excessive use of 'dry' biographical detail: Judy Crowder, 'Children's Literature', http://www.barnesandnoble.com/w/with-a-silent-companion-florida-ann-town/1012357837;jsessionid=1AAF56167B5FF793823F2D525B477240.

prodny_store02-atgap09?ean=9780889952119; Anon., 14 March 2004, http://www.amazon.com/With-Silent-Companion-Florida-Town/dp/B004GM5UEO; Jen, 20 March 2012, http://www.amazon.com/With-Silent-Companion-Florida-Town/dp/B004GM5UEO [all sources accessed 1 December 2015].

155. Florida Ann Town, *With a Silent Companion*, Northern Lights Young Novels series (1999; Alberta: Red Deer Press, 2000), p. 74.
156. Ibid., p. 118.
157. See the following passage in free indirect speech in which Margaret goes to considerable lengths to imagine their future marriage yet startlingly omits any kind of acknowledgement of the sexual relationship that this would presumably entail: 'Before Lord Charles had remarried, she had even allowed herself to consider the possibility of becoming the second Lady Somerset. The idea was not beyond the realm of possibility. They were good friends. They enjoyed each other's company. She got along well with Somerset's children. With Somerset as a husband she would have a highly ranked protector and a comfortable life. There would have been a flurry of gossip when she announced her sex, but that would die down eventually.' (Ibid., p. 118).
158. 'Était-ce donc cette dualité qui l'excitait tant? Était-ce la perspective de s'unir à un être qui, aux yeux du monde, semblait homme?' Sylvie Ouellette, *Le Secret du docteur Barry* (2012; Paris: Terres de femmes, De Borée, 2013), p. 127 (translation mine).
159. See Eve Kosofsky Sedgwick, 'Gender Asymmetry and Erotic Triangles', chapter 1 of *Between Men: English Literature and Male Homosocial Desire* (New York: Columbia University Press, 1985), pp. 21–27.
160. 'Her role clung to her skin', Ouellette, *Le Secret*, p. 309. Judith Butler, *Gender Trouble: Feminism and the Subversion of Identity* (London: Routledge, 1990), p. 33; see the opening discussion in the Introduction.
161. Andrew Pulver, 'Rachel Weisz to play real-life gender-fluid Victorian doctor', *Guardian,* 13 December 2016, https://www.theguardian.com/film/2016/dec/13/rachel-weisz-stars-james-barry-film-gender-fluid-victorian-doctor; Silas Lesnick, 'Rachel Weisz to Headline Dr. James Barry Biopic', *Movie News,* 12 December 2016; the other producers listed are Celine Rattray and Trudy Styler, http://www.comingsoon.net/movies/news/794263-james-barry-biopic; see also

'Rachel Weisz to star in Dr. James Barry biopic', *Female First*, 13 December 2016, http://www.femalefirst.co.uk/movies/movie-news/rachel-weisz-star-james-barry-biopic-1019991.html [all sources accessed 15 December 2016]. Rachel Weisz was originally listed as one of the support actors for the Barry feature film *Heaven and Earth*, see below.

162. *Heaven and Earth*, dir. Marleen Gorris, produced by Focus Films, lead roles to be played by Natascha McElhone and Pierce Brosnan; see *Movie Insider* (entry dated 5 February 2009), http://www.movieinsider.com/m2261/barry#plot [accessed 15 December 2016]. Rachel Weisz is here referenced as a former cast member. On the IMDb database two titles are listed, *Heaven and Earth* and *Barry*; http://www.imdb.com/title/tt0377458/ [accessed 17 April 2015]; the former is the English translation of the 'Hemel en Aarde' leper colony at the Cape whose mismanagement Barry exposed (Brennan, 'Pronunciations', *Tiger's Heart*, n.p.). For McElhone and the film's prospective plot see Vanessa Thorpe, 'Tragic star to play a legend of medicine', *Observer*, 21 September 2008, http://www.theguardian.com/film/2008/sep/21/medicine.mcelhone [accessed 17 April 2015]. See also 'Natascha to star as cross dressing doc', *Mirror*, 22 September 2008, updated 3 February 2012, http://www.mirror.co.uk/news/uk-news/natascha-to-star-as-cross-dressing-doc-340064 [accessed 28 October 2015]. A blog discussion on Barry for 'A Gender Variance Who's Who' suggests that funding for the film may have fallen through; see blog by Zagria, 18 October 2009, http://zagria.blogspot.co.uk/2008/01/james-miranda-stuart-barry-1795-1865.html#.Vl3EPL_ziNM [accessed 1 December 2015].
163. Du Preez and Dronfield, *Dr. James Barry*, p. 154.
164. Katriona Gilmore, Gilmore & Roberts, 'Doctor James', *The Innocent Left*, released by Navigator Records, 2012.
165. Garber, *Vested Interests*, p. 100.
166. *Saunders's News-Letter*, 14 August 1865, repr. in 'A Female Medical Combatant', *Medical Times and Gazette*, 26 August 1865, p. 227; also repr. in Percival R. Kirby, 'The Centenary of the Death of James Barry, M.D., Inspector-General of Hospitals (1795–1865)', *Africana Notes and News*, vol. 16:6 (June 1965), pp. 230–31, Wellcome Library, London, RAMC 455. The second quotation is attributed to General Chamberlayne in E[benezer] R[ogers], 'A

Female Member of the Army Medical Staff', *Lancet*, vol. 3768, 16 November 1895, p. 1269.

167. Jack Halberstam, *Trans: A Quick and Quirky Account of Gender Variability* (Oakland, CA: University of California Press, 2018), p. 3, pp. 5–6.
168. Halberstam raises probing questions about the practical complications of a 'genderless' identity given that 'there are few ways to interact with other human beings without being identified with some kind of gendered embodiment.' Ibid., p. 9.
169. The unspecified 'proofs' accepted by Rae (*Strange Story*, vi) for Bishop's claim consisted presumably in her reference to having found stretch marks, identified as such on the grounds of her experience as a mother of nine. (See McKinnon's letter to the Registrar General, 24 August 1865, Wellcome Library, London, RAMC 373; also quoted in Rose, *Perfect Gentleman*, p. 3). Holmes, however, queries how a body ravaged by 'two decades of tropical fever' might have yielded up this information, given that the charwoman further qualified her claim by referring to Barry having had a child 'when very young' (*Scanty Particulars* [1], p. 270).
170. Longford, 'James Barry', p. 213.
171. Garber, *Vested Interests*, p. 11. David J. Getsy, 'Capacity', special issue on 'Posttranssexual: Key Concepts for a Twenty-First Century Transgender Studies', *TSQ: Transgender Studies Quarterly*, vol. 1:1–2 (2014), p.47; see discussion in the introductory chapter of Rachel Caroll, *Transgender and the Literary Imagination: Changing Gender in Twentieth Century Writing* (Edinburgh: Edinburgh University Press, 2018).
172. Judith Halberstam, *Female Masculinity* (Durham: Duke University Press, 1998), p. 57.
173. Butler, *Gender Trouble*, p. 6 (emphases in original).
174. See her discussion of the early nineteenth-century French intersexual Finon D.: 'Despite her being dressed as a woman, her appearance was quite masculine. He shaved his beard every week, rode horseback, smoked, cursed, and got drunk. When he was too drunk … he sometimes assaulted women … She was also said to have played "the other part" in relations with the soldiers of a neighbouring garrison. She was an object of curiosity and was known in the area as the "bearded woman". Finon led an absolutely ambiguous life …'. Mak, *Doubting Sex*, p. 15, pp. 20–21.

175. As Halberstam notes, the very proliferation of terms and identity categories carries an uncomfortable reminder of the nineteenth-century drive for classification; see *Trans*, pp. 6–7). For varieties of transgender expression see Brubaker, *trans*, p. 98 and Jacqueline Rose, 'Who do you think you are', *London Review of Books*, vol. 38: 9, 5 May 2016, http://www.lrb.co.uk/v38/n09/jacqueline-rose/who-do-you-think-you-are [accessed 16 December 2016]. See also Katy Steinmetz, 'A Comprehensive Guide to Facebook's New Options for Gender Identity: An expert walks through what they mean, from transgender to pangender', *Time*, 14 February 2014, http://techland.time.com/2014/02/14/a-comprehensive-guide-to-facebooks-new-options-for-gender-identity/ [accessed 23 December 2017]. For further recommendations see Halberstam's discussion of 'they' in *Trans*, pp. 11–12. See also 'The Need for a Gender-Neutral Pronoun', *Gender Neutral Pronoun Blog*, https://genderneutralpronoun.wordpress.com/; also 'Language and Pronouns', *Gendered Intelligence*, http://genderedintelligence.co.uk/projects/kip/transidentities/language [both sources accessed 25 March 2017]. See further the University of Wisconsin-Milwaukee's LGTB Resource Center recommendation, as quoted in Avinash Chak, 'Beyond "he" and "she": The rise of non-binary pronouns', 'Magazine' section, *BBC News*, 7 December 2015, http://www.bbc.co.uk/news/magazine-34901704 [accessed 7 December 2015].
176. Emma Ramadan, 'Translator's Note' to Anne Garréta, *Sphinx*, trans. Emma Ramadan (Dallas, Texas: Deep Vellum Publishing, 2015), n.p. [p. 122]. Garrétta was invited to join Oulipo in 2000. Members of the French experimental Workshop for Potential Literature (Ouvroir de littérature potentielle) subject their work to deliberate constraints (such as the bypassing of gender in Garrétta's case or the omission of a letter, as in George Perec's *La Disparition*, a novel written without recourse to the letter e); see Ramadan's note for the language-specific decisions involved in the French original and those of the English translation.
177. See Jack Halberstam's blog 'On Pronouns', 3 September 2012, http://www.jackhalberstam.com/ [accessed 16 November 2015]. See also GLAAD's information sheet on 'What name and pronoun do I use', http://www.glaad.org/transgender/transfaq [accessed 15 November 2015].
178. Brubaker, *trans*, p. 10, p. 98.

179. See in the Introduction's opening epigraph section the extract from McKinnon's letter to the Registrar General, 24 August 1865. The longer letter establishes that McKinnon had known 'that gentleman for a good many years' and 'never had any suspicion that Dr. Barry was a female', a point that is reaffirmed at the end: there had been no need to examine the body 'as I could positively swear to the identity of the body as being that of a person whom I had been acquainted with as Inspector General of Hospitals for a period of eight or nine years.' Wellcome Library, London, RAMC 373. Except for the opening, the letter refers to Barry in gender-neutral terms.
180. *Saunders's News-Letter*, 14 August 1865, repr. in 'A Female Medical Combatant', *Medical Times and Gazette*, 26 August 1865, p. 227, and in Kirby, 'The Centenary of the Death of James Barry', p. 230.
181. General Chamberlayne, quoted in Rogers, 'A Female Member of the Army Medical Staff', *Lancet*, vol. 3768, 16 November 1895, p. 1269. The correspondence started with an enquiry to the editor on 12 October 1895 (vol. 3763, p. 959) and continued on 19 October (vol. 3764, p. 1021), 26 October (vol. 3765, p. 1086–7), 16 November 1895 (vol. 3768, p. 1269), through to 2 May 1896 (vol. 3792, p. 264).
182. Dr. G.W. Campbell, future dean of the McGill Medical School, quoted in James Ross MacMahon, 'Dr. James Barry: A Study in Deception', *McGill Medical Journal*, vol. 37:1 (February 1968), p. 31, Wellcome Library, London, RAMC 1264/6.
183. For Henderson see du Preez and Dronfield, *Dr. James Barry*, p. 342. For the letter see James Barry to Dr. Henderson, 5 October 1855, 'James Miranda Steuart Barry and the Crimean War', Archives@ University of Edinburgh, uploaded 6 June 2016, http://library-blogs.is.ed.ac.uk/edinburghuniversityarchives/2016/06/16/james-miranda-steuart-barry-and-the-crimean-war/ [accessed 5 August 2016]. The longer opening passage reads: 'I am (privately) starting for Sebastopol on Monday & please God shall return as soon as I shall have lionised or rather vagabondised & if you have any fancy to do the same on my return – well & Good…' (scans 3a and 3b).
184. Holmes, *Scanty Particulars* (1), pp. 240–1.
185. Photocopy of two pages of undated letter (August 1865?) headed '[but?] to Mama by Parthe's desire' and filed with a newspaper clip and transcript by John Guest, 'Sharp Encounter', *Sunday Times*, 9 November 1952, Wellcome Library, London, 'Letters by

Nightingale, 1864–1865', Ms. 9001/145. Guest writes that Sir Harry Verney, Nightingale's great-nephew, had 'recently c[o]me across' the letter, which is here dated to 'very shortly after Barry's death' (the date of which is recorded in handwriting other than Nightingale's at the top of the first extant page). The recipient is identified as 'Parthe', 'Nightingale's sister Parthenope, Lady Verney'. The first or earlier pages of the letter are not filed. The account of Nightingale's encounter with Barry is extracted in Lynn McDonald (ed.), *Florence Nightingale on Women, Medicine, Midwifery and Prostitution* (Waterloo, Ont.: Wilfrid Laurier University Press, 2005), p. 19. See also Holmes, *Scanty Particulars* (1), p. 271 and Rose, *Perfect Gentleman*, p. 141; also Brian Hurwitz and Ruth Richardson, 'Inspector General James Barry MD: Putting the Woman in her Place', *British Medical Journal*, vol.298: 6669, 4 February 1989, p. 305, n.49. In these references there is some variation in the text quoted that further confounds Nightingale's use of pronouns in the manuscript source. Nightingale's use of round parentheses and shifting use of pronouns is recorded correctly in McDonald.

186. See Sam Ward's equally remarkable act of transgendering George Sand in an 1840s letter to Longfellow: 'As for George Sand, nothing will be easier than for you to know him, should your travels lead you her way. I will furnish you with a warm letter to Janin who will have great pleasure in making you known to him, and I candidly think her worth seeking. Besides his genius for writing she has an impulse toward perfectibilitification [*sic*], and is intimate with that fiery apostle Lammenais who sympathises in his efforts to elevate people and recognizes in her a kindred spirit. Should it be your fortune to fall in with him do not fall in love with her. He will enchant you more in an evening, if the fit of Psychic inspiration be upon her, than any being you ever knew, & is a kind of moral hermaphrodite.' Quoted in Gary Williams, 'Speaking with the Voices of Others', introduction to Julia Ward Howe, *The Hermaphrodite*, ed. Gary Williams (Lincoln: University of Nebraska Press, 2004), pp.xvii–xviii.

187. For Barry's resentment of Nightingale see Rose, *Perfect Gentleman*, p. 141.

188. In a subsequent sentence Barry corrected his statement, clarifying that, 'there being no vacancy at the time for an officer of his rank he … endeavoured to … make himself as useful as possible … by obtaining permission for 500 sick & wounded men being sent to Corfu'; see 'The humble memorial of Dr. James Barry, Inspector General of

Hospitals', undated draft [1859], RAMC 373, Wellcome Library; Appendix 3. For other references see Holmes, *Scanty Particulars* (1), pp. 240–41.

189. The image reproduced here is of the first, hardcover edition. The (2017) paperback edition of the biography presents readers with a feminized portrait.
190. Du Preez and Dronfield, 'Authors' Note', *Dr. James Barry*, n.p.
191. Ibid., 389. Appendix A ('James Barry and the Physical Examination') notes that '[f]rom the eighteenth century through to the mid-Victorian period, men entering the British Army at the commissioned officer level were regarded as gentlemen, and taken at their word. … No man entering the Army at this level was required to prove his physical fitness by stripping for a medical examination.' A mandatory system of physical examination for all entrants was only introduced after 1870 (p. 388).
192. Ibid., p. 92.
193. Holmes, *Scanty Particulars* (1), n.p. For the quotation see also the slide on Leslie Feinberg, p. 27 in Danielle Audet, 'The "T" in LGBT: What CASAs Need to Know', http://nc.casaforchildren.org/files/public/site/conference/HO2015/E%20-%20The%20T%20in%20GLBT.pdf [accessed 18 September 2016].
194. Holmes, *Scanty Particulars* (1), p. 2. Crucially, while they also bypass Barry's gender, the Random House and Tempus editions omit the opening discussion and start with a passage that reverts to the convention: 'Dr. James Miranda Barry … lies dying'; *Scanty Particulars* (2), p.ix, and Rae, *Secret Life*, p. 7. For further discussion see Chapter 4.
195. Brennan, 'Notes on Staging', *Tiger's Heart*, n.p.
196. The doubling of characters is subject to casting decisions. Brennan outlines the 'Casting Requirements' for a cast of five; with a larger cast characters are each represented by one actor. See also 'Notes on a Larger Cast' and 'Production History', *Tiger's Heart*, n.p.
197. Mohr, *Barry*, *Five Solo Plays*, p. 45, p. 46.
198. 'It is …statements made by two persons who turn out to be the same person. One is in white and one is in black and it was hoped that the audience might not immediately recognise that to begin with and indeed the performers I have discussed it with said that did happen – there were sudden gasps when the more trusting … made the connection'; personal communication by David McKail, in an email to the author of 23 May 2015.

199. Racster and Grove, *Dr. James Barry*, Act I, p. 28, p. 33.
200. Marie-Luise Kohlke, 'Neo-Victorian Biofiction and the Special/Spectral Case of Barbara Chase-Riboud's *Hottentot Venus*', *Australasian Journal of Victorian Studies*, vol. 18:3 (2013), p. 6. Patricia Duncker, 'On Writing Neo-Victorian Fiction', *English*, vol. 63:243 (2014), p. 272.
201. Ouellette, *Le Secret du docteur Barry*, p. 392.
202. Elizabeth Freeman, 'Queer Belongings: Kinship Theory and Queer Theory', chapter 15 of *A Companion to Lesbian, Gay, Bisexual, Transgender and Queer Studies*, ed. Molly McGarry and George E. Haggarty (Maiden, MA: Blackwell, 2007), Blackwell Reference Online, http://www.blackwellreference.com/subscriber/tocnode.html?id=g9781405113298_chunk_g978140511329816 [accessed 16 December 2016].
203. Duncker, *James Miranda Barry*, p. 94.
204. Ibid., p. 113; Kilian, *GeschlechtSverkehrt*, p. 148.
205. Duncker, *James Miranda Barry*, p. 227.
206. Garber, *Vested Interests*, p. 122.
207. Ibid., p. 122.
208. Racster and Grove, *Journal*, p. 16.
209. 'A Mystery Still', p. 494. The scene is recreated in G.E.C., 'An Amazing Male Impersonation: The Strange Story of James Barry, Esq., M.D.', *Illustrated London News*, 16 March 1929, p. 148. Réné Juta's Barry, in *Cape Currey*, too has recourse to six towels (p. 91).

Chapter 3

1. *Saunders's News-Letter*, 14 August 1865, reproduced in 'A Female Medical Combatant', *Medical Times and Gazette*, 26 August 1865, p. 228, http://babel.hathitrust.org/cgi/pt?id=mdp.39015021328169;view=1up;seq=299 [accessed 2 December 2015]; also repr. in Percival R. Kirby, 'The Centenary of the Death of James Barry, M.D., Inspector-General of Hospitals (1795–1865)', *Africana Notes and News*, vol. 16:6 (June 1965), pp. 230–31.
2. Marie-Luise Kohlke, 'Neo-Victorian Biofiction and the Special/Spectral Case of Barbara Chase-Riboud's *Hottentot Venus*', *Australasian Journal of Victorian Studies*, vol.18:3 (2013), p. 13.
3. Hermione Lee, *Body Parts: Essays on Life-Writing* (London: Pimlico, 2008), p. 6, p. 8.

4. Judith Halberstam, *In a Queer Time and Place: Transgender Bodies, Subcultural Lives* (New York: New York University Press, 2005), p. 45. As previously noted, Halberstam is referred to as Jack in accordance with the author's preferred form of address; publications are referenced to the respective name in question.
5. Kathryn Hughes, *Victorians Undone: Tales of the Flesh in the Age of Decorum* (London: Fourth Estate, 2017), p. xv, p. xiv. This reader felt physically gripped throughout, but was distinctly troubled by increasing bodily (and mental) discomfort at the gratuitiousness of the carnage of a child's body parts in the last chapter (whether the particular corporeal response – a big filling coming loose, possibly from the unconscious grinding of teeth – is coincidental remains uncertain). If anything, this final chapter appears to indicate that the 'material turn' in life-writing embraces sensation – and sensationalism (even to the 'Fuck All' of the concluding words [p. xiv, p. 365]) – irrespective of whether transgender forms part of the textual and material body or not.
6. Kohlke, 'Neo-Victorian Biofiction', p. 4.
7. Ibid., p. 7.
8. Ibid., p. 8.
9. Ibid., pp. 9–10.
10. Ibid., p. 11. See Helen Davies's excellent book on *Gender and Ventriloquism in Victorian and Neo-Victorian Fiction: Passionate Puppets* (Basingstoke: Palgrave, 2012).
11. 'A Mystery Still', *All the Year Round*, XVII (1866–67), 18 May 1867, pp. 492–95.
12. General W. Chamberlayne, quoted in E[benezer] Rogers, 'A Female Member of the Army Medical Staff', *Lancet*, vol. 3768, 16 November 1895, p. 1269; E[benezer] Rogers, 'Introduction' to *A Modern Sphinx*, De luxe edition with seven illustrations (London: Maxwell, [1896]), p. v.
13. Max Saunders, *Self-Impression: Life-Writing, Autobiografiction & the Forms of Modern Literature* (Oxford: Oxford University Press, 2010), pp. 216–18.
14. For the cartoon's attribution to Lear (as having been sketched during his visit to Corfu in 1852) see Holmes, *Scanty Particulars: The Mysterious, Astonishing and Remarkable Life of Victorian Surgeon James Barry* (London: Penguin, 2002), p. 5, p. 238; hereafter *Scanty Particulars* (1). Holmes's US edition, which includes notes, does

not give a reference for Lear; see *Scanty Particulars: The Scandalous Life and Astonishing Secret of Queen Victoria's Most Eminent Military Doctor* (New York, Random House, 2002), p. 227; hereafter *Scanty Particulars* (2). According to Lear specialist Marco Graziosi it is unlikely that it was Lear who undertook the sketch: 'the picture does not really look like one of Lear's drawings, and the handwriting is also different, ... more formal than Lear usually wrote. Moreover, I think Lear did not visit Corfu in 1852: he was there in 1848, before moving on to Greece, and then again in 1855, when it became his base for some years. 1849–1853 he was in England, as far as I know. Finally, there is no indication in any of Lear's biographies that he met James Barry, neither does he mention him in any of the published letters; however, if Barry was in Corfu 1851–1857 ... they almost certainly met' (personal email correspondence, 27 August 2017). Barry did not leave Corfu until July 1857 (Holmes, *Scanty Particulars* [1], p. 247), but there is no convincing evidence that the cartoon was indeed Lear's work. See also Marco Graziosi's Lear website, 'A Blog of Bosh: Edward Lear and Nonsense Literature', https://nonsenselit.wordpress.com/ [accessed 26 August 2017].

15. 'A Mystery Still', pp. 492–93.
16. Ibid., p. 492.
17. The cartoon also serves as a satirical comment on a considerably more martial intervention on the part of the historical Barry than might be expected: in 1853, enraged by seeing a regiment being drilled in the searing sun, Barry protested vehemently on medical grounds, 'vigorously flourishing his horse hair whip' and accidentally (or perhaps not so accidentally) striking the commander, Lieutenant Colonel William Denny, in the face. Rachel Holmes, *Scanty Particulars: The Mysterious, Astonishing and Remarkable Life of Victorian Surgeon James Barry* (London: Penguin, 2002), pp. 238–39; hereafter *Scanty Particulars* (1); Michael du Preez and Jeremy Dronfield, *Dr. James Barry: A Woman Ahead of Her Time* (London: Oneworld Publications, 2016), p. 222, pp. 331–32.
18. Marjorie Garber, *Vested Interests: Cross-Dressing and Cultural Anxiety* (1992; London: Penguin, 1993), p. 55 (emphasis in original).
19. 'A Mystery Still' was published on 18 May 1867; for John Stuart Mill's speech before the House of Commons on 20 May 1867 see Hansard, *British Parliamentary Debates*, 187: 817–29, repr. as item

135 in the section 'Women and the Vote' in *Women, the Family, and Freedom: The Debate in Documents*, ed. Susan Groag Bell and Karen M. Offen, 2 vols (Stanford: Stanford University Press, 1983), I, pp. 482–88.

20. Mill, speech to the House of Commons, 20 May 1867, in Groag Bell and Offen, *Women, the Family, and Freedom*, p. 485.
21. Ibid., p. 487.
22. 'A Mystery Still', p. 493.
23. Ibid., p. 492.
24. Ibid., p. 493.
25. See G.E.C., 'An Amazing Male Impersonation: The Strange Story of James Barry, Esq., M.D.', *Illustrated London News*, 16 March 1929, p. 148. The piece is heavily reliant on 'A Mystery Still'.
26. 'A Mystery Still', p. 492.
27. Ibid., p. 492; O. Racster and J. Grove, *Dr. James Barry: A romantic play founded on South African history*, Lord Chamberlain's Office, British Library, LCP 1919/17 I No.2338, Act I, p. 28; Reginald Hargreaves, 'Dr. James Barry', *Women-at-Arms: Their Famous Exploits Throughout the Ages* (London: Hutchinson & Co, [1930]), p. 178; June Rose, *The Perfect Gentleman: The remarkable life of Dr. James Miranda Barry, the woman who served as an officer in the British Army from 1813 to 1859* (London: Hutchinson, 1977), p. 105. Florida Ann Town's *With a Silent Companion* (1999; Alberta: Red Deer Press, 2000) offers an extended adaptation (p. 158).
28. Edward Bradford referred to 'persons of high rank' who, having adopted Barry after the death of his parents, 'appeared to maintain an endearing interest in him to such an extent that, in his manifold military irregularities, the influence of members of that family was known to support and protect him.' See 'The Reputed Female Army Surgeon', *Medical Times and Gazette*, 9 September 1865, p. 293, http://babel.hathitrust.org/cgi/pt?id=mdp.39015021328169;view=1up;seq=299 [accessed 2 December 2015], also Wellcome Library, London, RAMC 373.
29. 'A Mystery Still', pp. 493–94. Having arrived at the Cape with a recommendation 'from a well-known eccentric Scottish nobleman' (i.e. the Earl of Buchan), Barry 'had a fair allowance from some source or other', p. 492.
30. See Racster and Grove's *Dr. James Barry*, Act I, p. 21: 'He is always forgiven and promoted, where others are turned down'. In Jean

Binnie's *Colours: James Barry – Her Story*, Barry is vindicated at his court-martial at the intervention of her former lover, the Duke of Wellington; play text, Act II, p. 83, Bristol Theatre Collection, WTC.PS/000047.

31. Holmes, *Scanty Particulars* (1), p. 225.
32. Havelock Ellis, *Eonism and Other Supplementary Studies*, vol. VII of *Studies in the Psychologies of Sex* (Philadelphia: F.A. Davies, 1928), p. 6; also in (extract of) 'Eonism' [from 1928 edition of *Studies in the Psychology of Sex*, vol. VII] in *Women and Cross-Dressing 1800–1939*, ed. Heike Bauer, 3 vols (London: Routledge, 2006), I, p. 159. George Thomas, Earl of Albemarle, *Fifty Years of My Life*, 2 vols (London: Macmillan, 1876), II, p. 100, and discussion in Chapter 2. For Barry's (as Dr. Fitzjames's) self-identified 'Scotch extraction' and high-born origins as the niece of a lord see Major E[benezer] Rogers, *A Modern Sphinx: A Novel*, British Library Historical Collection, 3 vols (London: John and Robert Maxwell, 1881), III, p. 289. The earlier quotation from Mark Twain is from the 'Conclusion' to *Following the Equator: A Journey Around the World* (1897), Project Gutenberg, Ebook ♯2895, http://www.gutenberg.org/files/2895/2895-h/2895-h.htm [accessed 8 April 2015].
33. George Edwin Marvell, 'The Mystery of the Kapok Doctor', *Cape Times Christmas Annual*, December 1904, pp. 13–17; this is followed, on p. 17, by a reproduction of Lord Albemarle's recollections of Barry in *Fifty Years of My Life* (II, pp. 100–101) and, on pp. 18–19, by a reprint of 'A Mystery Still'. For a synopsis of Marvell's story see G.E.C.'s 'An Amazing Male Impersonation', *Illustrated London News*, 16 March 1929, p. 148; see also James Bannerman, 'The Double Life of Dr. James Barry', *Macleans Magazine*, 1 December 1950, p. 50, Wellcome Library, London, RAMC 238.
34. 'Why has my life always been such a mystery', complains Lady Barrymore; 'Why was I taken from my mother, and never allowed to see her again? … What is it, who is it that has such power over me?' Lord Charles is not at liberty to tell, but intimates that his father, the Duke of Beaufort, 'has for many years been his Majesty's confidential friend' and that her father 'is a man of high rank', thus implying a royal connection. Racster and Grove, 'Prologue' of *Dr. James Barry*, pp. 7–8. See also Racster and Grove's novel, *The Journal of*

Dr. James Barry (London: Lane, 1932), p. 80; here, however, the royal link is less pronounced.

35. Colonel N.J.C. Rutherford, 'Dr James Barry: Inspector-General of the Army Medical Department', *Journal of the Royal Army Medical Corps*, vol. LXIII (July-Dec. 1939), p. 344; see also p. 119.
36. Rose, *Perfect Gentleman*, p. 31.
37. Mohr, *Barry: Personal Statements, Five Solo Plays* (Edinburgh: [David McKail], [1994]), p. 57.
38. Binnie, *Colours: James Barry – Her Story*. The play script held by Bristol Theatre Collection is dated 1989; another play text, held in the British Library (*Colours*), is dated 1988.
39. Barry was twenty when he took up his studies; according to the charwoman, the marks on the body indicated that the birth had happened at a young age; [Staff-Surgeon] McKinnon to [George Graham, the Registrar General], 24 August 1865, Wellcome Library, London, RAMC 373.
40. Du Preez and Dronfield, *Dr. James Barry*, p. 7 and p. 194 n.15. In her 11 April 1804 letter to her brother Mary Anne Bulkley refers to 'two Daughters'; June Rose Collection, RAMC 1264, Wellcome Library, London; see Appendix 1. For Juliana Bulkley, du Preez and Dronfield cite William Pressly, 'Portrait of a Cork Family: The Two James Barrys', *Journal of the Cork Historical and Archaeological Society*, vol. 90 (1985), p. 147 n.43.
41. Michael Lackey, 'Introduction: A narrative space of its own', in *Biographical Fiction: A Reader*, ed. Michael Lackey (New York: Bloomsbury, 2016), p. 10; Ina Schabert, *In Quest of the Other Person: Fiction as Biography* (Tübingen: Francke, 1990), p. 56. Schabert draws attention to the way in which biography has moved away from Leon Edel's injunction against fictionalization (in his 'Biography: A Manifesto' of 1978, see below) but sees a difference in the degree to which biography and biofiction shape life stories through imaginative means (pp. 60–61).
42. Du Preez and Dronfield, *Dr. James Barry*, pp. 7–9. Of little credibility, the story falters when Redmond is quoted pleading with his elder brother, James, 'to look back and Consider if you were in My Situation … how you would Approve of my behaviour' (p. 9); surely, however mentally unstable James Barry the painter was at that point, he would not have endorsed his brother's rape of their niece. Similarly, it is difficult to imagine that Jeremiah Bulkley would have

compounded the traumatic situation by throwing his wife and daughters out of the house, as Mary Anne claimed in her letter to James of January 1805; why, if his daughter had suffered violence, should he later write to say he had 'made up [his] mind to forgive' (quoted in *Dr. James Barry*, p. 57)? If the collapse of the Bulkley marriage was to do with a sexually reprehensible act, Juliana is more likely to have been an illegitimate child of Mary Anne's, and thus Margaret's actual (half)sister. The text here reads like an illustration of Edel's decree that the biographer should not 'imagine his facts'; Leon Edel, 'Biography: A Manifesto', *Biography*, vol. 1:1 (Winter 1978), p. 1.

43. See William Makepeace Thackeray's famous 'Foreword' to his 1848 novel, which sets the text up as a puppet show overseen by the show-man-puppeteer-author; *Vanity Fair* (New York: Norton, 1994), pp. ix-x: 'He is proud to think that his Puppets have given satisfaction to the very best company in this empire. The famous little Becky Puppet has been pronounced to be uncommonly flexible in the joints and lively on the wire: the Amelia Doll, though it has had a smaller circle of admirers, has yet been carved and dressed with the greatest care by the artist: the Dobbin Figure, though apparently clumsy, yet dances in a very amusing and natural manner ... And with this, and a profound box to his patrons, the Manager retires, and the curtain rises.'
44. 'A Mystery Still', p. 493.
45. In Jane Austen's *Emma* (1815; London: Penguin, 1996), Frank Churchill cultivates the air of a fop and contrives an extravagant trip to his hairdresser in town in order to purchase a piano for Jane Fairfax to whom he is secretly engaged. While Frank is as vain and inconsiderate to others as he makes out and Barry, though dandyish, is kind and caring, 'A Mystery Still' draws on the allusion to convey the sense of a secret.
46. James Barry, 'Memorandum of the Services of Dr. James Barry Inspector General of Hospitals' (undated, [1859]), Wellcome Library, London, RAMC 373; Appendix 4. See also Holmes, *Scanty Particulars* (1), pp. 182–84. In his 'Memorandum' Barry writes that he was 'recalled', but no such official order is recorded. Rose and Holmes suggest that Somerset's younger brother Fitzroy, then Military Secretary at the Horse Guards, had intervened on Barry's behalf, both in the new posting and in postponing the start date

(from January 1830 to 1 and then 25 September 1830). Barry remained in situ as Somerset's personal physician until his death in February 1831, and did not take up his post until June 1831. See Rose, *Perfect Gentleman*, pp. 93–95, and Holmes, *Scanty Particulars* (1), p. 189.

47. Rogers, *Modern Sphinx* (1881 ed.), II, p. 154; also in Major E[benezer] Rogers, *Madeline's Mystery: A Novel*, edited by the author of Lady Audley's Secret, etc. (London: John and Robert Maxwell, [1882]), p. 159, Harry Ransom Center, The University of Texas at Austin, WOLFF 752; Racster and Grove, *Dr. James Barry*, Act II, p. 48, and *Journal of Dr. James Barry*, p. 144; Rutherford, 'Dr. James Barry', p. 246; Anne and Ivan Kronenfeld, *The Secret Life of Dr. James Miranda Barry* (2000; Cambridge, MD: Write Words, ebooksonthenet, 2004), p. 271; Elizabeth Longford, 'James Barry', *Eminent Victorian Women* (1981; Stroud: History Press, 2008), p. 213. Further examples include Hargreaves's *Women-at-Arms* (p. 184), Robert Leitch's 'The Barry Room: The Tale Of A Pioneering Military Surgeon', US Medicine: The Voice of Federal Medicine, July 2001, http://web.archive.org/web/20070928030206/http://www.usmedicine.com/column.cfm?columnID=53&issueID=28 [accessed 13 December 2015], and Sydney Brandon's entry on James Barry in the *Oxford Dictionary of National Biography* (Oxford: Oxford University Press, 2004), online edn, http://www.oxforddnb.com/view/article/1563 [accessed 1 December 2015]; see also du Preez and Dronfield, *Dr. James Barry*, p. 231.
48. Binnie, *Colours: James Barry – Her Story*, Act II, pp. 82–83 (Bristol Theatre Collection play script). The happy outcome of the court-martial is further aided by the intervention of Arthur Wellington (one of Jane's former lovers), who ensures that the reforms for which she was taken to court are implemented and that the fiscal who stood in her way loses his position through the abolition of his office (a humorous reworking of Barry's loss of his post as Colonial Medical Officer at the Cape; the events at the Cape and Barry's court-martial following his appointment on St Helena are here telescoped together).
49. For a related observation see Edward Bradford's earlier 'Reputed Female Army Surgeon' (p. 293): 'The real marvel of [Barry's] history is, that a being of a frame so feeble, without domestic resources,

with a temper so irritable and even mischievous, in spite of frequent severe sickness in tropical climates, and constantly at variance with authority, should have attained the highest rank in the Medical Department, and have lived to the age of 65 years.'

50. 'A Mystery Still', p. 494. See Bradford's 'The Reputed Female Army Surgeon' (p. 293): 'When he was ill he invariably exacted from the officer who attended him a promise that, in the event of his death, strict precautions should be adopted to prevent any examination of his person.' A related incident in Trinidad 'about the year 1845 or '46' was later recounted by [Surgeon-General and Sir] T. Longmore who knew the family where Barry was staying: 'Dr B. exacted a promise from the lady of the house that if he died his body should be rolled in the sheets … and be buried without further disturbance.' Undated, Longmore Pamphlet Collection, vol. 4 (1863–1882), Wellcome Library, London, RAMC 423/4. In Racster and Grove's play and novel Barry asks Somerset to have her 'body sewn in canvas' if she should not survive her duel; *Dr. James Barry*, Act II, p. 58; see also *Journal*, p. 119.
51. 'A Mystery Still', p. 494. The inconsistencies in tone may indicate co-authorship.
52. Ibid., p. 494. See brief discussion at the end of the last chapter.
53. For the anonymous sodomy libel in Cape Town, 1826, as discussed in Chapter 2, see Holmes, *Scanty Particulars* (1), p. 138. The homosocial undertones would have appealed to the editor of *All the Year Round*, suggesting that Dickens might have had an editorial role in the story. For an exploration of Dickens's interest in homosocial and queer characters and plots see Holly Furneaux, *Queer Dickens: Erotics, Families, Masculinities* (Oxford: Oxford University Press, 2009).
54. 'A Mystery Still', p. 494; Holmes, *Scanty Particulars* (1), p. 97. The blood-letting passage is echoed in Racster and Grove's *Dr. James Barry* (Act I, p. 31).
55. 'A Mystery Still', p. 495.
56. J. C. M'Crindle, 'Dr James Barry', *Glasgow Herald* (December 1949), Wellcome Library, London, RAMC 238. Isobel Rae, *The Strange Story of Dr. James Barry: Army Surgeon, Inspector General of Hospitals, discovered on death to be a woman* (London: Longmans, Green & Co, 1958), p. 117. For the earlier reference see Hargreaves, *Women-at-Arms*, pp. 187–88.

57. Rose, *Perfect Gentleman*, p. 151.
58. On his 1860–61 trip to Jamaica, Barry had made friends with the McCrindle family in Kingston and had given them various gifts, including a signet ring with a crest and a memorial ring (these are referenced in J.C. M'Crindle's letter to the *Glasgow Herald*). There is, however, no reference to a black box in Holmes's account; see *Scanty Particulars* (1), p. 254.
59. Du Preez and Dronfield, *Dr. James Barry*, p. 376, p. 377, p. 382.
60. Du Preez and Dronfield cite a letter from Verran to Rutherford of April 1855 (*Dr James Barry*, p. 449 n.19); this source could not be traced in the Wellcome material. The reference may be an extrapolation from N.J.C. Rutherford's letter of 12 April [19]55, addressed to 'My dear Barnsley', with a separate note in a different hand and ink, 'acknowledged to Col. Rutherford & Miss Verran', Wellcome Library, London, RAMC 801/6/5/1, http://wellcomelibrary.org/item/b18495370 [accessed 13 September 2016]. In this letter Rutherford refers to Annie Verran, Barrie's daughter (by then in her 90s), who recollected being shown Barry's watch chain, and indicates that he has written to her. No reference is made to the trunk and its sensational contents in the letter.
61. Twain, 'Conclusion' to *Following the Equator*. For Twain's 'transvestite tales', like '1,002nd Arabian Night' (1883), 'Hellfire Hotchkiss' (1897) and *Pudd'nhead Wilson* (1894) see Garber's discussion in *Vested Interests*, p. 289.
62. Twain, 'Conclusion' to *Following the Equator*.
63. John Leigh, *Touché: The Duel in Literature* (Cambridge, MA: Harvard University Press, 2015), pp. 200–204.
64. All references are to Twain, 'Conclusion' to *Following the Equator* (emphasis in original).
65. Sarah Grand, *The Heavenly Twins* (1893; London: Heinemann, 1908), p. 456, p. 483.
66. Ibid., p. 456.
67. Ibid., p. 456.
68. Ménie Muriel Dowie, 'Introduction' to (ed.), *Women Adventurers: The Lives of Madame Velazquez, Hannah Snell, Mary Anne Talbot, and Mrs. Christian Davies* (London: Fisher Unwin, 1893), pp. xx-xxi.
69. Ibid., pp. xx–xxi.
70. Cicely Hamilton, *A Pageant of Great Women*, first produced (at the Scala Theatre, London) in 1909; 1948 edition reproduced in

Carolyn Christensen Nelson (ed.), *Literature of the Women's Suffrage Campaign in England* (Peterborough, Ontario: Broadview, 2004), pp. 221–32. For a recent reference to Barry in relation to the later Victorian women's movement see Jenni Murray's *Votes for Women! The Pioneers and Heroines of Female Suffrage* (London: Oneworld Publications, 2018); the chapter on Elizabeth Garrett Anderson starts with a discussion of that 'first' female-born doctor (see pp. 27–29).

71. In *Curtain Up! The Story of Cape Theatre* (Cape Town: Juta & Co, 1951) Olga Racster recalls that Thorndike, 'always flowing with enthusiasm was taken with the part of Barry' (p. 186).
72. See Dowie's introduction to *Women Adventurers*, p. xii: 'For to-day, women make war for themselves ... These in our book followed husbands and lovers – for love, so they say.'
73. Hargreaves, *Women-at-Arms*, p. 189.
74. Hargreaves, *Women-at-Arms*, p. 190. The layer-out's story of Barry's early motherhood seems here interpreted as an indication of the young 'female' Barry's 'natural' sexual abandon.
75. George Moore, 'Albert Nobbs', *Celibate Lives* (London: William Heinemann, 1927), repr. in Ann Heilmann and Mark Llewellyn (eds), *The Collected Short Stories of George Moore: Gender and Genre*, 5 vols (London: Pickering and Chatto, 2007), V, p. 198. First published in Moore's *A Story-Teller's Holiday* (1918) and a transposition of his earlier psychological tales about the sexual repression of a gay Catholic aesthete (*A Mere Accident*, 1887; 'John Norton', *Celibates*, 1895; 'Hugh Monfert', *In Single Strictness*, 1922/23), the novella was remediated in the later twentieth century by the feminist playwright Simone Benmussa (*The Singular Life of Albert Nobbs*, in *Benmussa Directs* [London: John Calder, 1979], pp. 22–121) and has more recently been adapted for a feature film starring Glenn Close, *Albert Nobbs*, dir. Rodrigo García (Mockingbird Films, Trillium Productions, Parallel Film Productions, 2011); see final shooting script by Gabriella Prekop, John Banville and Glenn Close, based on a treatment by Istvan Szabo and a short story by George Moore, WGA Registered #I00705-2, http://www.albertnobbs-the-movie.com/AlbertNobbs.pdf [accessed 17 April 2017]. For discussions of Moore's novella, Benmussa's play and/or the movie see Ann Heilmann, "Neither man nor woman'? Female Transvestism, Object Relations and Mourning in George Moore's "Albert Nobbs"', *Women: a cultural review*, vol. 14:3 (2003), pp. 248–62; Glenn Close, 'On Albert Nobbs' in *George Moore: Dublin, Paris, Hollywood*,

ed. Conor Montague and Adrian Frazier (Dublin: Irish Academic Press, 2012), pp. 197–201; Elizabeth Grubgeld, 'Framing the Body: George Moore's "Albert Nobbs" and the Disappearing Realist Subject', in *George Moore: Across Borders*, ed. Christine Huguet and Fabienne Dabrigeon-Garcier (Amsterdam, Rodopi, 2013), pp. 193–208. For a discussion of the way in which the 'transgender capacity' of the transmen Albert and Hubert of Moore's novella is reconfigured into a tragic story of loss, entrapment and self-alienation in second-wave feminist readings of Benmussa's play but recuperated in the film version, see chapters 1 and 6 of Rachel Caroll's *Transgender and the Literary Imagination: Changing Gender in Twentieth Century Writing* (Edinburgh: Edinburgh University Press, 2018).

76. Magnus Hirschfeld, *Transvestites: The Erotic Drive to Cross-Dress*, trans. Michael A. Lombardi-Nash (New York: Prometheus, 1991), p. 147 (first published in German in 1910); see also Vern L. Bullough's 'Introduction' to Hirschfeld's work, ibid., p. 12; [Magnus Hirschfeld], 'Transvestitism', chapter X in *Sexual Anomalies and Perversions: Physical and Psychological Development and Treatment. A Summary of the Works of the Late Professor Dr. Magnus Hirschfeld*, compiled as a humble memorial by his pupils (London: Torch Publishing Company, 1946), repr. in *Women and Cross-Dressing 1800–1939*, ed. Heike Bauer, 3 vols (London: Routledge, 2006), I, p. 288.
77. Hirschfeld, *Transvestites*, p. 411. Barry is presented as Lord Fitzroy Somerset's relative, 'through whose influence, she claimed, she was discharged from the army because of repeated disciplinary problems' (Lord Raglan died in 1855, ten years before Barry). Barry's ferocious temper is interpreted as fear of exposure: 'An officer who rode with her once suddenly said to her, "You truly look more like a woman than a man!" She whipped his face for it.' The story of Barry's anger at an irresponsible officer spilling over into an act of violence is here mixed up with Barry's fear of exposure. The anecdote is possibly adapted from Marvell's 'The Mystery of the Kapok Doctor'.
78. Ellis, *Eonism*, p. 6; 'Eonism', in Bauer, *Women and Cross-Dressing*, p. 159. Most of Ellis's brief account is paraphrased or directly borrowed from Albemarle's *Fifty Years of My Life*, II, pp. 100–101.
79. Ellis, *Eonism*, p. 3 (also in Bauer, *Women and Cross-Dressing*, p. 156). The reference is to the Chevalier D'Éon but could equally be applied to Barry.

80. Havelock Ellis, 'Eonism (Transvestism or Sexo-Aesthetic Inversion)', in section on 'Homosexuality', *The Psychology of Sex* [abbreviated one-vol. edition] (London: William Heinemann, 1948), p. 209; also repr. in extracts in Bauer, *Women and Cross-Dressing*, p. 281.
81. Ellis, 'Eonism (Transvestism or Sexo-Aesthetic Inversion)', ibid., p. 208 (also in Bauer, *Women and Cross-Dressing*, p. 280).
82. Ellis, *Eonism and Other Supplementary Studies*, pp. 1–2; also 'Eonism' in Bauer, *Women and Cross-Dressing*, p. 155. The Chevalier's swordsmanship inspired representations of Barry; in Marvell's 'The Mystery of the Kapok Doctor' Barry excels in the art of fencing (p. 15).
83. As Jacqueline Rose notes, the broad category of 'transgender' encompasses a variety of gender positions: '"transition" ("A to B")', i.e. transsexual; '"transitional" ("between A and B")', i.e. passing; 'A as well as B' or '"neither A nor B" – that's to say, "transcending", as in "above", or "in a different realm from", both'; see Rose's 'Who do you think you are', *London Review of Books*, vol. 38: 9, 5 May 2016, http://www.lrb.co.uk/v38/n09/jacqueline-rose/who-do-you-think-you-are [accessed 16 December 2016].
84. Garber, *Vested Interests*, p. 263.
85. Kohlke, 'Neo-Victorian Biofiction', p. 8 (emphases in original). Colm Toíbín's *The Master* (London: Picador, 2004) and Barbara Chase-Riboud's *The Hottentot Venus* (New York: Anchor, 2003) might serve as examples to differentiate between the two variants, illustrating the ways in which readers are given greater, or first, insight into the biofictional characters' inner lives.
86. The quotations deriving from George Moore's 'Albert Nobbs' (*The Collected Short Stories of George Moore*, V, p. 198, p. 201) might be applied to Margaret's perceived longing for her 'lost' femininity as depicted in du Preez and Dronfield's biography.
87. Binnie, *Colours*, Act II, p. 90 (Bristol Theatre Collection).
88. Kohlke, 'Neo-Victorian Biofiction', p. 12.
89. Marvell, 'The Mystery of the Kapok Doctor', p. 14.
90. Ibid., p. 15.
91. Ibid., p. 15, p. 16.
92. Racster and Gove, *Dr. James Barry*, Act II, p. 22. The stage directions are not italicized in the photocopy of the script, but their fainter font suggests that the original typescript had colour coding.
93. Réné Juta, *Cape Currey* (1920; Memphis: General Books, 2010), p. 86.

94. Ibid., p. 91.
95. The name of Juta's Aletta van Breda may have been inspired by Aletta Kueneppe in Marvell's 'The Mystery of the Kapok Doctor'.
96. Ibid., p. 83.
97. Ibid., p. 91.
98. A century after Rogers, Anne Garrétta chose the same title for her narrative *mise-en-scène* of gender circumvention, *Sphinx*, trans. Emma Ramadan (Dallas, Texas: Deep Vellum Publishing, 2015).
99. Kohlke, 'Neo-Victorian Biofiction', pp. 12–13.
100. Ebenezer Rogers [to T. Longmore], 22 January 1882, Longmore Pamphlet Collection (1863–1882), Wellcome Library, London, RAMC 423/4. E. Rogers, Lieutenant-Colonel (late Staff Officer of Pensioners and formerly Captain 3rd West India Regiment), 'A Female Member of the Army Medical Staff', 'Notes, Comments, and Answers to Correspondents' section, *Lancet*, vol. 3764, 19 October 1895, p. 1021. A typed copy of the ensuing *Lancet* correspondence is available in the Wellcome Library, London, RAMC 801/6/5/1, http://wellcomelibrary.org/item/b18495370 [accessed 13 September 2016]. E[benezer] Rogers, 'Introduction' to *A Modern Sphinx*, De luxe edition with seven illustrations (London: Maxwell, [1896]), pp. v–vi.
101. Ebenezer Rogers [to T. Longmore], 22 January 1882, Longmore Pamphlet Collection.
102. Letter of 22 January 1882, Longmore Pamphlet Collection (emphasis in original). See opening epigraph section. Rogers refers to the French translation of the original *Saunders's News-Letter* report of 1865 in the *Revue Étrangère.*
103. Most of the passages dropped are (at times lengthy) digressions that deflect from the plot. Some of the changes are stylistic in nature; thus a male 'witch' becomes a 'conjuror' (*Modern Sphinx* [1881 ed.], II, p. 204; *Madeline's Mystery*, p. 178), and the prose of awkward sentences is improved: 'for she is ever pale, pale to excess, no blush, or crimson tints flush her downy cheeks, or light up, with animation, that faultless countenance in repose' (*Modern Sphinx*, I, p. 150) turns into: 'for she is ever pale, pale to excess; no crimson tints flush her downy cheeks, or give animation to that faultless countenance' (*Madeline's Mystery*, p. 54). All the chapters bar one (chapter I of vol. II) are retained; the one exception, 'The Doctor's Experiences', is a digression on Fitzjames being used as a decoy by the same society lady who also compromised Whitlington. Part of

this chapter is moved to the end of the previous one (which in *Modern Sphinx* breaks off abruptly at the end of vol. I and is continued in vol. II). Braddon did, however, anglicize Creoline's name; see discussion below.

104. In *Madeline's Mystery* (p. 66) the entire episode, which takes up several pages in *A Modern Sphinx* (1881 ed., I, pp. 187–91; the quotation is from p. 191), is contracted to the following passage: 'the three officers, annoyed at the doctor's arrogance and selfishness [at refusing to allow them access], resigned all claims to the state-room, and, after a social evening, they determined to patrol the deck till day light in company of the Commander'.
105. A passage that describes a Creole heiress' 'crisping locks rippl[ing] over a darksome but voluptuous bust' is removed in *Madeline's Mystery*. See Rogers, *Modern Sphinx* (1881 ed.), I, p. 97.
106. E. Rogers, 'A Female Member of the Army Medical Staff', *Lancet*, vol. 3792, 2 May 1896, p. 264. In his 19 October 1895 contribution to the reader correspondence in the *Lancet* (vol. 3764, p. 1021) on the subject of 'A Female member of the Army Medical Staff', Rogers claimed that *Modern Sphinx* was out of print but that *Madeline's Mystery* 'may still, I fancy, be obtained' and that he 'retained a few copies' of *Modern Sphinx* which he should 'have pleasure in placing ... at [readers'] disposal.' However, in his 'Introduction' to the 1896 edition of *Modern Sphinx* (p. iii) he refers to 'a few hundred unbound copies' of his original novel that 'lay *perdu*' at the bookbinders, and which he had bound for the purpose of the illustrated edition. That these copies had been left unbound in 1881 suggests that the initial three decker was considered to have little sales potential.
107. Julia Thomas, 'Illustrations and the Victorian Novel', in *The Oxford Handbook of Victorian Literary Culture*, ed. Juliet John (Oxford: Oxford University Press, 2016), p. 622.
108. Rogers, *Modern Sphinx* (1881 ed.), I, p. 40; *Madeline's Mystery*, p. 19. The character is introduced in a chapter entitled 'Who Is He?'.
109. Rogers, *Modern Sphinx* (1881 ed.), I, p. 210; *Madeline's Mystery*, p. 72.
110. Rogers, 'Introduction' to *Modern Sphinx* (1896 ed.), p. x; see also E. Rogers, 'A Female Member of the Army Medical Staff', *Lancet*, vol. 3768, 16 November 1895, p. 1269.
111. Rogers, *Modern Sphinx* (1881 ed.), I, p. 199; *Madeline's Mystery*, p. 69. The goat became a staple of the myth in Barry's lifetime: a

handwritten extract from a letter 'from Dr. Linton to Dr. Hall, Scutari, 6 November 1855', filed in RAMC 801/5/1 in the Wellcome Library, London, refers to Barry being reported to have 'left [Corfu] on a pleasure trip to the Crimea accompanied by his Horse, his Goat, his Dogs, & Servants'; however, 'he did not honor us with any of the animals.' See http://wellcomelibrary.org/item/b18495370 [accessed 13 September 2016]. The goat makes an appearance also in Rutherford's fictionalized article 'Dr James Barry', p. 242.

112. The original press is now under the remit of Pearson UK, and the publisher 'has no objection in principle' to granting permission to reproduce this image, but 'because of the age of this title, the contractual details are no longer available' and the publisher holds 'no record of this title'. The designer of the image is not referenced in the book. Correspondence from the Rights and Permissions Team, Pearson UK, Cape Town, 25 April 2017.
113. Rogers, *Modern Sphinx* (1881 ed.), II, p. 12; *Madeline's Mystery*, p. 106.
114. Rogers, *Modern Sphinx* (1881 ed.), I, p. 198; *Madeline's Mystery*, p. 68.
115. Rogers, *Modern Sphinx* (1881 ed.), II, p. 239; *Madeline's Mystery*, p. 190.
116. See the title of chapter 5 of Elaine Showalter's *Sexual Anarchy: Gender and Culture at the Fin de Siècle* (London: Bloomsbury, 1991), pp. 76–104.
117. Rogers, *Modern Sphinx* (1881 ed.), I, p. 78, p. 266, *Madeline's Mystery*, p. 32, p. 88. For the link with Fitzjames see pp. 266–67, *Madeline's Mystery*, p. 88: 'Light, gauzy fabrics, padded and tight-laced, feathers and furbelows, with the tiniest best-fitting boots and gloves … combin[ed] to present as unreal and as unsubstantial a creature as art and artifice could possibly produce.' Lucy Audley and Jean Muir are the villainous protagonists of Mary Braddon's best-selling *Lady Audley's Secret* (1861) and Louisa May Alcott's pseudonymous novella *Behind a Mask, or A Woman's Power* (1866).
118. Rogers, *Modern Sphinx* (1881 ed.), I, pp. 103–104; *Madeline's Mystery*, p. 41.
119. Rogers, 'Introduction' to *Modern Sphinx* (1896 ed.), pp. xiii-xiv, p. xvi.
120. Rogers, 'Introduction' to *Modern Sphinx* (1896 ed.), p. xi (emphasis in original).

121. The implicit imputation here, too, is that Barry was just too high-born to risk lifting her cover any further by too close an association with honours bestowed by royalty. Rogers, 'Introduction' to *Modern Sphinx* (1896 ed.), pp. xi-xii (emphases in original).
122. Rogers, 'Introduction' to *Modern Sphinx* (1896 ed.), p. vi, p. ix.
123. Rogers, *Modern Sphinx* (1881 ed.) III, p. 284; *Madeline's Mystery*, p. 310. See the title pages of Hannah Snell's *The Female Soldier* and *The Life and Surprising Adventures of Mary Anne Talbot*, in Dowie's *Women Adventurers*, p. 53, p. 133.
124. Rogers, *Modern Sphinx* (1881 ed.), III, p. 287; *Madeline's Mystery*, p. 311.
125. Rogers, *Modern Sphinx* (1881 ed.), III, p. 281; *Madeline's Mystery*, p. 309.
126. Rogers, *Modern Sphinx* (1881 ed.), III, pp. 297–98; *Madeline's Mystery*, p. 314.
127. Rogers, *Modern Sphinx* (1881 ed.), I, p. 204, p. 205. This passage is omitted in *Madeline's Mystery*, as is a later passage from *Modern Sphinx* that also references the first biotale: 'it must surely remain a mystery still' (*Modern Sphinx*, III, p. 282).
128. Ebenezer Rogers to T. Longmore, 25 February 1882, Longmore Pamphlet Collection (1863–1882), Wellcome Library, London, RAMC 423/4. For the longer published account discussed below see E. Rogers, 'A Female Member of the Army Medical Staff', *Lancet*, vol. 3768, 16 November 1895, p. 1269. See also Holmes, *Scanty Particulars* (1), p. 276; Rae, *Strange Story*, pp. 93–94, and Rose, *Perfect Gentleman*, p. 124.
129. Rogers, *Modern Sphinx* (1881 ed.), I, p. 150; *Madeline's Mystery*, p. 54. For a recent academic study of the parallels between transgender and transracial identity formation and performance, see Rogers Brubaker, *trans: Gender and Race in an Age of Unsettled Identities* (Princeton: Princeton University Press, 2016).
130. Rogers, *Modern Sphinx* (1881 ed.), I, p. 97, p. 98. As mentioned above, this is a reference dropped in *Madeline's Mystery.*
131. Rogers, *Modern Sphinx* (1881 ed.), I, pp. 96–98; *Madeline's Mystery*, pp. 38–39.
132. Rogers, *Modern Sphinx* (1881 ed.), III, p. 104; *Madeline's Mystery*, p. 216.
133. See the reference to Creoline having 'become quite creolized and objectionable' since the discovery of her origins; Rogers, *Modern Sphinx* (1881 ed.), II, p. 270; *Madeline's Mystery*, pp. 201–2.

134. Kit Brennan, *Tiger's Heart* (1996; Vancouver: Scirocco Drama, revised edn 1998), Act II, Scene 24, p. 108.
135. Brubaker, *trans*, p. 92.
136. Jay Prosser, *Second Skins: The Body Narratives of Transsexuals* (New York: Columbia University Press, 1998), p. 101.
137. Ibid., p. 116.
138. Ibid., pp. 100–101.
139. The classic example is the opening sentence of Jan Morris's *Conundrum* (London: Faber and Faber, 1974), p. 1: 'I was three or perhaps four years old when I realized that I had been born into the wrong body, and should really be a girl. I remember the moment well, and it is the earliest memory of my life.'
140. Prosser, *Second Skins*, p. 69.
141. Monique Rooney, 'Grave endings: the representation of passing', *Australian Humanities Review*, vol. 23 (Sept. 2001), http://australianhumanitiesreview.org/2001/09/01/grave-endings-the-representation-of-passing/ [accessed 22 December 2016].
142. Halberstam, title of chapter 4, *In a Queer Time and Place*, pp. 76–96.
143. See films like Kimberley Peirce's *Boys Don't Cry* (Fox Searchlight Pictures, The Independent Film Channel Productions, Killer Films, 1999), as discussed in Rooney, 'Grave endings: the representation of passing', and Halberstam, *In a Queer Time and Place*, pp. 83–92.
144. For an illustration of this double gaze see the cover of Florida Ann Town's *With a Silent Companion* (Fig. 3.7).
145. 'A Mystery Still', p. 493.
146. See Elizabeth Longford's account of how, in Cape Town, Barry always presented himself in 'her plumed hat, unwieldy sword, three-inch false soles and high-heeled boots', accompanied by 'black Sambo' or 'black John' and her dog Psyche; 'James Barry', *Eminent Victorian Women*, p. 218.
147. While in this case Barry's depiction in the medium of illustration is clearly remediated from earlier textual sources, it is important to remain aware of the complex relationship in the nineteenth century of illustration and text. As Julia Thomas reminds us, illustrations can operate independently from the text and can precede a textual depiction; the 'original' can be either in the pictorial or textual medium. See Julia Thomas, 'Illustrations and the Victorian Novel', in *The Oxford Handbook of Victorian Literary Culture*, ed. Juliet John (Oxford: Oxford University Press, 2016), pp. 617–36; see also the

introduction to Thomas's *Nineteenth-Century Illustration and the Digital* (Basingstoke: Palgrave, 2017), p. 3.

148. In *Curtain Up! The Story of the Cape Theatre* (Cape Town: Juta and Co, 1951), Olga Racster recalled seeing 'a natty young Georgian officer, as stiff as a telegraph pole. His red uniform coat was skin-tight, his breeches ended in dandified top-boots with red heels; the hand holding the reins of his dapple-grey horse was gloved in white, and by his side walked a Malay holding an immense orange umbrella over him.' This sight, she wrote, inspired her to write Barry's life (p. 100, p. 101). The pageant was held in celebration of the Act of Union and filmed by Frank Lascelles; Holmes, *Scanty Particulars* (1), p. 179. For Rutherford's portrait see 'Dr. James Barry', p. 118. Here, too, the influence of 'A Mystery Still' is noticeable: 'Faint memories in the spoken word recall the picture of a small, dandified figure, always in high-collared tunic and high black riding boots with exaggeratedly high heels, passing through the town riding a Basuto pony covered to the hocks by a fine net and led by a black servant, Barry sitting easily in the saddle holding a green-lined umbrella over his head.'
149. Rose, *Perfect Gentleman* (p. 32); see also Rae, *Strange Story* (p. 29).
150. Jean Binnie, *Colours*, dir. Joan Harrison (Leeds Playhouse, October 1988). See the photograph from the production in J. L. Reyner's review of the play, 'Visible difference', *The Stage and Television Today*, vol. 5613, 10 November 1988, p. 16. For the play text see *Colours: James Barry – Her Story*, Act II:1, p. 49 (Bristol Theatre Collection).
151. Edward Bradford [Deputy-Inspector-General of Hospitals], 'The Reputed Female Army Surgeon: Letter from Deputy-Inspector Bradford', *Medical Times and Gazette*, vol. 2, 9 September 1865, p. 293, http://babel.hathitrust.org/cgi/pt?id=mdp.39015021328169;view=1up;seq=299 [accessed 2 December 2015]; also Wellcome Library, London, RAMC 373. For the anecdote about the shoulder pads of the 'Kapok Doctor' see Rae, *Strange Story*, p. 22.
152. Ellen Moers, 'Brummell', *The Dandy: Brummell to Beerbohm* (Lincoln: University of Nebraska Press, 1978), p. 21. See also Nigel Rodgers's reference to Brummel's use of 'highly starched' cravats in *The Dandy: Peacock or Enigma?* (London: Bene Factum Publishing, 2012), p. 35.
153. The slave trade was abolished in 1807 in the British Empire, but this did not affect the status of existing slaves; full abolition did not come into effect until 1834.

154. Edouard Manet, *Olympia* (1863), Musée d'Orsay, Paris, http://www.musee-orsay.fr/en/collections/works-in-focus/search/commentaire_id/olympia-7087.html [accessed 22 December 2015].
155. Brubaker, *trans*, p. 94.
156. Kronenfeld, *The Secret Life*, p. 137.
157. Ibid., p. 204.
158. Ibid., p. 127.
159. Ibid., p. 128. The factual Miranda's eldest son with his English lover Sarah Andrews was called Leandro; see Robert Harvey, *Liberators: Latin America's Struggle for Independence 1810–1830* (London: John Murray, 2000), p. 50.
160. Du Preez and Dronfield, *Dr. James Barry*, p. 59.
161. Ibid., p. 61. Shortly after her first outing as a man, Margaret is, however, described as having 'discovered the delights of being a man': the freedom of movement bestowed by breeches to stride out and enjoy 'unfettered walking' (p. 65). Biographers who, like Rachel Holmes, see Barry as the agent of a fulfilled and self-identified life, focus on these 'delights', presenting a Barry who enthusiastically adopted the dandy's dress code: 'James Barry was captivated by the possibilities of this new fashion. … Careful attention was to be paid to colours and cuts. … Knitted breeches, a suit, a hat and laced ruffles were essential wear for the young pupil dressers. It was regulation to remove the hat "with the courtesy of a gentleman" when walking the wards. This was a theatrically pronounced formality of gesture that Barry – a great lover of hats – relished. …. Th[e] flame of hair falling over "large, tender blue eyes" must have given Barry the look of a truly dandified Adonis.' (*Scanty Particulars* [1], p. 51). See also p. 53: 'The chest and upper sleeves of Barry's dress and frock coats were stuffed with malleable wadding that enabled reshaping of the upper body. His day boots and evening shoes were worn with stacked heels … Stays held up his sharply tailored jackets, and like every self-respecting dandy he employed the services of a stay-maker to shape his corsetry. He strove to realign the shape of his body through the artifice of his clothes. And in doing so he was conforming to the most avant-garde male fashion. He was … typical of the very apotheosis of male fashion of the time.'
162. Sebastian Barry, *Whistling Psyche* (London: Faber and Faber, 2004), p. 31; for Psyche see p. 15.
163. Florida Ann Town, *With a Silent Companion* (1999; Alberta: Red Deer Press, 2000), p. 78, p. 87; for her renunciation of romance see p. 74.

164. Ibid., pp. 44–47.
165. Mohr, *Barry: Personal Statements, Five Solo Plays*, p. 52; also 1984 play script, p. 10, National Library of Scotland, Edinburgh, Traverse Theatre Inventory, Acc. 9285/8.
166. Town, *With a Silent Companion,* pp. 47–48.
167. Garber, *Vested Interests*, p. 122, p. 126.
168. Town, *With a Silent Companion,* p. 49.
169. Ibid., p. 46.
170. Ibid., pp. 61–62.
171. Ibid., p. 119.
172. See Jacques Lacan, 'The Mirror Stage as Formative of the Function of the I as Revealed in Psychoanalytic Experience', *Écrits: A Selection,* trans. Alan Sheridan (London: Tavistock, 1989), pp. 1–8.
173. Sylvie Ouellette, *Le Secret du docteur Barry* (2012; Paris: Terres de femmes, De Borée, 2013), p. 25 ('assumer pleinement le rôle qui lui était dévolu'); p. 31 ('He had to play the grand game'); translations mine. I am grateful to Nathalie Saudo-Welby for advising on all the French translations.
174. Ibid., p. 22 ('you are truly becoming a man'), p. 25 ('James joue son rôle à la perfection'); translations mine.
175. Ibid., p. 50: 'Barry se plantait volontiers devant son miroir pendant de longues minutes pour s'exercer à prendre les poses de mise. – "J'ai réussi, je suis exactement comme eux, à présent …" songeait-il chaque fois qu'on lui adressait quelque compliment … En toutes circonstances, le dandy devait étonner et susciter l'envie de celui qui le regardait, chose à laquelle Barry prenait un immense plaisir.' (Translation mine.)
176. Ibid., p. 63: 'Pour moi, Margaret Bulkley n'existe plus. Elle est morte lorsque James Miranda Barry est né!'; 'vous ne pourrez jamais renier votre féminité'; 'Mais aux yeux du monde, je suis un homme! ... Depuis plusieurs années, j'ai appris à parler comme eux, à marcher comme eux et même à m'asseoir comme eux! Surtout, … j'agis comme un homme, je pense comme un homme et désormais je me considère tout à fait comme un homme' (translation mine).
177. Ibid., p. 64 ('presque surprise'), translation mine.
178. Ibid., p. 168: 'Barry aperçut finalement son visage dans la glace. Elle tressaillit violemment, surprise de se voir en femme…. Somerset vint se placer derrière elle et l'enlaça' (translation mine).
179. Given the novel's play with queer relations, it is intriguing that the option of cohabitation in male guise is not raised, presumably

because this would replicate Barry's purely sexual affair with Somerset. Consensual homosexual relations were, of course, prohibited by law.

180. Ouellette, *Le secret*, p. 213: 'Ses gestes n'avaient plus à être étudiés or empruntés; tout lui venait naturellement' (translation mine). While this sentence leaves the sex open, the framing sentences use the female pronoun.
181. Ibid., p. 262: 'Chacune était un monde isolé en soi, mais au sein duquel une énorme complexité était représentée. En dépit de leurs dimensions restraintes, elles pouvaient offrir des contrastes surprenants à qui savait les découvrir. En un sens, elles étaient tout à fait semblables à James Miranda Barry. … *Leur beauté masque les horreurs qu'elles renferment; leur géographie précise et leurs bordures immuables marquent un fort contraste avec la liberté qu'elles peuvent aussi offrir.*' (Emphases in original; translation mine). A similar point is made in Holmes's biography, *Scanty Particulars* (1), p. 208. See also Rachel Carroll's discussion of the use of tropes of colonialism as a 'metaphor for the life history of the transgender subject', *Transgender and the Literary Imagination*, chapter 3.
182. Racster and Grove, *Journal*, p. 81.
183. Ibid., p. 16. This sentiment is echoed in Duncker's *James Miranda Barry* (London: Serpent's Tail, 1999), p. 94: 'Now you're really a man. Soon you'll be a real doctor. You can be a gentleman. … You've got to change your way of thinking. That's all.'
184. Ibid., p. 121, emphases in original; for an earlier scene when she talks courage to herself to brave the confrontation with her husband-commissioner, see p. 58.
185. Ibid., p. 52.
186. Ibid., p. 21. Barry's outfit is reproduced, as factual information, in Rae's *Strange Story*, p. 22, Rose's *Perfect Gentleman*, p. 39, Holmes's *Scanty Particulars* (1), p. 67, and du Preez and Dronfield's *Dr. James Barry*, p. 178.
187. Ibid., p. 23, p. 21.
188. Ibid., p. 29, p. 34.
189. Ibid., p. 54, p. 14 (emphasis mine).
190. *Saunders's News-Letter*, 14 August 1865, repr. in 'A Female Medical Combatant', *Medical Times and Gazette*, 26 August 1865, p. 228.
191. Bradford, 'The Reputed Female Army Surgeon', p. 293.
192. E[benezer] Rogers, 'A Female Member of the Army Medical Staff', *Lancet*, vol. 3764, 19 October 1895, p. 1021. Cloete / Cleote:

Barry's more recent biographers, Rose, Holmes, du Preez and Dronfield, use the oe spelling, which also appears on family heritage sites like Geni and MyHeritage.

193. Quoted in E[benezer] Rogers, 'A Female Member of the Army Medical Staff', *Lancet*, vol. 3792, 2 May 1896, p. 264.
194. Ibid.
195. For an inflated narrative see Hargreaves, *Women-at-Arms*, pp. 180–81 (Cleoté); for more serious biographies see Rae, *Strange Story*, p. 29 (Cleote); Rose, *Perfect Gentleman*, p. 44 (Cloete); Holmes, *Scanty Particulars* (1), p. 86 (Cloete); du Preez and Dronfield, *Dr. James Barry*, pp. 155–59 (Cloete). In the latter, the scene is fictionalized (see also the start of the chapter, p. 150). Heavily adapted from Rutherford's 'Dr. James Barry' (pp. 174–75), the passage depicts Barry suffering a wound in the thigh which he is able to attend to himself, thus narrowly escaping exposure (p. 158).
196. R.C. Bellenger, letter to Major-General A. MacLennan, O.B.E., 17 November 1969, Wellcome Library, London, RAMC 238 (emphasis in original). The letter heading of the typescript is 'Empire History, R C Bellenger, 198 Old Brompton Road, London SW5, Books Bought and Sold.'
197. Holmes, *Scanty Particulars* (1), pp. 88–89.
198. Leigh, *Touché*, p. 256. As Pushkin's *Eugene Onegin* (1833) indicates, literary duels could also foreshadow later events in a writer's life; Pushkin died in a duel in 1837 (Leigh, ibid., p. 116).
199. Leigh, *Touché*, p. 173, p. 254.
200. Miranda was awarded the title of baron by the French revolutionary army in 1792; see Harvey, *Liberators*, p. 36; see also passim discussion in Chapter 1.
201. 'The Duel fought by the Duke of Wellington and the Duke of Winchelsea – 23 March 1829', *British Newspaper Archive*, http://blog.britishnewspaperarchive.co.uk/2013/03/23/the-duel-fought-by-duke-of-wellington-and-the-earl-of-winchilsea-23-march-1829/ [accessed 29 December 2015]; Leigh, *Touché*, p. 180; for the embourgeoisement of the duel see p. 109.
202. Leigh, *Touché*, p. 110, p. 165, p. 173.
203. For details of Cloete's family background see Holmes, *Scanty Particulars* (1), p. 85, du Preez and Dronfield, *Dr. James Barry*, p. 155.

204. For Barry's self-construction as an officer and gentleman see the terms of his court-martial, as discussed in Chapter 2, and his defence (epigraph 1, Chapter 1). Leigh, *Touché*, p. 14, p. 110.
205. For duel as 'set piece' see Leigh, *Touché*, p. 14.
206. Binnie, *Colours*, Act I:8, pp. 38–47 (Bristol Theatre Collection).
207. Marvell, 'The Mystery of the Kapok Doctor', pp. 15–16.
208. Hargreaves, *Women-at-Arms*, p. 48, p. 86, pp. 180–81.
209. 'A Mystery Still', p. 492, p. 493; Racster and Grove, *Dr. James Barry*, Act I, p. 31; Rose, *Perfect Gentleman*, p. 43; Mohr, *Barry: Personal Statements*, *Five Solo Plays*, p. 62, and 1984 play script, p. 23, National Library of Scotland, Edinburgh, Traverse Theatre Inventory, Acc. 9285/8.
210. Hargreaves, 'Dr. James Barry', *Women-at-Arms*, pp. 181–82. The scene is adapted and embellished in du Preez and Dronfield, *Dr. James Barry*, p. 158.
211. Leigh, *Touché*, p. 261.
212. 'A Mystery Still', p. 492.
213. Leigh, *Touché*, p. 280.
214. 'Mais ... mais ... bégaya-t-il d'une faible voix, complètement soufflé par la vision de ce qui s'offrait à lui. Mais vous êtes une femme!', Ouellette, *Le Secret*, p. 137 (translation mine).
215. Anne and Ivan Kronenfeld, *The Secret Life*, p. 186.
216. Patricia Duncker, *James Miranda Barry* (London: Serpent's Tail, 1999), p. 239, p. 219, p. 366.
217. Juta, *Cape Currey*, p. 38.
218. Ibid., pp. 52–53.
219. Ibid., p. 29.
220. Ibid., p. 61, p. 72.
221. Garber, *Vested Interests*, p. 202.
222. Ibid., p. 202.
223. Garber argues that 'it is the doctor or mortician as the ultimate agent of discovery, the bed as a deathbed rather than a place of sexuality and procreation, that is a recurrent feature of the cross-dressing story as it is told ... in biography and newspaper reports' (*Vested Interests*, p. 203).
224. The layer-out's expectation that she be paid for her services is often interpreted as an attempt at blackmail, but Holmes suggests that her 'angry employer' had confiscated 'Barry's money to cover his rental' and, '[m]ost probably ... did not regard herself as responsible for

settling her dead lodger's laying-out fees'; *Scanty Particulars* (1), p. 260.

225. Fenton died ten years after Barry, in 1875; her journal was not published until 1901. See Holmes, *Scanty Particulars* (1), p. 278.
226. Mrs. Bessie [Elizabeth] Knox Fenton, *The Journal of Mrs. Fenton: The Narrative of Her Life in India, the Isle of France (Mauritius), and Tasmania During the Years 1826–1830*, with a Preface by Sir Henry Lawrence (London: Edward Arnold, 1901), entry dated 18 June 1829, p. 324 (emphases in original). Also discussed in Holmes, *Scanty Particulars* (1), pp. 276–78, and in James Ross MacMahon, 'Dr. James Barry: A Study in Deception', *McGill Medical Journal*, vol. 37:1 (February 1968), p. 28, Wellcome Library, London, RAMC 1264/6.
227. Fenton, *Journal*, p. 324.
228. Ibid., pp. 323–24. Barry claimed the officers had neglected their hospital duties for private practice, but her nurse testified to calling them after office hours. For further details see Rose, *Perfect Gentleman*, pp. 90–92.
229. Rutherford, 'Dr. James Barry', p. 175. For Rogers's story see *A Modern Sphinx* (1881 edition), I, pp. 198–99; also in *Madeline's Mystery*, pp. 68–69.
230. Racster and Grove, *Journal*, p. 110.
231. Ibid., *Journal*, p. 88.
232. Kronenfeld, *Secret Life*, p. 213.
233. See Dr. G.W. Campbell, quoted in MacMahon, 'Dr. James Barry: A Study in Deception', p. 31; [Staff Surgeon Major] McKinnon to [George Graham, the Registrar General], 24 August 1865, Wellcome Library, London, RAMC 373.
234. Rogers, 'A Female Member of the Army Medical Staff', *Lancet*, vol. 3768, 16 November 1895, p. 1269: see also Rogers's 'Introduction' to *Modern Sphinx* (1896 ed.), p. x. Rogers's second-hand account is presented as based on his own experience in June Rose's 'Quest for Dr. James Barry' (BBC, 1973), typescript, pp. 17–18, Wellcome Library, London, RAMC 1069. In *Perfect Gentleman*, however, Rose places Rogers's account in the context of his endeavour to reissue his novel (p. 124). Elizabeth Longford's *Eminent Victorian Women* refers to the incident as factual (p. 226). The scene is pictured in a cover illustration to James Bannerman's 'The Double Life of Dr. James Barry', *Maclean's Magazine*, 1 December 1950, p. 49,

Wellcome Library, London, RAMC238. Barry's body is hidden under the bedclothes, but the officer in the foreground who is whispering to his colleague appears to have discovered his secret. Barry's 'real' identity is hinted at by the painting of a lady that hangs over the mirror facing the figure in the bed.

235. Handwritten copy (by Rogers) of J. de Montmarency's letter [addressed to 'My dear Major'], 16 February 18[9]2, and commentary (n.d.) by T. Longmore, dating the incident to '1845 or '46' [1845 would be the more likely date since Barry returned to Britain in December 1845 and from there travelled to Malta in November 1846; Rose, *Perfect Gentleman*, p. 125, p. 126]; Longmore Pamphlet Collection, vol. 4 (1863–1882), Wellcome Library, London, RAMC 423/4. Montmarency wrote that he 'was not actually in the room when Dr. James Barry's sex was discovered in 1841, the matter was confidentially told me immediately after the discovery by one of the party present, so I would not wish that either his name, nor mine, to be brought before the public in the matter.' [*Sic*] The wording suggests that some kind of discovery or at least supposition *was* made.
236. Binnie, *Colours*, Act II, p. 90 (Bristol Theatre Collection).
237. '[J]e vous voie comme un pionnier de la médecine, et de plus d'une façon, à partir de ce soir.' Ouellette, *Le Secret*, p. 281 (translation mine).
238. E. Rogers, 'A Female Member of the Army Medical Staff', *Lancet*, vol. 3764, 19 October 1895, p. 1021; for further details see Chapter 2.
239. Rogers, *A Modern Sphinx* (1881 ed.), I, p. 191. This scene, as discussed above, was stripped of its allusive elements in *Madeline's Mystery*.
240. Rutherford, 'Dr. James Barry', p. 242. The story borrows heavily from Rogers's *Modern Sphinx* (1881 edition) and lifts pages from that novel's chapter IX about Dr. Fitzjames ('Who is He?') and the scandalous rumours that circulate about the doctor's unmanly conduct (see Rutherford, pp. 243–45; *Modern Sphinx*, pp. 193–205, also in *Madeline's Mystery*, pp. 67–70).
241. 'En lisant le dégoût sur le visage de la femme, elle sut qu'il ne lui serait plus nécessaire de se soucier d'elle, à l'avenir.' Ouellette, *Le Secret*, p. 221 (translation mine).
242. Racster and Grove, *Journal*, p. 167.
243. Ibid., pp. 167–68.

244. Duncker, *James Miranda Barry*, pp. 234–35.
245. Ibid., p. 367 (emphasis in original).
246. The standard response for wives of exposed gender impersonators was to feign ignorance; see Julie Wheelwright, *Amazons and Military Maids: Women Who Dressed as Men in Pursuit of Life, Liberty and Happiness* (London: Pandora, 1989), pp. 1–4.

Chapter 4

1. James Barry's final speech at his court-martial in November/December 1836, as quoted in June Rose, *The Perfect Gentleman: The remarkable life of Dr. James Miranda Barry, the woman who served as an officer in the British Army from 1813 to 1859* (London: Hutchinson, 1977), p. 112. The sentence is also quoted in Rachel Holmes, *Scanty Particulars: The Mysterious, Astonishing and Remarkable Life of Victorian Surgeon James Barry* (London: Penguin, 2002), hereafter *Scanty Particulars* (1), p. 220. In Holmes's US edition the source is referenced to the General Court Martial, 24 November to 3 December 1836, 'The Trial of Dr. Barry', Public Records Office (National Archives), CO 247/52; see *Scanty Particulars: The Scandalous Life and Astonishing Secret of Queen Victoria's Most Eminent Military Doctor* (New York: Random House, 2002), hereafter *Scanty Particulars* (2), p. 341. My search in the National Archives, file CO 247/52, did not locate this document. The file contains correspondence used in the court-martial and the final verdict (copies of these documents are filed in the June Rose Collection in the Wellcome Library London, RAMC 1264).
2. Kit Brennan, 'Foreword', *Tiger's Heart* (Vancouver: Scirocco Drama, revised edn 1998), p. 16. The play was first published in 1996.
3. Judith Butler, *Gender Trouble: Feminism and the Subversion of Identity* (London; Routledge, 1990), p. 25.
4. Judith Halberstam, *In a Queer Time & Place: Transgender Bodies, Subcultural Lives* (New York: New York University Press, 2005), p. 61.
5. For 'miniature man' see Sebastian Barry, *Whistling Psyche*, in *Whistling Psyche. Fred and Jane* (London: Faber and Faber, 2004), p. 50.

6. For quotations see Judith Butler, 'Preface (1999)' to *Gender Trouble* (New York: Routledge, 1999), p. xv, and Andrew Parker and Eve Kosofsky Sedgwick, 'Introduction: Performativity and Performance', in *Performativity and Performance*, ed. Andrew Parker and Eve Kosofsky Sedgwick (London: Routledge, 1995), p. 2. For further explication see Sara Salih, *Judith Butler* (London: Routledge, 2002), pp. 62–64.
7. Butler's gender performativity has come under attack by contemporary transgender scholars concerned with embodiment and the 'natural' ontology of the reconstructed, transsexual body, but in Barry's pre-operative period, it is gender performance, not gender reassignment, that shapes and affirms identification processes. See Jay Prosser, *Second Skins: The Body Narratives of Transsexuality* (New York: Columbia University Press, 1998), pp. 21–45; Jacqueline Rose, 'Who do you think you are?', *London Review of Books*, vol. 38:9, 5 May 2016, http://www.lrb.co.uk/v38/n09/jacqueline-rose/who-do-you-think-you-are [accessed 16 December 2016].
8. Max Saunders, *Self-Impression: Life-Writing, Autobiografiction, and the Forms of Modern Literature* (Oxford: Oxford University Press, 2010).
9. Ansgar Nünning, 'Fictional Metabiographies and Metaautobiographies: Towards a Definition, Typology and Analysis of Self-Reflexive Hybrid Metagenres', in *Self-Reflexivity in Literature*, ed. Werner Huber, Martin Middeke, and Hubert Zapf (Würzburg: Königshausen & Neumann, 2005), p. 199.
10. E[benezer] Rogers, 'Introduction' to *A Modern Sphinx*, De luxe edition with seven illustrations (London: John and Robert Maxwell, [1896]), p. ix.
11. Benjamin Poore, *Heritage, Nostalgia and Modern British Theatre: Staging the Victorians* (Basingstoke: Palgrave, 2012), p. 100.
12. 'Empathetic unsettlement' has been conceptualized by trauma theorist Dominick LaCapra as the act of 'put[ting] oneself in the other's position while recognizing the difference of that position', thus making it possible to 'counteract[t] victimization, including self-victimization'; see his *Writing History, Writing Trauma* (Baltimore: Johns Hopkins University Press, 2001), p. 36, p. 38, p. 40, p. 78.
13. Sebastian Barry, *Whistling Psyche*, p. 50.
14. Olga Racster and Jessica Grove's *Dr. James Barry* has fourteen main and a number of subsidiary characters. Frederic Mohr's *Barry:*

Personal Statements, in *Five Solo Plays* (Edinburgh: [David McKail], [1994]) features Barry on his own; the young 'female' and older 'male' Barry may be played by the same or two separate actors. Sebastian Barry's *Whistling Psyche* juxtaposes Barry with Florence Nightingale. The 'Casting Requirements' for Brennan's *Tiger's Heart* (n.p.) specify five actors, with four playing double roles; its second production, at the Frederick Wood Theatre, University of British Columbia, 1996, however, saw a fuller cast of thirteen and further supportive actors; see 'Production History' (n.p.).

15. For details of the large cast and the actors' multiple roles see the Abbey Theatre Archive records of Jean Binnie's *Colours*, https://www.abbeytheatre.ie/archives/production_detail/702/ [accessed 2 August 2017] and Robin Thornber, 'Double firsts', *Guardian*, 30 September 1988, p. 31. Subsequent references are to the play text, *Colours: James Barry – Her Story* (1989), Bristol Theatre Collection, WTC.PS/000047.
16. Ina Schabert, *In Quest of the Other Person: Fiction as Biography* (Tübingen: Francke, 1990), p. 103.
17. Sebastian Barry, *Whistling Psyche*, p. 57.
18. Ibid., p. 57.
19. Ibid., p. 56.
20. David Cregan, '"Everyman's story is the whisper of God": Sacred and secular in Barry's Dramaturgy', in *Out of History: Essays on the Writing of Sebastian Barry*, ed. Christina Hunt Mahony (Dublin: Carysfort Press, 2004), pp. 70–71; Poore, *Heritage, Nostalgia and Modern British Theatre,* p. 100.
21. For the doubling effect see Poore, *Heritage, Nostalgia and Modern British Theatre,* p. 99. The quotation is sourced from Parker and Kosofsky Sedgwick, 'Introduction' to *Performativity and Performance,* p. 2 (emphases in original).
22. Thornber, 'Double firsts', p. 31; J.R.L. Reyner, 'Visible Difference', *The Stage and Television Today*, vol. 5613, 10 November 1988, p. 16; Abbey Theatre Archive, Dublin, https://www.abbeytheatre.ie/archives/production_detail/702/ [accessed 5 August 2017].
23. Mohr, 'Preface' to *Five Solo Plays*, n.p.
24. Sebastian Barry, *Whistling Psyche*, p. 37.
25. Stephen Reynolds, 'Autobiografiction', *Speaker*, new series, vol. 15: 366, 6 October 1906, p. 28, https://blogs.kcl.ac.uk/maxsaunders/

autobiografiction/autobiografiction-scan/ [accessed 27 February 2018]. Saunders, *Self-Impression*, p. 171.

26. Saunders, *Self-Impression*, p. 171.
27. Ibid., p. 171.
28. Ibid., p. 206.
29. Ibid., p. 1.
30. Glennis Byron, *Dramatic Monologue* (London: Routledge, 2003), p. 2, p. 32; Cornelia D.J. Pearsall, 'The dramatic monologue', in *The Cambridge Companion to Victorian Poetry*, ed. Joseph Bristow (Cambridge: Cambridge University Press, 2000), p. 69.
31. Pearsall, 'Dramatic monologue', p. 74. See also Byron, *Dramatic Monologue*, p. 65.
32. Sebastian Barry, *Whistling Psyche*, p. 25, p. 52.
33. Byron, *Dramatic Monologue*, pp. 6–7, p. 15.
34. Pearsall, 'Dramatic monologue', pp. 68–69, p. 72, p. 79; see also Byron's reference to the dramatic monologue's 'social critique' (*Dramatic Monologue*, p. 6).
35. Pearsall, 'Dramatic monologue', p. 68; Dorothy Mermin, *The Audience in the Poem: Five Victorian Poets* (New Brunswick: Rutgers University Press, 1983), p. 11.
36. The quotation is from Brennan, *Tiger's Heart*, Act 1, Scene 15, p. 73. Binnie's *Colours* cannot easily be categorized as a postmodernist play; my subsequent discussion therefore focuses on the other three contemporary plays.
37. Mohr, stage directions to *Barry*, parts one and two, *Five Solo Plays*, p. 45 p. 64; also 1984 play script, p. 2, p. 23, National Library of Scotland, Edinburgh, Traverse Theatre Inventory, Acc. 9285/8.
38. Mary Brennan, 'Barry', *Glasgow Herald*, 17 May 1984; see also Joyce McMillan, 'Barry', *Guardian*, 14 May 1984: 'the Barry of this first half appears simply as another mask, a bright, articulate and well-adjusted young woman who sees her life as a man as a grand adventure, and her position as a pregnant woman quite undisturbing despite 10 years of masquerading as a man.' National Library of Scotland, Edinburgh, Traverse Theatre Inventory Acc. 9285/8.
39. Mohr, *Barry*, *Five Solo Plays*, p. 64; play script, p. 23.
40. A reference to the charge in Barry's court-martial; see Chapter 2. See also Mohr, *Barry*, *Five Solo Plays*, p. 72; play script, p. 32.
41. Mohr, *Barry*, *Five Solo Plays*, p. 55; play script, p. 14.
42. Mohr, *Barry*, *Five Solo Plays*, p. 52, p. 57; play script, p. 11, p. 15.

43. Mohr, *Barry*, *Five Solo Plays*, p. 71; play script, p. 31.
44. Patricia Duncker, *James Miranda Barry* (London: Serpent's Tail, 1999), p. 281. For the earlier quotation see Brennan, 'Barry', National Library of Scotland, Edinburgh, Traverse Theatre Inventory Acc. 9285/8. The original text reads 'sexuality', but the slippage in Barry's identity in the play revolves around his sex, not his sexual orientation.
45. In personal email exchange (23 May 2015) McKrail commented that 'The "buggery" joke is a real occurrence which happened to the brother of an aged Scottish actor I was working with, who was a Medical Officer in India during the second world war in conversation with a sergeant major in his (Scottish) regiment.' The quotations are from Mohr, *Barry*, *Five Solo Plays*, p. 64, p. 69, p. 74; play script, p. 24 (slight variation), p. 29, p. 34.
46. Frederic Mohr [David McKail], *Barry.* A dramatization for television of the life of Inspector General of Army Hospitals, MAJOR-GENERAL JAMES MIRANDA BARRY, 1795–1865: The first woman doctor of modern western medicine, p. 58, Scottish Theatre Archive, STA MN57/1, University of Glasgow. The ageing Barry of Binnie's *Colours: James Barry – Her Story*, too, is overcome by a sense of loneliness; see play text (1989), Act II, p. 90 (Bristol Theatre Collection).
47. Mohr, *Barry*, *Five Solo Plays*, p. 72; play script, p. 32.
48. Mohr, *Barry*, *Five Solo Plays*, p. 72; play script, p. 32.
49. Mohr, *Barry*, *Five Solo Plays*, p. 76; play script, p. 37.
50. Mohr, *Barry*, *Five Solo Plays*, p. 66, p. 74; play script, p. 25, p. 35.
51. Claire Gleitman, '"In the dank margins of things": *Whistling Psyche* and the Illness of Empire', in *Out of History: Essays on the Writings of Sebastian Barry*, ed. Christina Hunt Mahony (Dublin: Carysfort Press, 2006), p. 214.
52. Freud's quip is apocryphal; see 'Sometimes a Cigar Is Just a Cigar', Quote Investigator, http://quoteinvestigator.com/2011/08/12/just-a-cigar/ [accessed 23 January 2016].
53. Pearsall, 'Dramatic monologue', p. 79.
54. Gleitman, 'In the dank margins of things', p. 216.
55. Sebastian Barry, *Whistling Psyche*, p. 35, p. 36.
56. No Man's Land exhibition, Martin Tilley Gallery, Cardiff, 28 February to 24 March 2018, http://www.artwales.com/exhibition-mtg-en.php?locationID=263. For Sebastian Barry's *Whistling Psyche*, see p. 9, p. 3.
57. Sebastian Barry, *Whistling Psyche*, p. 52.
58. Mohr, *Barry*, *Five Solo Plays*, p. 74; play script, p. 35. Barry, *Whistling Psyche*, p. 10, p. 11.

59. Practical considerations of taking care of a dog onstage and the greater force of the imagination is referenced by Mohr as the reason for ruling out Psyche's presence; undated handwritten manuscript filed with correspondence on and reviews of 1984 production, p. 3, National Library of Scotland, Edinburgh, Traverse Theatre Inventory Acc. 9285/8.
60. Sebastian Barry, *Whistling Psyche*, p. 50, p. 51.
61. Ibid., p. 61. Pearsall, 'Dramatic monologue', p. 72.
62. Gleitman, 'In the dank margins of things', p. 226.
63. Ibid.
64. Rogers, 'A Female Member of the Army Medical Staff', *Lancet*, vol. 3768, 16 November 1895, p. 1269: see also Rogers's 'Introduction' to *Modern Sphinx* (1896 ed.), p. x. See discussion of this scene in Chapter 3.
65. Sebastian Barry, *Whistling Psyche*, p. 49. The invocation of *The Tempest* here associates Barry with Caliban as a fallen 'Miranda'. See Prospero's denunciation of Caliban as 'Filth as thou art' and a 'thing of darkness I acknowledge mine' in Shakespeare's *The Tempest*, Act I, Scene 1 and Act V, Scene 1. Nightingale's music box may be another reference to Shakespeare's island.
66. Sebastian Barry, *Whistling Psyche*, p. 43.
67. See discussion by Gleitman, 'In the dank margins of things', pp. 210–12. For Virginia Woolf's famous dictum that 'on or about December 1910, human character changed', see 'Mr. Bennett and Mrs. Brown' (1924), repr. in *The Gender of Modernism: A Critical Anthology*, ed. Bonnie Kime Scott (Bloomington: Indiana University Press, 1990), p. 634.
68. Matthew Arnold, 'Stanzas from the Grande Chartreuse' (1855), Stanza 15, l.85-86, in *Victorian Poetry: An Annotated Anthology*, ed. Francis O'Gorman (Oxford: Blackwell, 2004), p. 308.
69. Sebastian Barry, *Whistling Psyche*, p. 15.
70. Gleitman, 'In the dank margins of things', p. 213.
71. 'A Mystery Still', *All the Year Round*, XVII (1866–67), 18 May 1867, p. 494.
72. Rachel Carroll, *Transgender and the Literary Imagination: Changing Gender in Twentieth Century Writing* (Edinburgh: Edinburgh University Press, 2018), chapter 3. For a contemporary version of the companionate master/servant relationship, see for example Sylvie Ouellette's *Le Secret du docteur Barry* (2012; Paris: Terres de femmes, De Borée, 2013).

73. Michael du Preez and Jeremy Dronfield, *Dr. James Barry: A Woman Ahead of Her Time* (London: Oneworld Publications, 2016), pp. 172–73, p. 222.
74. Binnie, *Colours*, Act I:8, p. 35 (Bristol Theatre Collection).
75. Ibid., Act II, p. 91.
76. Sebastian Barry, *Whistling Psyche*, p. 15, p. 43, p. 10.
77. Ibid., p. 11.
78. Ibid., p. 51.
79. Ibid., p. 46.
80. Ibid., p. 64. Nightingale's satirical description of Barry's appearance is reminiscent of the *Cape Town* and *London Illustrated News* illustration of the portrait in 'A Mystery Still'; see Fig. 3.6.
81. Brennan, *Tiger's Heart*, Act I, Scene 5, p. 38 (emphasis in original).
82. Ibid., Act I, Scene 16, p. 82.
83. Ibid., Act I, Scene 16, p. 81.
84. Ibid., Act I, Scene 13, p. 64.
85. Ibid., Act I, Scene 11, p. 57; Scene 2, p. 29.
86. Ibid., Act I, Scene 16, p. 80.
87. Ibid., Act II, Scene 28, p. 123, emphases in original.
88. Rogers Brubaker, *trans: Gender and Race in an Age of Unsettled Identities* (Princeton: Princeton University Press, 2016), p. 72 (emphases in original).
89. Saunders, *Self-Impression*, p. 216.
90. Ibid., p. 216, p. 218; see also brief outline in my introductory chapter.
91. Ina Schabert, 'Fictional Biography, Factual Biography, and their Contamination', *Biography*, vol. 5:1 (Winter 1982), p. 13.
92. Saunders, *Self-Impression*, p. 218.
93. Laura E. Savu, *Postmortem Postmodernists: The Afterlife of the Author in Recent Narrative* (Madison: Fairleigh Dickinson University Press, 2009).
94. A.S. Byatt, *The Biographer's Tale* (London: Quality Paperbacks Direct, 2000), p. 236. See also Julian Barnes's *Flaubert's Parrot* (London: Jonathan Cape, 1984). For a more teasing example see Vladimir Nabokov's *Pale Fire* (New York: Vintage International, 1989).
95. Ibid., p. 237; see also p. 214.
96. Schabert, 'Fictional Biography, Factual Biography, and their Contamination', p. 6.

97. Ibid. This is echoed in Michael Lackey's 'Introduction: A narrative space of its own', in *Biographical Fiction: A Reader*, ed. Michael Lackey (New York: Bloomsbury, 2016), p. 10: 'It is this art of transforming the biographical subject into a literary symbol that most distinguishes authors of biographies and biofiction.'
98. In some instances, Barry biofiction ends before Barry's death, thus circumventing posthumous disgrace for a 'happy ending' that sees Barry enjoying his retirement. This is the case in Anne and Ivan Kronenfeld's *The Secret Life of Dr. James Miranda Barry* (Cambridge, MD: Write Words, 2000), which ends with Barry/Pandora and her lover Leander preparing to attend Elizabeth Garrett's graduation ceremony, in May 1865 (two months before the historical Barry died – and factually five years before Garrett completed her medical studies). This counterfactual ending is, however, an exception in the Barry canon.
99. Schabert, 'Fictional Biography, Factual Biography, and their Contamination', pp. 5–7.
100. Ira B. Nadel, 'Narrative and the Popularity of Biography', *Mosaic*, vol. 20:4 (1987), p. 135.
101. Schabert, *In Quest of the Other Person*, p. 48, p. 60.
102. Ibid., 48. See also Martin Middeke, 'Introduction: Life-writing, Historical Consciousness, and Postmodernism', *Biofictions: The Rewriting of Romantic Lives in Contemporary Fiction and Drama*, ed. Martin Middeke and Werner Huber (London: Camden House, 1999), p. 22.
103. Colonel N.J.C. Rutherford, 'Dr. James Barry: Inspector-General of the Army Medical Department', *Journal of the Royal Army Medical Corps*, vol. LXIII (July–Dec. 1939), pp. 106–24, pp. 173–78, pp. 240–48. In *Dr. James Barry*, du Preez and Dronfield refer to the piece as a 'biographical essay', noting that, 'profoundly frustrated by the gaps and mysteries' in the documentary evidence, Rutherford had 'invented details quite literally to fill the empty spaces and solve the puzzles' (p. 383). They thus read Rutherford's text as a 'biography' in miniature (p. 388) when it is more accurately to be identified as a patchwork of anecdotes and mostly fictional earlier sources.
104. Rae's biography lists sources used for each chapter in a bibliography (*Strange Story*, pp. 118–20); Rose's *Perfect Gentleman* provides an annotated bibliography (but no chapter references) and an index; Holmes's *Scanty Particulars* (1) has a 'Select Bibliography' and an index but no references. Selected references are, however, supplied

in the US edition of *Scanty Particulars* (2) and the second UK edition, *The Secret Life of Dr. James Barry: Victorian England's Most Eminent Surgeon* (Stroud: Tempus, 2007); these versions, on the other hand, lack the self-reflexive discussion of the first edition's Preface; for further details see below and Chapter 2. Densely referenced, the most recent biography, *Dr. James Barry* by du Preez and Dronfield, adheres most closely to academic conventions.

105. Du Preez and Dronfield, *Dr. James Barry*, chapter 1, p. 3; chapter 6, p. 38; chapter 9, p. 94; chapter 21, p. 229; chapter 23, p. 254.
106. Holmes, *Scanty Particulars* (1), p. 93.
107. Ibid., pp. 126–27; see also pp. 59–60.
108. Ibid., p. 2.
109. By dropping the conceptual frame, the US and second UK editions of Holmes's biography also lose the opening to the paragraph that draws attention to the trope ('The outline of that attempt at an ending in Barry's case runs as follows …'; *Scanty Particulars* [1], p. 3). What in the first edition is presented as a deliberate and ironic mimicry of the conventional beginning (Barry's death, attended by the doctor, 'Black John' and Psyche) in the later editions becomes a replica of the very structure Holmes sets out to critique: 'July 1865. London sweats beneath a heat wave. The central streets of the city are a den of infection. Dr. James Miranda Barry, Inspector General of Hospitals and one of the most senior medical officers in the British military, lies dying at Margaret Street.' (Holmes, *Secret Life*, p. 7, and *Scanty Particulars* [2], p. ix; first line italicized). In contradistinction to the other biographies, however, this paragraph is followed by an overview of Barry's life rather than a disclosure of his sex.
110. Holmes, *Scanty Particulars* (1), p. 1. See the opening epigraph to this chapter. For Lewis Carroll's *Alice's Adventures in Wonderland* see *Alice in Wonderland*, ed. Donald J. Gray (New York: Norton, 1992), p. 94: '"Begin at the beginning," the King said, very gravely, "and go on until you come to the end: then stop."'
111. See Jacques Derrida, 'Of an Apocalyptic Tone Recently Adopted in Philosophy', *Oxford Literary Review*, vol. 6:2 (1984), p. 36.
112. Schabert, 'Fictional Biography, Factual Biography, and their Contamination', p. 6, see also above.
113. In the US and second UK editions the present tense is turned into the past, thus distancing the reader from the events.

114. Holmes, *Scanty Particulars* (1), pp. 8–11. Ouellette's novel *Le Secret du docteur Barry* offers a related reflection: Barry was 'né au moment de son admission à l'université', born in the moment of his admission to university (p. 11).
115. Holmes, *Scanty Particulars* (1), p. 298.
116. Ibid., p. 312.
117. Schabert, 'Fictional Biography, Factual Biography, and their Contamination', pp. 4–5.
118. Holmes, *Scanty Particulars* (1), p. 3.
119. Duncker's *James Miranda Barry* shows the young Barry taking one of Mr. Fyfe's dissection lessons, though here the corpse is male and Barry is inadvertently distracted by one of his friends having a fainting spell (pp. 66–68). The friend is Jobson, the factual fellow student who unsuccessfully tried to teach Barry boxing; in the novel, too, Jobson fails in this task, but is more successful in coaching Barry in the art of shooting, hence Barry's later reputation as a duellist. Du Preez and Dronfield's biography also contains a fictionalized dissection scene of a female corpse; here, however, it is the sexist jokes of his instructor that teach Barry that he needs to disconnect himself from the female flesh on which he operates. Severing off the dead woman's breasts in the process of dissecting the thorax, while Mr. Fyfe drops coarse remarks about the erotic qualities of the female nipple, Barry steels himself to the conviction that it 'was a mere organ, a formation of tissue; the passions of the mind had no place here, nor indeed its frailties. He lowered the blade, and began to cut' (*Dr. James Barry*, p. 72). The scene creates a vivid impression of the slippage of medical practice and sexual assault – the very reason why the historical Barry would so instantly and sharply intervene when he found syphilitic female patients subjected to abuse by male attendants on St Helena in 1836.
120. Jacques Derrida and Avital Ronell, 'The Law of Genre', *Critical Inquiry* (On Narrative), vol. 7:1 (1980), p. 57, p. 74.
121. Rae, *Strange Story*, p. v.
122. Ibid., p. vi. For her use of 'A Mystery Still's' story about the footman who after Barry's death settled all accounts see my earlier discussion in Chapter 2. For her adaptation of passages from Rogers's *A Modern Sphinx* see p. 90, where she quotes a passage about Dr. Fitzjames's kind treatment of a soldier's wife, arguing that 'it must surely bear the mark of truth'. Similarly, she draws on Racster and

Grove's fictional scenario when she describes Barry's dandified appearance: 'When off duty Dr. Barry went to balls wearing "a coat of the latest pea-green Hayne, a satin waistcoat, and a pair of tight-fitting 'inexpressibles'"' (p. 22). See Olga Racster and Jessica Grove, *The Journal of Dr. James Barry* (London: Lane, 1932), p. 21.

123. Rae, *Strange Story*, p. 29. For a similar influence of the cartoon on Rose's *Perfect Gentleman*, see p. 32 (as quoted in Chapter 3).
124. See Rae, *Strange Story*, p. 22, as above; Rose's *Perfect Gentleman* (p. 39), Holmes's *Scanty Particulars* (1, p. 67), and du Preez and Dronfield's *Dr. James Barry* (p. 178). The 'pea-green Hayne' coat also makes an appearance in Duncker's *James Miranda Barry*, p. 190.
125. 'A Mystery Still', p. 493; Rae, *Strange Story*, p. 82; Rose, *Perfect Gentleman*, p. 115; du Preez and Dronfield, *Dr. James Barry*, p. 282.
126. See Chapter 2 for Marjorie Garber's discussion, in *Vested Interests: Cross-Dressing and Cultural Anxiety* (1992; London: Penguin, 1993), of the 'normalization of the story of the transvestite' as a strategy of neutralizing the threat of gender transgression by reference to economic or emotional prerogatives (p. 69).
127. J. C. M'Crindle, 'Dr. James Barry', *Glasgow Herald* (December 1949), Wellcome Library, London, RAMC 238; Rose, *Perfect Gentleman*, p. 150. (The name is rendered elsewhere as McCrindle). Du Preez and Dronfield speculate that this ring was one of the mourning rings Mrs. Bulkley had made in 1809 when she had her will drawn up because of her failing health (*Dr. James Barry*, p. 56, p. 350).
128. 'The humble memorial of Dr. James Barry, Inspector General of Hospitals', undated draft [1859], Wellcome Library, London, RAMC 373; see Appendix 3.
129. Brennan, 'Foreword' to *Tiger's Heart*, p. 17; for the earlier parenthetical quotation see Rose, *Perfect Gentleman*, p. 150.
130. Binnie, *Colours*, Act I, p. 15 (Bristol Theatre Collection).
131. Holmes, *Scanty Particulars* (1), p. 281. The reference is to Lieutenant Colonel R.C. Francis writing in *Guy's Hospital Gazette* (27 September 1986). For parallels drawn with Mrs. Gamp see also Rutherford's 'Dr. James Barry', pp. 247–48. Du Preez and Dronfield note that the 'confident, irascible and bold' charwoman who insisted on seeing McKinnon to demand payment for her services 'could almost be Mrs. Gamp to the life' ('Appendix B: Who Discovered Dr. Barry's Secret?', *Dr. James Barry*, p. 391).
132. Holmes, *Scanty Particulars* (1), p. 19. Janet Carphin, letter to *Lancet*, 19 October 1895, p. 1021.

133. James Barry to General Miranda, 7 January 1810, reproduced in vol. 23 of the *Archivo del General Miranda*, ed. José Nucete Sardi, Antonio Alamo, Jacinto Fombona Pachano and Eduardo Arroyo Lamela, Academia Nacional de la Historia (CARACAS) (Caracas, 1929–50), pp. 265–67, British Library, London, Reference Collection 9774.h.1. Duncker, *James Miranda Barry*, pp. 65–66. The letter is quoted by Holmes, *Scanty Particulars* (1), pp. 28–29; Rose, *Perfect Gentleman,* pp. 24–25, and Rae, *Strange Story*, pp. 4–5.
134. Holmes, *Scanty Particulars* (1), p. 292. The early letter is dated 11 April 1804 and is signed Margaret Anne Bulkley; it was written at the dictation of her mother; June Rose Collection, RAMC 1264, Wellcome Library; see Appendix 1. Compare with James Barry, 'Memorandum of the Services of Dr. James Barry Inspector General of Hospitals', stamped 30 Jan 1859, Wellcome Library file RAMC 373; see Appendix 4.
135. See W. L. Pressly, 'Portrait of a Cork Family: The Two James Barrys', *Journal of the Cork Historical and Archaeological Society*, vol. 90 (1985), pp. 137–49. This article reproduces samples of Margaret Bulkley's and Barry's handwriting. A similar lacuna can be observed in Florida Ann Town's *With a Silent Companion* (1999; Alberta: Red Deer Press, 2000), the 'Epilogue' of which details the author's substantial archival research that led to her discovery of James Barry's birth identity but which omits any reference to Pressly as well as to two of the previous biographers, June Rose and Rachel Holmes.
136. Rose, *Perfect Gentleman*, p. 46. By contrast, Rose (p. 46), Rae (*Strange Story*, p. 27) and du Preez and Dronfield (*Dr. James Barry*, p. 162) note that Barry was sent to the island on official orders to deal with a cholera epidemic. Holmes draws on Rose's account to highlight the fact that news of the cholera outbreak in Mauritius in late 1819 did not reach the Cape Colony until early 1820, which makes it unlikely that Barry was sent there on formal business (*Scanty Particulars* [1], pp. 90–91).
137. Holmes, *Scanty Particulars* (1), p. 90. See also later discussion, p. 270.
138. Rose, *Perfect Gentleman*, p. 103.
139. Holmes, *Scanty Particulars* (1), p. 211.
140. Ibid., p. 309.
141. Garber, *Vested Interests,* p. 201, p. 202.

142. Quoted from the back cover of Holmes's *Scanty Particulars* (1).
143. Holmes, *Scanty Particulars* (1), pp. 2–3.
144. Ibid., p. 132; for the earlier quotation see p. 129.
145. Ibid., p. 57, p. 144.
146. Holmes cites the malicious rumours spread by Somerset and Barry's enemies in the British Parliament; *Scanty Particulars* (1), p. 143. For previous quotations see p. 57, p. 144.
147. Carroll, *Transgender and the Literary Imagination*, chapter 3. The earlier reference is to Barbin's autobiographical narrative, published posthumously by Ambroise Tardieu in 1874 and reproduced, originally in 1980, in *Michel Foucault présente Herculine Barbin dite Alexina B.* (1978; [Paris]: Gallimard, 2014); English edition: Michel Foucault [ed.], *Herculine Barbin: Being the Recently Discovered Memoirs of a Nineteenth-Century French Hermaphrodite*, trans. Richard McDougall (1980; New York: Vintage, 2010). Barbin anticipated his later dispossession on the dissection table: 'When that day comes a few doctors will make a little stir around my corpse; they will shatter all the extinct mechanisms of its impulses, will draw new information from it, will analyze all the mysterious sufferings that were heaped up on a single human being.' (Vintage, p. 103; Gallimard, p. 127). By choosing this passage for her epigraph to chapter 10, Holmes draws implicit analogies with the contemporary response to Barry's death, though Barry was more fortunate in that the sensation broke after his burial. For a brief synopsis of Barbin's case, see Alice Domurat Dreger, *Hermaphrodites and the Medical Invention of Sex* (Cambridge, Massachusetts: Harvard University Press, 1998), pp. 16–19. See also my discussion in the concluding chapter.
148. Holmes, *Scanty Particulars* (1), p. 320.
149. Ibid., p. 320.
150. Ibid., p. 321, p. 326.
151. Ibid., p. 320.
152. Ibid., p. 326.
153. Schabert, 'Fictional Biography, Factual Biography, and their Contamination', p. 1.
154. Ibid., p. 4, p. 5, p. 7.
155. Saunders, *Self-Impression*, p. 216, emphasis in original.
156. Holmes, *Scanty Particulars* (1), p. 34.
157. Binnie, *Colours*, Act II, p. 91 (Bristol Theatre Collection).
158. Duncker, *James Miranda Barry*, p. 3.
159. Ibid., p. 294.

160. Saunders, *Self-Impression*, p. 1.
161. Ibid., p. 221 (emphases in original).
162. Patricia Duncker, 'James Miranda Barry', *Monsieur Shoushana's Lemon Trees* (London: Serpent's Tail, 1997), 37.
163. Ibid., p. 37.
164. Ibid., p. 37.
165. Ibid., p. 38.
166. Ibid., p. 40. The painting depicts the 'Rape of the Sabines' myth; the real-life James Barry did not produce a painting on this motif.
167. Ibid., p. 31.
168. Ibid., p. 40.
169. Ibid., p. 40.
170. Ibid., p. 40.
171. Ibid., p. 40.
172. Ibid., p. 41.
173. Ibid., p. 41.
174. Ibid., p. 42.
175. Anna Livia (ed.), *The Pied Piper: Lesbian Feminist Fiction* (London: Onlywomen Press, 1989).
176. Depending on how the closing scene of *Whistling Psyche* is performed, the embrace of Barry and Nightingale can be given lesbian meaning. Olga Racster and Jessica Grove's *Journal of Dr. James Barry* tentatively gestures at female same-sex desire only to normalize any impulse toward sexual transgression: Sophie and Lavinia find happiness in suitable marriages, Barry spends the rest of her life secretly pining for Cloete, and rebellious and sexually unrestrained female characters like Mary die in childbirth. For the previous reference see Judith Halberstam, *Female Masculinity* (Durham: Duke University Press, 1998), p. 46: 'Such a presumption … funnels female masculinity into models of sexual deviance rather than accounting for the meanings of early female masculinity within the history of gender definition and gender relations.'
177. Lucia Boldrini, '"Allowing it to speak out of him": The Heterobiographies of David Malouf, Antonio Tabucci and Marguerite Yourcenar', in 'Autobiografictions: Comparatist Essays', ed. Lucia Boldrini and Peter Davies, special issue of *Comparative Critical Studies*, vol. 1:3 (2004), p. 252; Lucia Boldrini, *Autobiographies of Others: Historical Subjects and Literary Fiction* (London: Routledge, 2012), p. 5.

178. Schabert, *In Quest of the Other Person*, p. 35, p. 28.
179. The novel in question was *Hallucinating Foucault* (London: Bloomsbury, 1996), a pseudo-biofiction and heterobiography in which a PhD student working on a prominent (invented) queer French poststructuralist writer, whose own identity is tied to his passionate, textually embodied reader-writer relationship with Foucault, seeks out the object of his study, now confined to a psychiatric hospital in the French provinces. The information about the protracted composition of *James Miranda Barry* derives from Patricia Duncker's response to audience questions about biofictional working practices following her keynote lecture on 'Re-Imagining George Eliot' at the BAVS 2016: 'Consuming (the) Victorians' conference at Cardiff University on 31 August 2016.
180. Patricia Duncker, 'The Lunatic, the Lover and the Poet: On Writing *Hallucinating Foucault*', in *Spatial Representations of British Identities*, ed. Merle Tönnies and Heike Buschmann (Heidelberg, Winter: 2012), p. 24.
181. Duncker, *James Miranda Barry*, pp. 5–6.
182. Ibid., p. 298: 'The stone sarcophagus is cracked across. There is a huge fissure in the lid of her grave, as if the last day has already been announced and her spirit has escaped. I peer surreptitiously into the crack, but see only lichen, earth and broken stone.'
183. Ibid., p. 274. The factual Mary Anne is in Duncker's novel rendered as Mary Ann.
184. Ibid., p. 4, p. 27.
185. See Plates 28 and 98 in William L. Pressly, *The Life and Art of James Barry* (New Haven: Yale University Press, 1981).
186. National Portrait Gallery, London, c.1767, http://www.npg.org.uk/collections/search/portrait/mw00371/James-Barry-Dominique-Lefevre-James-Paine-the-Younger?LinkID=mp03421&role=sit&rNo=0 [accessed 8 April 2016]; Plate 4 in Pressly, *The Life and Art of James Barry*, p. 12. For other editions of the translated novel see Duncker's website, http://patriciaduncker.com/books/james-miranda-barry.html [accessed 27 August 2016].
187. In her portrayal of the painter's dilapidated house and neighbourhood, Duncker draws on contemporary accounts reproduced in chapter 9 ('The Late Years') of Pressly's *The Life and Art of James Barry*, such as W.H. Curran's contemporary account (cited by Pressly, p. 189): '[the area in front of the house was] bestrewn with skeletons of cats and dogs, marrow-bones, waste-paper, fragments

of boys' hoops, and other playthings, and with the many kinds of missiles, which the pious brats of the neighb[ou]rhood had hurled against the unhallowed premises. A dead cat lay upon the projecting stone of the parlour window, immediately under a sort of appeal to the public, or a proclamation setting forth, that a dark conspiracy existed for the wicked purpose of molesting the writer, and injuring his reputation, and concluding with an offer of some pounds as a reward to any one, who should give such information as might lead to the detection and conviction of the offenders. This was in Barry's handwriting, and occupied the place of one pane of glass. The rest of the framework was covered with what I had once imagined to be necromantic devices – some of his own etchings, but turned upside down, of his great paintings at the Adelphi'. See Duncker, *James Miranda Barry*, pp. 124–27.

188. See Holmes's opening point that 'It is a vexing prospect for any biographer to attempt to write about a subject who appears to have had no childhood.' (*Scanty Particulars* [1], p. 1).
189. Rose, *Perfect Gentleman*, p. 31; Holmes, *Scanty Particulars* (1), p. 143. Racster and Grove's *Journal* repeatedly alludes to a mysterious family secret that put Somerset in charge of Barry's fortunes. Somerset engineered her disastrous marriage to the Baronet Thomas Barrymore, then helped her escape, and expresses a sense of responsibility for her well-being. Rose's *Perfect Gentleman* draws attention to the fact that 'All through her life [Barry's] attachment to Charles Somerset was undoubtedly her most important human contact'; 'In as far as [Lord Charles] was concerned he was the only man who knew her secret and her family background. Whatever passed between them, it seems clear that he represented father, brother, protector – and even lover. In fact whatever "normal" emotions she allowed herself to feel for a man were expressed in her relationship with him.' (*Perfect Gentleman*, p. 49, p. 45). In *Scanty Particulars* Holmes suggests that Barry's first spaniel named Psyche was a lover's present: 'Psyche's presence is an invocation of the absent, elusive figure of Cupid, a continual reference to the mysterious coupling in darkness whose product was Pleasure' ([1], p. 83). Somerset's Romantic disregard for conventions (he had eloped with his first wife), his strong erotic drive combined with his widowerhood, Barry's need of a confidant and an intimate relationship, his position as Somerset's favourite, even the jealous fit that resulted in the duel

with Cloete, as well as Barry's withdrawal to Mauritius when Somerset decided to look out for a new wife: all 'the evidence … points towards a strange, compelling and erotic relationship' (p. 65). Du Preez and Dronfield also suggest a passionate mutual attachment, but their biography is surprisingly reticent about the nature of the relationship, in contradistinction to other parts of Barry's emotional and sexual life, where they allow free reign to the imagination (such as speculations about Margaret's teenage rape and pregnancy, her ever resurgent femininity and the revelations of her travelling trunk).

190. Rachel Carroll reads this as an 'erasure of [Barry's] colonial history' that parallels the 'erasure of Barry's Irish heritage' since the novel anglicizes the childhood settings and also relocates Lord Erskine's Scottish estate to Shropshire; see *Transgender and the Literary Imagination*, chapter 3. The island setting, on the other hand, draws on the historical Barry's postings to Mauritius and Malta; at the same time, Barry's Greek assistant and the prominence of Greek names among the islanders suggest Corfu. It was in Corfu that Barry struck an officer in the face with his whip for parading his men in the full glare of the midday sun; the novel's Captain Boaden is modelled on the real-life Colonel Denny. See Holmes, *Scanty Particulars* (1), pp. 238–39.
191. Jay Prosser, *Second Skins: The Body Narratives of Transsexuality* (New York: Columbia University Press, 1998), p. 5.
192. Eveline Kilian, *GeschlechtSverkehrt: Theoretische und literarische Perspektiven des gender-bending* (Königstein: Ulrike Helmer Verlag, 2004), p. 138.
193. See Mary Hammond's review of the novel, 'The Enigma of James Barry', *Women: A Cultural Review*, vol. 13:1 (2010), pp. 104–106.
194. Georges Letissier, 'Nomadic Transgender Identity: Patricia Duncker's *James Miranda Barry* and Wesley Stace's *Misfortune*', *Neo-Victorian Studies*, vol. 9:2 (2017), p. 16, p. 31.
195. Jana Funke, 'Obscurity and Gender Resistance in Patricia Duncker's *James Miranda Barry*', *European Journal of English Studies*, vol. 16:3 (2012), p. 224.
196. Letissier, 'Nomadic Transgender Identity', p. 15.
197. Judith Halberstam, *In a Queer Time and Place: Transgender Bodies, Subcultural Lives* (New York: New York University Press, 2005), p. 153.
198. Bianca Leggett, 'Teaching Translit: An Unsettled and Unsettling Genre', in *Teaching twenty-first Century Genres*, ed. Katy Shaw

(Basingstoke: Palgrave, 2016), p. 149, p. 150. 'Translit' is, however, primarily applied to novels that 'cross history without being historical' by 'insert[ing] the contemporary reader into other locations and times, while leaving no doubt that [the] viewpoint is relentlessly modern and speaks entirely of our extreme present'; see Douglas Coupland's review of Hari Kunzru's *Gods Without Men* in which he coined the term, 'Convergences', *New York Times*, 8 March 2012, http://www.nytimes.com/2012/03/11/books/review/gods-without-men-by-hari-kunzru.html [accessed 1 August 2017].

199. See above for pointers to Corfu. Barry first visited Mauritius in 1819–20 and was formally posted there in 1928. Both Malta and Corfu have Turkish forts and monasteries, settings that are referenced in the novel.
200. Duncker, *James Miranda Barry*, p. 256. The historical Barry witnessed the eruption of cholera in Mauritius in November 1819 (Rose, *Perfect Gentleman*, p. 46).
201. The only exception are Parts Five and Six, both narrated in the first person; but any sense of continuity is disrupted by the temporal distance of over two decades.
202. Nünning, 'Fictional Metabiographies and Metaautobiographies', p. 203, p. 205. For the earlier quotations, in sequential order, see Nünning, 'Fictional Metabiographies and Metaautobiographies', p. 201; Ansgar Nünning, 'An Intertextual Quest for Thomas Chatterton: the Deconstruction of the Romantic Cult of Originality and the Paradoxes of Life-Writing in Peter Ackroyd's Fictional Metabiography *Chatterton*', in *Biofictions: The Rewriting of Romantic Lives in Contemporary Fiction and Drama*, ed. Martin Middeke and Werner Huber (London: Camden House, 1999), p. 29.
203. Nünning, 'Fictional Metabiographies and Metaautobiographies', p. 207.
204. Ibid., p. 202, p. 203.
205. Duncker, *James Miranda Barry*, p. 107.
206. Ibid., p. 151.
207. 'Comedy of Masks' references *Commedia dell'Arte*, from which this image is adapted; Giacomo Oreglia, *The Commedia dell'Arte*, trans. Lovett F. Edwards (London: Methuen,1968), p. 1.
208. For a reproduction of the Scaramucia and Fricasso pairing from Jacques Callot's *Balli di Sfessania* see Oreglia, *The Commedia dell'Arte*, p. 147. The etching is also featured in 'Balli di Sfessania',

Giornale Nuovo, 11 June 2004, http://www.spamula.net/blog/2004/06/balli_di_sfessania.html [accessed 19 April 2017]. I am grateful to Chris Balme for drawing my attention to Callot's ballet.

209. Holmes, *Scanty Particulars* (1), p. 44.
210. Ibid., p. 63; Rae, *Strange Story*, p. 21.
211. Holmes, *Scanty Particulars* (1), p. 237. As Kathryn Hughes notes in *Victorians Undone: Tales of the Flesh in the Age of Decorum* (London: 4th Estate, 2017), shaving was *de rigeur* up to the late 1850s: 'Throughout the first half of the nineteenth century a hairy chin had been the badge of the political dissident or one of those other figures from a nightmare, the Frenchman, the Irishman, artist or tramp' (p. 99).
212. Holmes, *Scanty Particulars* (1), p. 237. See Hughes's discussion of the impact of the mid-century's Beard movement on Carlyle, Collins, Darwin, Dickens, Lear and Tennyson in chapter 2 of *Victorians Undone*, particularly pp. 99–107.
213. Duncker, *James Miranda Barry*, p. 216.
214. Ibid., p. 219.
215. John Leigh, *Touché: The Duel in Literature* (Cambridge, MA: Harvard University Press, 2015), p. 293.
216. This image, entitled 'Murray Miniature' in the Wellcome Library file of the holdings of the Museum of Military Medicine, RAMC 801.6.5.3, is referenced as a 'watercolour painting of Dr James Barry executed at the Cape some time before 1828' in Percival R. Kirby's 'Dr James Barry, Controversial South African Medical Figure: A Recent Evaluation of His Life and Sex', *South African Medical Journal*, 25 April 1970, p. 511, Wellcome Library, RAMC 658.
217. Duncker, *James Miranda Barry*, p. 102.
218. Ibid., p. 229.
219. Ibid., p. 264; for previous quotations see p. 243, p. 263.
220. Ibid., p. 35; for earlier quotation see p. 48.
221. Duncker, *James Miranda Barry*, p. 94; Funke, 'Obscurity and Gender Resistance in Patricia Duncker's *James Miranda Barry*', p. 218.
222. Butler, *Gender Trouble*, p. 47; Kilian, *GeschlechtSverkehrt,* p. 66.
223. Duncker, *James Miranda Barry*, p. 277.
224. Carroll, *Transgender and the Literary Imagination*, chapter 3. See also Holmes, *Scanty Particulars* (1), p. 293: 'Much has been made of the assistance the young Barry received from august male patrons. … But Mary Anne Bulkley's maternal persistence and determination

were equally important.' In Town's novel, while Mary Anne is a considerably less forceful character and is not the moving force behind her daughter's transformation, she does assert herself when she breaks with husband and son to focus all her energies on helping Margaret succeed. When after Miranda's death Margaret wants to give up, it's her mother whose encouragement makes her determined to persevere.

225. Duncker, *James Miranda Barry*, p. 368. See Simone de Beauvoir's famous dictum, 'One is not born, but rather becomes, a woman', *The Second Sex*, ed. and trans. H. M. Parshley (1949; London: Picador, 1988), p. 296.
226. Duncker, *James Miranda Barry*, p. 368 (emphases in original).
227. Ibid., p. 358.
228. Binnie, *Colours*, Act II, p. 78 (Bristol Theatre Collection).
229. Duncker, *James Miranda Barry*, p. 257.
230. Derrida and Ronell, 'The Law of Genre', p. 57.
231. Ibid., p. 57; Hayden White, 'Anomalies of Genre: The Utility of Theory and History for the Study of Literary Genres', *New Literary Theory*, 34:3 (Summer 2003), p. 600.

Chapter 5

1. Patricia Duncker, *Hallucinating Foucault* (London: Serpent's Tail, 1996), p. 112. *Hallucinating Foucault* constitutes an intertext for *James Miranda Barry* since it was written when Duncker hit difficulties with her novel-in-progress. (Question and answer session following Duncker's keynote on 'Re-Imagining George Eliot', 'BAVS 2016: Consuming [the] Victorians' conference, Cardiff University, 31 August 2016.)
2. Ansgar Nünning, 'Fictional Metabiographies and Metaautobiographies: Towards a Definition, Typology and Analysis of Self-Reflexive Hybrid Metagenres', in *Self-Reflexivity in Literature*, ed. Werner Huber, Martin Middeke, and Hubert Zapf (Würzburg: Königshausen & Neumann, 2005), p. 199.
3. Anne Garréta, *Sphinx*, trans. Emma Ramadan (Dallas, Texas: Deep Vellum Publishing, 2015), p. 117.
4. Marjorie Garber, *Vested Interests: Cross-Dressing and Cultural Anxiety* (1992; London: Penguin, 1993), p. 11.

5. Jack Halberstam, *Trans: A Quick and Quirky Account of Gender Variability* (Oakland, CA: University of California Press, 2018), p. 8. As Halberstam notes, initiatives like trans artist Chris E. Vargas's MOTHA (Museum of Transhirstory and Art) seek to address this lacuna. See http://www.sfmotha.org/
6. Judith Halberstam, *In a Queer Time and Place: Transgender Bodies, Subcultural Lives* (New York: New York University Press, 2005), p. 55.
7. Trev Broughton, 'Life Writing and the Victorians', in *The Oxford Handbook of Victorian Literary Culture*, ed. Juliet John (Oxford: Oxford University Press, 2016), p. 46.
8. Ethel Smyth's 'The March of the Women' (1910) was adopted as their anthem by the Women's Social and Political Union.
9. See Juliet Jacques, *Trans: A Memoir* (London: Verso, 2015), p. 309: 'fiction is a field in which trans people have not been well represented. In literary fiction, trans characters tend to be written by outsiders [non-trans authors] – to illustrate their wider points about gender, or to make things more exotic.'
10. Julia Novak, 'The Notable Woman in Fiction: The Afterlives of Elizabeth Barrett Browning', *a/b: Auto/Biography Studies*, vol. 31:1 (2016), p. 88.
11. Marie-Luise Kohlke, 'Sexsation and the Neo-Victorian Novel: Orientalising the Nineteenth Century in Contemporary Fiction', in *Negotiating Sexual Idioms: Image, Text, Performance*, ed. Marie-Luise Kohlke and Luisa Orza (Amsterdam: Rodopi, 2008), p. 67.
12. Sebastian Barry, *Whistling Psyche,* in *Whistling Psyche. Fred and Jane* (London: Faber and Faber, 2004), p. 43.
13. 'James Miranda Barry', Commemorative Plaques, University of Edinburgh, 16 October 2015, http://www.ed.ac.uk/about/people/plaques/barry [accessed 5 August 2016].
14. Michael du Preez and Jeremy Dronfield, *Dr. James Barry: A Woman Ahead of Her Time* (London: Oneworld Publications, 2016), p. 150.
15. Kit Brennan, 'Foreword' to *Tiger's Heart* (1996; Vancouver: Scirocco Drama, revised edn 1998), p. 17.
16. June Rose, *The Perfect Gentleman: The remarkable life of Dr. James Miranda Barry, the woman who served as an officer in the British Army from 1813 to 1859* (London: Hutchinson, 1977), p. 32; Rachel Holmes, *Scanty Particulars: The Mysterious, Astonishing and Remarkable Life of Victorian Surgeon James Barry* (London: Penguin,

2003), p. 320, hereafter *Scanty Particulars* (1). See also my previous discussion in Chapter 4.

17. The metaphor of the rear-view mirror as a marker of the neo-Victorian desire to reconstruct the nineteenth century originates from Simon Joyce's *The Victorians in the Rearview Mirror* (Athens: Ohio University Press, 2007). For the 'desire to speak with the dead' see Holmes's 'Epilogue', which muses about whether Barry wished to be discovered by the afterworld, and starts with an epigraph that cites the opening of Stephen Greenblatt's *Shakespearean Negotiations: The Circulation of Energy in Renaissance England* (Oxford: Oxford University Press, 2001), p. 1: 'I began with the desire to speak with the dead.' (*Scanty Particulars*, p. 320).
18. See Mary Shelley's 'Introduction' to the 1831 edition of *Frankenstein*, ed. Johanna M. Smith (Boston: Bedford/St. Martin's, 2000), p25.
19. Caroline Lusin, 'Writing Lives and "Worlds": English Biographical Fiction at the Turn of the 21st Century', in *Mediation, Remediation and the Dynamics of Cultural Memory*, ed. Astrid Erll and Ann Rigney in collaboration with Laura Basu and Paulus Bijl (Berlin: de Gruyter, 2009), pp. 265–67; Lusin's reference point is Nelson Goodman's *Ways of Worldmaking* (1978; Indianapolis: Hackett Publishing, 1992).
20. Max Saunders, *Self-Impression: Life-Writing, Autobiografiction, and the Forms of Modern Literature* (Oxford: Oxford University Press, 2010).
21. Marie-Luise Kohlke, 'Neo-Victorian Biofiction and the Special/Spectral Case of Barbara Chase-Riboud's *Hottentot Venus*', *Australasian Journal of Victorian Studies*, vol. 18:3 (2013), pp. 4–21. The notion of 'ex-centricity' originates from Linda Hutcheon's discussion of historiographic metafiction's interest in characters marginalized in official history; see *A Poetics of Postmodernism: History, Theory, Fiction* (London: Routledge, 1988), p. 95.
22. Kohlke, 'Neo-Victorian Biofiction', p. 5.
23. For references in this paragraph see ibid., p. 11, p. 13.
24. Nünning, 'Fictional Metabiographies and Metaautobiographies', p. 198, see opening epigraph to Chapter 1; for discussion of his typology of biofiction see Chapter 4.
25. Jacques Derrida and Avital Ronell, 'The Law of Genre', *Critical Inquiry* (On Narrative), vol. 7:1 (1980), p. 57.

26. Hermione Lee, *Body Parts: Essays on Life-Writing* (London: Pimlico, 2008), p. 8. Jay Prosser, *Second Skins: The Body Narratives of Transsexuality* (New York: Columbia University Press, 1998). Rogers Brubaker, *trans: Gender and Race in an Age of Unsettled Identities* (Princeton: Princeton University Press, 2016).
27. Ansgar Nünning, 'Making Events – Making Stories – Making Worlds: Ways of Worldmaking from a Narratological Point of View', in *Mediation, Remediation and the Dynamics of Cultural Memory*, ed. Astrid Erll and Ann Rigney in collaboration with Laura Basu and Paulus Bijl (Berlin: de Gruyter, 2009), p. 209.
28. As Elaine Showalter comments in her biography, the novel reflects Howe's 'feelings of loneliness, rejection, and uncertainty, as a woman and an artist' and can be read as 'a metaphor for her own feelings of androgyny and a mediation on her husband's emotional and sexual absence'; it discloses 'a wildly unconventional side of her imagination, with hidden depths of sexual fantasy, anger and protest'. Showalter, *The Civil Wars of Julia Ward Howe: A Biography* (New York: Simon & Schuster, 2016), p. 88. For the composition period of the text see Gary Williams, 'Speaking with the Voices of Others', introduction to Julia Ward Howe, *The Hermaphrodite*, ed. Gary Williams (Lincoln: University of Nebraska Press, 2004), p. x.
29. Howe, *The Hermaphrodite*, p. 195.
30. Ibid., p. 19.
31. 'One long gaze of tearless anguish, one mute appeal to heaven, and Ronald was gone, and the beautiful monster sat as before on the heap of stones, in the ancient forum, himself as mute and dead as any thing there'; Howe, *The Hermaphrodite*, p. 193; for earlier quotation see p. 19.
32. Howe, *The Hermaphrodite*, p. 22. This statement resonates with the protagonist's self-assessment in George Moore's novella 'Albert Nobbs'; see my discussion in Chapter 3.
33. Ibid., p. 131.
34. Ibid., p. 136.
35. 'Laurence, do not hold your head so stiffly erect. Let me see you sit down, slowly and softly. For heaven's sake, do not put back your hand to divide your skirts, it is not a feminine custom. Your legs are too far apart, your knees must touch each other. Let me see you rise … now, walk – petticoats en avant, mince your steps, and undulate a little more in your movements. Let me hear you laugh – not so loud, if you

please, and pray make a more gradual disclosure of your teeth. You will do exceedingly well, I think – upon my soul, you are a handsome creature!' Howe, *The Hermaphrodite*, p. 136.

36. Ibid., p. 187.
37. Ibid., p. 197.
38. Intense groin pains, which were caused by a descending testicle.
39. Chesnet, 'Question d'identité: vice de confirmation des organes génitaux externes; hypospadias; erreur sur le sexe', *Annales d'hygiène publique et de medicine légale*, vol. XIV (1860), repr. in *Michel Foucault présente Herculine Barbin dite Alexina B.* ([Paris]: Gallimard, 2014), p. 150; English-language edition: Michel Foucault [ed.], *Herculine Barbin*, trans Richard McDougall (New York: Vintage, 2010), p. 128.
40. The 'Dossier' contains biographical, periodical press and medical material as well as a satirical biofiction: Oscar Panizza's German-language story of 1893, 'Ein skandalöser Fall' [in *Visionen der Dämmerung* (München: G. Müller, 1914)], repr. as 'A Scandal at the Convent' (1893), trans. Sophie Wilkins, in *Herculine Barbin*, [ed.] Michel Foucault (New York: Vintage, 2010), pp. 154–99; 'Un scandale au couvent', trans Jean Bréjoux, in *Michel Foucault présente Herculine Barbin dite Alexina B.* ([Paris]: Gallimard, 2014), pp. 173–220. The story satirizes female professional rivalry between the low-born and ambitious Head Sister of a convent and the wealthy aristocratic Mother Superior, whose protégée is discovered in bed with her favourite and most gifted school girl Alexina. In the course of the witch hunt the Head Sister instigates, all the exposed parties are forced to leave and the Head Sister succeeds in her plan of assuming the Mother Superior's role.
41. *Mes souvenirs*, in *Michel Foucault présente Herculine Barbin dite Alexina B.* (1978; [Paris]: Gallimard, 2014), p. 127, p. 77, also p. 133; English-language edition: *My Memoirs*, in *Herculine Barbin*, [ed.] Michel Foucault, trans Richard McDougall (1980; New York: Vintage, 2010), p. 103, p. 54, also p. 110. These editions will hereafter be referenced as 'Gallimard edition' and 'Vintage edition'.
42. '[C]omme si le changement d'état civil n'avait pas eu lieu. En fait, Abel disparaît ainsi tout à fait avec son suicide, laissant derrière lui, en même temps qu'un manuscript, la jeune femme qu'il a été.' Eric Fassin, 'Postface: Le vrai genre', *Michel Foucault présente Herculine Barbin dite Alexina B.* ([Paris]: Gallimard, 2014), p. 243. This postscript is not available in the 2010 English-language edition.

43. See references to 'Monsieur', 'son ami' (not 'son amie') and 'mon [not 'ma'] pauvre Camille', Gallimard edition, p. 110, p. 115, p. 121. Apart from the male title (Vintage edition, p. 86), male address is difficult to render in English.
44. Michel Foucault, 'Préface: Le vraie sexe', *Michel Foucault présente Herculine Barbin dite Alexina B.* ([Paris]: Gallimard, 2014), p. 17; [English-language edition] 'Introduction', *Herculine Barbin*, [ed.] Michel Foucault (New York: Vintage, 2010), p. xiii.
45. 'Peut-être cet soif de l'inconnu, si naturelle à l'homme.' (Gallimard, p. 138; Vintage, p. 115) Arguably, 'man' here can be taken to stand for humanity, but the closure on masculinity is surely significant, even if, given the edited nature of the text, we cannot be certain that this is how the manuscript actually concluded.
46. 'She enjoyed being "other" without ever having to be "of the other sex"' (Foucault, 'Préface: Le vrai sexe', Gallimard edition, p. 18). This sentence is missing from the English-language edition.
47. For an in-depth critique of the 'constitutive contradiction' of Foucault's instrumentalization of Barbin's narrative in his 'anti-emancipatory call for sexual freedom', see Judith Butler, *Gender Trouble: Feminism and the Subversion of Identity* (New York: Routledge, 1990), p. 97, pp. 93–106.
48. Foucault, 'Postface: Le vrai genre', Gallimard edition, p. 17; Vintage, p. xiii. Rogers Brubaker, *trans: Gender and Race in an Age of Unsettled Identities* (Princeton: Princeton University Press, 2016), p. 10.
49. 'If I were to write a novel, I could … produce pages that would be as dramatic, as gripping, as any that have ever been created by Alexandre Dumas or Paul Féval!' (Vintage edition, p. 35; Gallimard edition, p. 58). The hero's name is given as 'Camille' and the emotional intensity of the text is heightened by hyperbolic use of exclamation marks, creating the impression of an over-excited, almost feverish narrative voice.
50. *Herculine Barbin*, Vintage edition, p. 32; Gallimard edition, p. 55. For the parallel with *Jane Eyre*, see Vintage edition, p. 9; Gallimard edition, pp. 31–32: at eleven, Barbin falls in love 'at first sight' with Lea, a girl of 'modest grace' and frail health who is marked out for an early and tragic death.
51. Jay Prosser, *Second Skins: The Body Narratives of Transsexuality* (New York: Columbia University Press, 1998), p. 119.

52. For the first doctor's 'extraordinary excitement' see *Herculine Barbin*, Vintage edition, p. 68; Gallimard edition, p. 92.
53. See Chesnet above and E. Gujon, 'Étude d'un cas d'hermaphrodisme imparfait chez l'homme', *Journal de l'anatomie et de la physiology de l'homme* (1869), pp. 609–39, repr. in *Michel Foucault présente Herculine Barbin dite Alexina B.* ([Paris]: Gallimard, 2014), pp. 151–64; English-language edition: 'A study of a case of incomplete hermaphroditism in a man', *Herculine Barbin*, [ed.] Michel Foucault, trans Richard McDougall (New York: Vintage, 2010), pp. 128–44.
54. Fassin, 'Postface: Le vrai genre', p. 256, p. 258.
55. *Herculine Barbin*, Vintage edition, p. 109; Gallimard edition, p. 133.
56. *Herculine Barbin*, Vintage edition, p. 90; Gallimard edition, p. 114.
57. Virginia Woolf, *A Room of One's Own*, in *A Room of One's Own/Three Guineas*, ed. Michèle Barrett (London: Penguin, 1993), p. 32.
58. See the epigraph from Patricia Duncker's *Hallucinating Foucault* that opens this chapter, and Katriona Gilmore, Gilmore & Roberts, 'Doctor James', *The Innocent Left*, released by Navigator Records, 2012.

The Barry Archive

Chronology of Selected Primary Sources on James Barry in Victorian and Neo-Victorian Life-Writing

1804	Mary Anne Bulkley to James Barry RA, 11 April 1804, letter written and co-signed by Margaret Anne Bulkley, Wellcome Library, London, RAMC 373 [Appendix 1]
1805	Mary Anne Bulkley to James Barry RA, 14 January 1805, Wellcome Library, London, RAMC 373
1810	James Barry to General Miranda, 7 January 1810, Archivo del general Miranda, 24 vols, (Caracas, 1929–50), vol. 23, ed. José Nucete Sardi, Antonio Alamo, Jacinto Fombona Pachano and Eduardo Arroyo Lamela, pp. 265–67. British Library, General Reference Collection 9774.h.1.
1812	Jacobus Barry, 'Disputatio Medica Inauguralis, de Merocele, vel Hernia Crurali' (June 1812), Edinburgh Research Archive, https://www.era.lib.ed.ac.uk/handle/1842/417 [accessed 8 November 2015].
[1859]	James Barry, 'The humble memorial of Dr. James Barry, Inspector General of Hospitals', undated draft [1859], Wellcome Library, London, RAMC 373. [Appendix 3]
1859	James Barry, 'Memorandum of the Services of Dr. James Barry Inspector General of Hospitals', stamped 30 Jan 1859, Wellcome Library, London, RAMC 373. [Appendix 4]

A. Heilmann, *Neo-/Victorian Biographilia and James Miranda Barry*, https://doi.org/10.1007/978-3-319-71386-1

1865 'From our own correspondent', *Saunders's News-Letter and Daily Advertiser*, 14 August 1865, repr. in Percival R. Kirby, 'The Centenary of the Death of James Barry, M.D., Inspector-General of Hospitals (1795–1865)', *Africana Notes and News*, vol. 16:6 (June 1965), pp. 230–31, Wellcome Library, London, RAMC 455.

1865 'A Strange Story', *Manchester Guardian*, 21 August 1865.

1865 George Graham, Registrar General, to Staff Surgeon Major D.R. McKinnon, 23 August 1865, Wellcome Library, London, RAMC 373.

1865 Staff Surgeon [David Reid] McKinnon to the Registrar General of Somerset House, 24 August 1865, Wellcome Library, London, RAMC 373.

1865 'A Female Medical Combatant', *Medical Times and Gazette*, 26 August 1865, pp. 227–28.

1865 Edward Bradford, Deputy-Inspector-General of Hospitals, 'The Reputed Female Army Surgeon: Letter from Deputy-Inspector Bradford', *Medical Times and Gazette*, 9 September 1865, p.293.

[1865/1952] Nightingale, Florence, undated fragment of letter headed 'to Mama by Parthe's desire' [August 1865?], filed with a newspaper clip and transcript by John Guest, 'Sharp Encounter', *Sunday Times*, 9 November 1952, 'Letters by Nightingale, 1864–1865', Wellcome Library, London, Ms. 9001/145.

1867 'A Mystery Still', *All the Year Round*, XVII (1866–67), 18 May 1867, pp. 492–95.

1881 Major E[benezer] Rogers, *A Modern Sphinx*, 3 vols (London: John and Robert Maxwell, 1881). British Library Historical Print editions.

1882 Major E. Rogers, *Madeline's Mystery.* Edited by the author of Lady Audley's Secret [*sic*] (London: J. and R. Maxwell, [1882]). Harry Ransom Center, The University of Texas at Austin, WOLFF 752.

1895 George A. Bright, M.D., U.S. Navy, 'A Female Member of the Army Medical Staff', 'Notes, Comments, and Answers to Correspondents' section, *Lancet* [letter dated

30 September 1895, followed by editor's note], vol. 3763, 12 October 1895, p.959.

1895 Janet Carphin, 'To the Editors of *The Lancet*', 'Notes, Comments, and Answers to Correspondents' section, *Lancet* [letter dated 14 October 1895], vol. 3764, 19 October 1895, p.1021.

1895 H. Laing Gordon, M.D. Edin., 'To the Editors of *The Lancet*', 'Notes, Comments, and Answers to Correspondents' section, *Lancet* [letter dated 14 October 1895], vol. 3764, 19 October 1895, p.1021.

1895 C. F. Moore, M.D., F.R.C.S., Ireland, 'To the Editors of *The Lancet*', 'Notes, Comments, and Answers to Correspondents' section, *Lancet* [letter dated 14 October 1895], vol. 3764, 19 October 1895, p.1021.

1895 E. Rogers, Lieutenant-Colonel, late Staff Officer of Pensioners and formerly Captain 3rd West India Regiment, 'A Female Member of the Army Medical Staff', 'Notes, Comments, and Answers to Correspondents' section, *Lancet* [letter dated 15 October 1895], vol. 3764, 19 October 1895, p.1021.

1895 A.M.S., 'To the Editors of *The Lancet*', 'Notes, Comments, and Answers to Correspondents' section, *Lancet* [letter dated 16 October 1895], vol. 3764, 19 October 1895, p.1021.

1895 'Captain', 'To the Editors of *The Lancet*', 'Notes, Comments, and Answers to Correspondents' section, *Lancet* [letter dated 17 October 1895], vol. 3765, 26 October 1895, p.1087. [This entry is followed by an editor's note.]

1895 E. Rogers, Lieutenant-Colonel, 'A Female Member of the Army Medical Staff', 'Notes, Comments, and Answers to Correspondents' section, *Lancet* [letter dated 21 October 1895], vol. 3765, 26 October 1895, pp. 1086–87.

1896 E. Rogers, Lieutenant Colonel, 'A Female Member of the Army Medical Staff', 'Notes, Comments, and Answers to Correspondents' section, *Lancet* [letter dated 28 April 1896], vol. 3792, 2 May 1896, p.264.

1896	Lieut.-Colonel E. Rogers, *A Modern Sphinx: A Novel.* Edition de luxe, with seven illustrations. In one volume (London: n.p. [1896]). British Library General Reference Collection, C.194.a.672.
1904	George Edwin Marvell, 'The Mystery of the Kapok Doctor'. Section on 'Romances of the Cape'. *Cape Times Christmas Annual*, December 1904, pp. 13–19. National Library of South Africa, General Reference Collection 1876–1910.
1919	Olga Racster and Jessica Grove, *Dr. James Barry: A romantic play founded on South African history* (1919), Lord Chamberlain's Office, British Library, LCP 1919/17 I No.2338.
1920	Réné Juta, *Cape Currey* (1920; Memphis: General Books, 2010).
1929	G.E.C., 'An Amazing Male Impersonation: The Strange Story of James Barry, Esq., M.D.', *Illustrated London News*, 16 March 1929, p.148.
1932	Olga Racster and Jessica Grove, *The Journal of Dr. James Barry* (London: Lane, 1932).
1932	Olga Racster and Jessica Grove, *Dr. James Barry: Her Secret Story* (London: Gerald Howe, 1932). With five illustrations.
1939	Colonel N[athaniel] J[ohn] C[rawford] Rutherford, 'Dr James Barry: Inspector-General of the Army Medical Department', *Journal of the Royal Army Medical Corps*, vol. LXIII (July-Dec. 1939), pp. 106–24, pp. 173–78, pp. 240–48.
1949	J. C. M. M'Crindle, 'Dr James Barry', *Glasgow Herald* (December 1949), Wellcome Library, London, RAMC 238.
1958	Isobel Rae, *The Strange Story of Dr. James Barry: Army Surgeon, Inspector-General of Hospitals, Discovered on Death to be a Woman* (London: Longmans, Green and Co, 1958).
1969	R. C. Bellenger, letter to Major-General A. MacLennan, O.B.E., 17 November 1969, Wellcome Library, London, RAMC 238.

1973	June Rose, *Quest for Dr. James Barry*, prod. Madeau Stewart (BBC radio broadcast, 27 June 1973), Wellcome Library, London, RAMC 1089.
1977	June Rose, *The Perfect Gentleman: The remarkable life of Dr. James Miranda Barry, the woman who served as an officer in the British Army from 1813 to 1859* (London: Hutchinson, 1977).
1984	Frederic Mohr [David McKail], 'Barry: Personal Statements', 1984 play script, National Library of Scotland, Edinburgh, Traverse Theatre Inventory, Acc. 9285/8; also Scottish Theatre Archive, Glasgow, STA Mn 63/7.
[1985?]	Frederic Mohr [David McKail], 'Barry'. A dramatization for television of the life of Inspector General of Army Hospitals, MAJOR-GENERAL JAMES MIRANDA BARRY, 1795–1865: The first woman doctor of modern western medicine [Unfinished script, undated]. Scottish Theatre Archive, STA MN57/1, University of Glasgow.
1988/89	Jean Binnie, *Colours*. Play produced (with the subtitle *Jean Barry Esq*) at the Abbey Theatre, Dublin, and at Leeds Playhouse, October 1988. Play scripts held by the British Library, MPS 3993 (dated 1988), and (with the subtitle *James Barry – Her Story*, dated 1989) by Bristol Theatre Collection, WTC.PS/000047.[1]
1989/97	Patricia Duncker, 'James Miranda Barry'. First published in *The Pied Piper*, ed. Anna Livia and Lilian Mohin (London: Onlywomen Press, 1989), repr. in *Monsieur Shoushana's Lemon Trees* (London: Serpent's Tail, 1997), pp. 37–42.
1992	Jean Binnie, 'Dr Barry'. Radio play, broadcast by BBC *Who Sings the Hero?* series, 19 August 1992.
1994	Frederic Mohr, *Barry: Personal Statements. Five Solo Plays* (Edinburgh: [David McKail], [1994]), pp. 43–76.
1994	'An Experiment', *A Skirt through History*, dir. Philippa Lowthorpe (BBC, 1994), http://explore.bfi.org.uk/4ce2b7d7be08e
1996	Kit Brennan, *Tiger's Heart* (1996; Vancouver: Scirocco Drama, revised edn 1998).

1999	Patricia Duncker, *James Miranda Barry* (London: Serpent's Tail, 1999).
2000	Ann Kronenfeld and Ivan Kronenfeld, *The Secret Life of Dr. James Miranda Barry* (2000; Cambridge, MD: Write Words, ebooksonthenet, 2004).
2002	Patricia Duncker, *The Doctor* (New York: Harper Perennial, 2002) [US edition of *James Miranda Barry*].
2002	Rachel Holmes, *Scanty Particulars: The Mysterious, Astonishing and Remarkable Life of Victorian Surgeon James Barry* (London: Penguin, 2002)
2002	Rachel Holmes, *Scanty Particulars: The Scandalous Life and Astonishing Secret of Queen Victoria's Most Eminent Military Doctor* (New York: Random House, 2002).
2004	Sebastian Barry, *Whistling Psyche*. In *Whistling Psyche. Fred and Jane* (London: Faber and Faber, 2004), pp. 7–61.
2007	Rachel Holmes, *The Secret Life of Dr. James Barry: Victorian England's Most Eminent Surgeon* (Stroud: Tempus/The History Press, 2007).
2011	Patricia Duncker, *James Miranda Barry* (London: Bloomsbury, 2011).
2012	Gilmore & Roberts, 'Doctor James', *The Innocent Left*, released by Navigator Records, 2012. [Lyrics by Katriona Gilmore.]
2012	Sylvie Ouellette, *Le Secret du docteur Barry* (2012; Paris: Terres de femmes, De Borée, 2013).
2016	Michael du Preez and Jeremy Dronfield, *Dr. James Barry: A Woman Ahead of Her Time* (London: Oneworld, 2016).
2017	Kate Milsom, 'James Barry 1789–1865', *No Man's Land* exhibition, Martin Tinney Gallery, Cardiff, 28 February to 24 March 2018, http://www.artwales.com/exhibition-mtg-en.php?locationID=263 [accessed 10 March 2018].

Archives Consulted

Archivo del general Miranda, ed. Vicente Dávila (vols 1–14), Commission of the Academia Nacional de la Historia (vol.15); José Nucete Sardi, Antonio Alamo, Jacinto Fombona Pachano and Eduardo Arroyo Lamela

(vols 16–24) (Caracas, 1929–50). British Library, General Reference Collection 9774.h.1.
Bristol Theatre Collection, University of Bristol
British Library, London
Harry Ransom Center, The University of Texas at Austin, USA
James Barry papers, National Archives, Kew, Richmond. Files CO 247/49, CO 247/52, PRO 30/46/18.
Museum of Military Medicine, Keogh Barracks, Ash Vale, Aldershot
National Library of Scotland, Edinburgh
National Library of South Africa, Cape Town, South Africa
Royal Society of Arts, London
Scottish Theatre Archive, Special Collections, University of Glasgow
Wellcome Library, London: James Barry papers, files RAMC 238, RAMC 373, RAMC 423/4, RAMC 455, RAMC 658, RAMC 748, RAMC 801.6.5 (801.6.5.1, 801.6.5.2, 801.6.5.3), RAMC 992, RAMC 1069, RAMC 1264

Note

1. The title is recorded as given on the Abbey Theatre Archive website, https://www.abbeytheatre.ie/archives/production_detail/702/ [accessed 5 August 2017].

Bibliography

Ackroyd, Peter, *The Last Testament of Oscar Wilde* (London: Penguin, 1993).

Albert Nobbs, dir. Glenn Close (Mockingbird Films, Trillium Productions, Parallel Film Productions, 2011). Final shooting script by Gabriella Prekop, John Banville and Glenn Close, based on a treatment by Istvan Szabo and a short story by George Moore, WGA Registered #I00705-2, http://www.albert-nobbs-themovie.com/AlbertNobbs.pdf [accessed 17 April 2017].

Alcott, Louisa May, *Behind a Mask*, in *Alternative Alcott*, ed. Elaine Showalter (1866; New Brunswick: Rutgers University Press, 1988), pp. 97–202.

A.M.S., 'To the Editors of *The Lancet*', 'Notes, Comments, and Answers to Correspondents' section, *Lancet* [letter dated 16 October 1895], vol. 3764, 19 October 1895, p.1021.

Angela *[sic]*, 'Margaret Ann Bulkley: The extraordinary Doctor James Barry', *A Silver Voice from Ireland* blog, 17 July 2011, https://thesilvervoice.wordpress.com/2011/07/17/the-most-hardened-creaturedoctor-james-barry/ [accessed 14 August 2016].

Archivo del general Miranda, ed. Vicente Dávila (vols 1–14), Commission of the Academia Nacional de la Historia (vol.15); José Nucete Sardi, Antonio Alamo, Jacinto Fombona Pachano and Eduardo Arroyo Lamela (vols 16–24) (Caracas, 1929–50). British Library, General Reference Collection 9774.h.1.

Arias, Rosario and Patricia Pulham (eds), *Haunting and Spectrality in Neo-Victorian Fiction: Possessing the Past* (Basingstoke: Palgrave Macmillan, 2010).

Arnold, Gaynor, *Girl in a Blue Dress* (Birmingham: Tindal Street Press, 2008).

Arnold, Matthew, 'Stanzas from the Grande Chartreuse' (1855), in *Victorian Poetry: An Annotated Anthology*, ed. Francis O'Gorman (Oxford: Blackwell, 2004), pp. 305–12.

A. Heilmann, *Neo-/Victorian Biographilia and James Miranda Barry*, https://doi.org/10.1007/978-3-319-71386-1

Arnold, René, 'A Female Medical Combatant – Le médecin militaire femelle', *Revue Étrangère*, vol. and date unknown, p.112, in Longmore Pamphlet Collection, vol. 4 (1863–1882), Wellcome Library, London, RAMC 423/4.

Audet, Danielle, 'The "T" in LGBT: What CASAs Need to Know', http://nc.casaforchildren.org/files/public/site/conference/HO2015/E%20-%20The%20T%20in%20GLBT.pdf [accessed 18 September 2016].

Austen, Jane, *Emma*, ed. Fiona Stafford (1815; London: Penguin, 1996).

Avery, Simon, 'Tighe [née Blanchford], Mary', in *The Cambridge Guide to Women's Writing in English*, ed. Lorna Sage (Cambridge: Cambridge University Press, 1999), p.625.

Bailey, Peter J., '"Why Not Tell the Truth?": The Autobiographies of Three Fiction Writers', *Critique*, vol. 32: 4 (1991), pp. 211–223.

Baillie, Joanna, *Plays on the Passions,* ed. Peter Duthie (Peterboro: Broadview, 2001), pp. 67–388.

Baker, Sarah, *Transgender Behind Prison Walls* (Hook, Hampshire: Waterside Press, 2017).

Baldor, Lolita C., 'Pentagon says transgender troops will be able to enlist in military next month despite Trump's opposition', *Independent*, 11 December 2017, http://www.independent.co.uk/news/world/americas/us-politics/transgender-troops-enlist-trump-ban-pentagon-go-ahead-latest-a8104481.html [accessed 23 December 2017].

'Balli di Sfessania', *Giornale Nuovo*, 11 June 2004, http://www.spamula.net/blog/2004/06/balli_di_sfessania.html [accessed 19 April 2017]

Bannerman, James, 'The Double Life of Dr. James Barry', *Maclean's Magazine*, 1 December 1950, pp. 49–55, Wellcome Library, London, RAMC238.

Barbin, Abel, 'Mes souvenirs', in *Michel Foucault présente Herculine Barbin dite Alexina B., suivi de Un scandale au couvent d'Oscar Panizza* (1978; [Paris]: Gallimard, 2014), pp. 23–138.

Barbin, Abel, 'My Memoirs', in Michel Foucault [ed.], *Herculine Barbin: Being the Recently Discovered Memoirs of a Nineteenth-Century French Hermaphrodite*, trans Richard McDougall (1980; New York: Vintage, 2010), pp. 1–115.

Barnes, Julian, *Flaubert's Parrot* (London: Jonathan Cape, 1984).

Barry, Jacobus, 'Disputatio Medica Inaugralis, de Merocele, vel Hernia Crurali' (June 1812), Edinburgh Research Archive, https://www.era.lib.ed.ac.uk/handle/1842/417 [accessed 8 November 2015].

Barry, James, 'The humble memorial of Dr James Barry, Inspector General of Hospitals', undated draft [1859], Wellcome Library, London, RAMC 373.

Barry, James, 'Memorandum of the Services of Dr. James Barry Inspector General of Hospitals', stamped 30 Jan 1859, Wellcome Library, London, RAMC 373.

Barry, Sebastian, *Whistling Psyche,* in *Whistling Psyche. Fred and Jane* (London: Faber and Faber, 2004), pp. 7–61.

Baskerville, Stephen W., 'Barry, James, fourth earl of Barrymore (1667–1748)', *Oxford Dictionary of National Biography* (Oxford: Oxford University Press, 2004), online edn, http://www.oxforddnb.com/view/article/65188 [accessed 1 December 2015].

Bauer, Heike (ed.), *Women and Cross-Dressing 1800–1939*, 3 vols (London: Routledge, 2006).

Baynes, Chris, 'Britain's first pregnant man gives birth to girl', *Independent*, 8 July 2017, http://www.independent.co.uk/news/uk/home-news/britains-first-pregnant-man-gives-birth-to-girl-hayden-cross-a7830346.html [accessed 9 July 2017].

'#BBCtrending: Meet my transgender kid', *BBC News Magazine*, 7 March 2015, http://www.bbc.co.uk/news/magazine-31697046 [accessed 7 December 2015].

'BBC Afternoon Plays, 1984–2002', http://www.suttonelms.org.uk/lost10.html [accessed 29 November 2015].

Beauvoir, Simone de, *The Second Sex*, ed. and trans. H. M. Parshley (1949; London: Picador, 1988).

Bell, Susan Groag and Karen M. Offen (eds), *Women, the Family, and Freedom: The Debate in Documents*, 2 vols (Stanford: Stanford University Press, 1983).

Bellenger, R. C. to Major-General A. MacLennan, O.B.E., 17 November 1969, Wellcome Library, London, RAMC 238.

Benmussa, Simone, *The Singular Life of Albert Nobbs*, in *Benmussa Directs* (London: John Calder, 1979), pp. 22–121.

Binnie, Jean, *Colours*, play text (1988), British Library, London, MPS3993.

Binnie, Jean, *Colours: James Barry – Her Story*, play text (1989), Bristol Theatre Collection, Bristol, WTC/PS/000047.

Binnie, Jean, 'Dr Barry'. Radio play, *Who Sings the Hero?* series, BBC, 19 August 1992. Listed under 'BBC Afternoon Plays, 1984–2002', http://www.suttonelms.org.uk/lost10.html [accessed 29 November 2015].

Binnie, Jean, 'First among women', letter to *British Medical Journal*, vol. 304, 25 January 1992, p.257.

Blair, Olivia, 'Vogue model Hanne Gaby Odiele comes out as intersex', *Independent*, 24 January 2017, http://www.independent.co.uk/life-style/health-and-families/vogue-model-hanne-gaby-odiele-intersex-comes-out-gender-belgian-sex-x-y-chromosome-chanel-prada-a7542851.html [accessed 25 January 2017].

Blake, Catriona, *The Charge of the Parasols: Women's Entry to the Medical Profession* (London: Women's Press, 1990).

Boccardi, Mariadele, *The Contemporary British Historical Novel: Representation, Nation, Empire* (Basingstoke: Palgrave Macmillan, 2009).

Boehm-Schnitker, Nadine and Susanne Gruss, 'Introduction' to 'Spectacles and Things: Visual and Material Culture and/in Neo-Victorianism', ed. Nadine

Boehm-Schnitker and Susanne Gruss, special issue of *Neo-Victorian Studies*, vol. 4:2 (2011), pp. 1–23.

Boehm-Schnitker, Nadine and Susanne Gruss, 'Introduction: Fashioning the Neo-Victorian – Neo-Victorian Fashions', in *Neo-Victorian Literature and Culture: Immersions and Revisitations*, ed. Nadine Boehm-Schnitker and Susanne Gruss (London: Routledge, 2014), pp. 1–20.

Boehm-Schnitker, Nadine and Susanne Gruss (eds), *Neo-Victorian Literature and Culture: Immersions and Revisitations* (London: Routledge, 2014).

Boldrini, Lucia, '"Allowing it to speak out of him": The Heterobiographies of David Malouf, Antonio Tabucchi and Marguerite Yourcenar', in 'Autobiografictions: Comparatist Essays', ed. Lucia Boldrini and Peter Davies, special issue of *Comparative Critical Studies*, vol. 1:3 (2004), pp. 243–63.

Boldrini, Lucia, *Autobiographies of Others: Historical Subjects and Literary Fiction* (London: Routledge, 2012).

Boldrini, Lucia and Peter Davies (eds), 'Autobiografictions: Comparatist Essays', special issue of *Comparative Critical Studies*, vol. 1:3 (2004).

Bornstein, Kate, *Gender Outlaw: On Men, Women, and the Rest of Us* (New York: Random House, Vintage, 1995).

Bowser, Rachel A. and Brian Croxall (eds), 'Steampunk, Science, and (Neo) Victorian Technologies', special issue of *Neo-Victorian Studies*, vol. 3:1 (2010).

Boys Don't Cry, dir. Kimberly Peirce (Fox Searchlight Pictures, The Independent Film Channel Productions, Killer Films, 1999).

Braddon, Mary, *Lady Audley's Secret*, ed. David Skilton (1862; Oxford: Oxford University Press, 1992).

Bradford, Edward, Deputy-Inspector-General of Hospitals, 'The Reputed Female Army Surgeon: Letter from Deputy-Inspector Bradford', *Medical Times and Gazette*, 9 September 1865, p.293.

Brandon, Sydney, 'Barry, James', *Oxford Dictionary of National Biography* (Oxford: Oxford University Press, 2004), online edn, http://www.oxforddnb.com/view/article/1563 [accessed 1 December 2015].

Brandreth, Gyles, *Oscar Wilde and the Candlelight Murders* (London: John Murray, 2007).

Brandreth, Gyles, *Oscar Wilde and the Ring of Death* (London: John Murray, 2008).

Brandreth, Gyles, *Oscar Wilde and the Dead Man's Smile* (London: John Murray, 2009).

Brandreth, Gyles, *Oscar Wilde and the Nest of Vipers* (London: John Murray, 2010).

Brandreth, Gyles, *Oscar Wilde and the Vatican Murders* (London: John Murray, 2011).

Brandreth, Gyles, *Oscar Wilde and the Murders at Reading Gaol* (London: John Murray, 2012).

Brennan, Kit, *Tiger's Heart* (1996; Vancouver: Scirocco Drama, revised edn 1998).

Brennan, Mary, 'Barry', *Glasgow Herald*, 17 May 1984, National Library of Scotland, Edinburgh, Traverse Theatre Inventory Acc. 9285/8.

Bright, George A., M.D, U.S. Navy, 'A Female Member of the Army Medical Staff', 'Notes, Comments, and Answers to Correspondents' section, *Lancet* [letter dated 30 September 1895], vol. 3763, 12 October 1895, p.959.

Brontë, Charlotte, *Jane Eyre*, ed. Richard Dunn (New York: Norton, 2001), pp. 5–308.

Broughton, Trev, 'Life Writing and the Victorians', in *The Oxford Handbook of Victorian Literary Culture*, ed. Juliet John (Oxford: Oxford University Press, 2016), pp. 45–61.

Brown, Mark, 'Secret transgender Victorian surgeon feted by Historic England', *Guardian* online, 25 July 2017, https://www.theguardian.com/society/2017/jul/25/secret-transgender-victorian-surgeon-feted-by-heritage-england [accessed 25 July 2017].

Brubaker, Rogers, *trans: Gender and Race in an Age of Unsettled Identities* (Princeton: Princeton University Press, 2016).

Bulman, May, 'Almost half of all trans pupils have tried to take own lives, study finds', *Independent*, 28 June 2017, http://www.independent.co.uk/news/uk/home-news/trans-pupils-attempt-suicide-take-own-lives-lgbt-education-schools-study-stonewall-cambridge-a7809841.html [accessed 29 June 2017].

Bulman, May, 'Mr, Ms, or Mx? HSBC bank offers trans customers gender-neutral titles', *Independent*, 31 March 2017, http://www.independent.co.uk/news/uk/home-news/hsbc-bank-transgender-customers-neutral-titles-mx-ind-mre-a7659686.html [accessed 1 April 2017].

Buncombe, Andrew, 'Donald Trump's transgender ban criticised by 56 former generals and admirals', *Independent*, 1 August 2017, http://www.independent.co.uk/news/world/americas/us-politics/donald-trump-transgender-ban-us-military-56-generals-admirals-criticise-palm-center-a7871641.html [accessed 1 August 2017].

Burns, Robert, 'Trump officially directs Pentagon to ban transgender recruits', *Independent*, 25 August 2017, http://www.independent.co.uk/news/world/americas/us-politics/trump-transgender-ban-trans-troops-medical-treatment-latest-a7913686.html [accessed 26 August 2017].

Butler, Judith, *Gender Trouble: Feminism and the Subversion of Identity* (London: Routledge, 1990).

Butler, Judith, 'Preface' to *Gender Trouble: Feminism and the Subversion of Identity* (New York: Routledge, 1999), pp. vii-xxviii.

Byatt, A.S., *The Biographer's Tale* (London: Quality Paperbacks Direct, 2000).

Byron, Glennis, *Dramatic Monologue* (London: Routledge, 2003).

Cacciottolo, Mario and Monica Soriano, 'Transgender child: The boy putting his female puberty on hold', *BBC News* online, 1 December 2016, http://www.bbc.co.uk/news/health-38132301 [accessed 1 December 2016]

'Caitlin Jenner on Donald Trump's failure to protect trans people: "This is a disaster"', *Independent*, 24 February 2017, http://www.independent.co.uk/news/world/americas/caitlyn-jenner-donald-trump-transgender-bathroom-row-twitter-video-lgbt-rights-a7596816.html [accessed 14 April 2017].

'Captain', 'To the Editors of *The Lancet*', 'Notes, Comments, and Answers to Correspondents' section, *Lancet* [letter dated 17 October 1895], vol. 3765, 26 October 1895, p.1087.

Cardwell, Sarah, *Adaptation revisited: Television and the classic novel* (Manchester: Manchester University Press, 2002).

Carphin, Janet, 'To the Editors of *The Lancet*', 'Notes, Comments, and Answers to Correspondents' section, *Lancet* [letter dated 14 October 1895], vol. 3764, 19 October 1895, p.1021.

Carroll, Lewis, *Alice's Adventures in Wonderland*, in *Alice in Wonderland*, ed. Donald J. Gray (New York: Norton, 1992), pp. 1–99.

Carroll, Rachel, *Transgender and the Literary Imagination: Changing Gender in Twentieth Century Writing* (Edinburgh: Edinburgh University Press, 2018).

Castle, Terry, *The Apparitional Lesbian: Female Homosexuality and Modern Culture* (New York: Columbia University Press, 1993).

Caulfield, James, *Portraits, Memoirs and Characters of Remarkable Persons from the Reign of Edward the Third to the Revolution*, 2 vols (London: James Caulfield, 1794).

Chak, Avinash, 'Beyond "he" and "she": The rise of non-binary pronouns', *BBC News Magazine*, 7 December 2015, http://www.bbc.co.uk/news/magazine-34901704 [accessed 14 April 2017].

'Changing the rules: Breaking transgender taboos at work', *BBC News* online, 6 May 2016, http://www.bbc.co.uk/news/business-36194759 [accessed 31 December 2016].

Chase-Riboud, Barbara, *The Hottentot Venus* (New York: Anchor Books, 2003).

Chesnet, 'Question d'identité: vice de confirmation des organes génitaux externes; hypospadias; erreur sur le sexe', *Annales d'hygiène publique et de medicine légale*, vol. XIV (1860), repr. in *Michel Foucault présente Herculine Barbin dite Alexina B.* ([Paris]: Gallimard, 2014), pp. 147–50.

Chesnet, 'The question of identity; the malformation of the external genital organs; hypospadias; an error about sex', repr. in *Herculine Barbin*, [ed.] Michel Foucault, trans Richard McDougall (New York: Vintage, 2010), pp. 124–28.

Chidzoy, Sally, 'Transgender inmate found dead in Woodhill prison cell', *BBC News* online, 1 December 2015, http://www.bbc.co.uk/news/uk-england-beds-bucks-herts-3497222 [accessed 14 April 2017].

Close, Glenn, 'On Albert Nobbs', in *George Moore: Dublin, Paris, Hollywood*, ed. Conor Montague and Adrian Frazier (Dublin: Irish Academic Press, 2012), pp. 197–201.

Coleridge, Samuel Taylor, 'The Rime of the Ancient Mariner', *The Norton Anthology of Poetry*, 4th edn, ed. Margaret Ferguson, May Jo Salter and John Stallworthy (New York: Norton, 1996), pp. 744–59.

Collins, Wilkie, *The Woman in White* (1860; London: Penguin, 2009).

Copley, Hamish, 'Dr. James Miranda Barry', *The Drummer's Revenge: LGTB history and politics in Canada*, 2 December 2007, https://thedrummersrevenge.wordpress.com/2007/12/02/dr-james-miranda-barry/ [accessed 29 October 2015].

'Colours – Jean Barry Esq. 1988 [Abbey] by Jean Binnie', *Abbey Theatre Archives* database, https://www.abbeytheatre.ie/archives/production_detail/702/ [accessed 2 August 2017].

Coupland, Douglas, 'Convergences', *New York Times*, 8 March 2012, http://www.nytimes.com/2012/03/11/books/review/gods-without-men-by-hari-kunzru.html [accessed 1 August 2017].

Crawford, Elizabeth, 'Women and The First World War: The Work of Women Doctors', originally published in *Ancestors* (July 2006), repr. on Crawford's website 'Woman and Her Sphere', http://womanandhersphere.com/2014/05/06/women-and-the-first-world-war-the-work-of-women-doctors/ [accessed 18 April 2015].

Cregan, David, '"Everyman's story is the whisper of God": Sacred and secular in Barry's Dramaturgy', in *Out of History: Essays on the Writing of Sebastian Barry*, ed. Christina Hunt Mahony (Dublin: Carysfort Press, 2004), pp. 61–82.

Crellin, Olivia, 'The transgender family where the father gave birth', *BBC Magazine* online, 23 September 2016, http://www.bbc.co.uk/news/magazine-37408298 [accessed 24 September 2016].

Crowder, Judy, 'Children's Literature' [reader reviews of *With a Silent Companion*], http://www.barnesandnoble.com/w/with-a-silent-companion-florida-ann-town/1012357837;jsessionid=1AAF56167B5FF793823F2D525B477240.prodny_store02-atgap09?ean=9780889952119 [accessed 14 April 2017].

The Danish Girl, dir. Tom Hooper (Working Title Films, Pretty Pictures, ReVision Pictures, 2015).

DasGupta, Sayantani, 'Downcast, Decapitated and Dead: Why Don't Women in Book Covers and Ads Stare Back?', *Adios Barbie: the body image site for everybody*, 22 March 2012, http://www.adiosbarbie.com/2012/05/downcast-decapitated-and-dead/ [accessed 18 April 2017].

Da Silva, Chantal, 'Jennifer Lopez lauded for use of gender-neutral pronouns', *Independent*, 24 July 2017, http://www.independent.co.uk/arts-entertainment/music/news/jennifer-lopez-gender-neutral-pronouns-they-nibling-the-fosters-a7856941.html [accessed 25 July 2017].

[Davies, Mrs Christian], *The Life and Adventures of Mrs. Christian Davies, commonly called Mother Ross* (London: R. Montagu, 1740), repr. in *Women Adventurers: The Lives of Madame Velazquez, Hannah Snell, Mary Anne Talbot, and Mrs. Christian Davies*, ed. Ménie Muriel Dowie (London: Fisher Unwin, 1893), pp. 55–119.

Davies, Helen, *Gender and Ventriloquism in Victorian and Neo-Victorian Fiction: Passionate Puppets* (Basingstoke: Palgrave Macmillan, 2012).

Deacon, Harriet, 'Medical Gentlemen and the Process of Professionalisation before 1860', in *The Cape Doctor in the Nineteenth Century: A Social History*, ed. Harriet Deacon, Howard Phillips and Elizabeth van Heyningen (Amsterdam: Rodopi, 2004), pp. 85–103.

Deacon, Harriet and Elizabeth van Heyningen, 'Opportunities Outside Private Practice before 1860', in *The Cape Doctor in the Nineteenth Century: A Social History*, ed. Harriet Deacon, Howard Phillips and Elizabeth van Heyningen (Amsterdam: Rodopi, 2004), pp. 133–168.

Defoe, Daniel, *A General History of the Pyrates, from their first Rise and Settlement in the Island of Providence to the present Time. With the remarkable Actions and Adventures of the two Female Pyrates Mary Read and Anne Bonny* (London: T. Warner, 1724), Project Gutenberg ebook, http://www.gutenberg.org/files/40580/40580-h/40580-h.htm [accessed 29 March 2016].

Derbyshire, Victoria, 'The story of two transgender children', *BBC News Magazine* online, 7 April 2015, http://www.bbc.co.uk/news/magazine-32037397 [accessed 15 January 2016].

Derrida, Jaques, 'Of an Apocalyptic Tone Recently Adopted in Philosophy', *Oxford Literary Review*, vol. 6:2 (1984), pp. 3–37.

Derrida, Jacques and Avital Ronell, 'The Law of Genre', *Critical Inquiry* ('On Narrative'), vol. 7:1 (1980), pp. 55–81.

Dickson Wright, A., 'Caesarian Section', St Mary's Hospital Gazette, vol. 74 (January to February 1968), pp. 22–23. Wellcome Library, London, RAMC 748.

Dillon, Henry William, Sir, *A Narrative of My Professional Adventures* (1790–1839), ed. Michael A. Lewis, 2 vols (n.p.: Navy Records Society, 1956).

Dilworth, Miles, 'Single sex schools "failing in their legal duties to accommodate transgender pupils"', *Independent*, 9 April 2017, http://www.independent.co.uk/news/education/education-news/single-sex-schools-failing-legal-duties-accommodate-transgender-pupils-stonewall-women-equalities-a7674896.html [accessed 10 April 2017].

Ditum, Sarah, 'I'm not surprised that the BBC chastised Jenni Murray over her transgender comments – this is what institutional sexism looks like', *Independent*, 7 March 2017, http://www.independent.co.uk/voices/jenni-murray-sunday-times-transgender-india-willoughby-a7616151.html [accessed 14 April 2017].

Dowie, Ménie Muriel, 'Introduction' to *Women Adventurers: The Lives of Madame Velazquez, Hannah Snell, Mary Anne Talbot, and Mrs. Christian Davies*, ed. Ménie Muriel Dowie (London: Fisher Unwin, 1893), pp. v–xxiii.

'Dr. James Barry', *The Secret Histories Project* blog, 12 December 2012, http://secrethistoriesproject.tumblr.com/post/37785045159/17-dr-james-barry-when-dr-james-barry-died-in [accessed 1 December 2015].

'Dr. James Miranda Barry (1789–1855): Transgender British Surgeon', *The Legacy Project*, http://www.legacyprojectchicago.org/James_Miranda_Barry/imag000.jpg [accessed 12 August 2017].

Dreger, Alice Domurat, *Hermaphrodites and the Medical Invention of Sex* (Cambridge: Harvard University Press, 1998).

'The Duel fought by the Duke of Wellington and the Duke of Winchelsea – 23 March 1829', British Newspaper Archive, http://blog.britishnewspaperarchive.co.uk/2013/03/23/the-duel-fought-by-duke-of-wellington-and-the-earl-of-winchilsea-23-march-1829/ [accessed 29 December 2015].

Duncker, Patricia, *The Doctor* (New York: Harper Perennial, 2002).

Duncker, Patricia, *Hallucinating Foucault* (London: Bloomsbury, 1996).

Duncker, Patricia, 'James Miranda Barry', originally published in *The Pied Piper: Lesbian Feminist Fiction*, ed. Anna Livia (London: Onlywomen Press, 1989), repr. in *Monsieur Shoushana's Lemon Trees* (London: Serpent's Tail, 1997), pp. 37–42.

Duncker, Patricia, *James Miranda Barry* (London: Serpent's Tail, 1999).

Duncker, Patricia, *James Miranda Barry* (London: Bloomsbury, 2011).

Duncker, Patricia, 'The Lunatic, the Lover and the Poet: On Writing *Hallucinating Foucault*', in *Spatial Representations of British Identities*, ed. Merle Tönnies and Heike Buschmann (Heidelberg: Winter, 2012), pp. 19–32.

Duncker, Patricia, 'On Writing Neo-Victorian Fiction', *English*, vol. 63:243 (2014), pp. 253–74.

Ebershoff, David, *The Danish Girl* (London: Weidenfeld & Nicolson, 2000).

Edel, Leon, 'Biography: A Manifesto', *Biography*, vol. 1:1 (Winter 1978), pp. 1–3.

Effie Gray, dir. Richard Laxton, writer Emma Thompson (Sovereign Films, 2014).

Ellis, Havelock, *Eonism and Other Supplementary Studies*, vol. VII of *Studies in the Psychologies of Sex* (Philadelphia: F.A. Davies, 1928).

Ellis-Petersen, Hannah, 'BBC film on child transgender issues worries activists', *Independent*, 11 January 2017, https://www.theguardian.com/society/2017/jan/11/bbc-film-on-child-transgender-issues-worries-activists [accessed 11 January 2017].

Encyclopaedia of South African Theatre, Film, Media and Performance (ESAT), http://esat.sun.ac.za [accessed 14 April 2017].

England, Charlotte, 'US Supreme Court throws out transgender bathroom case after Donald Trump retracts anti-discrimination law', *Independent*, 7 March 2017, http://www.independent.co.uk/news/world/americas/us-supreme-court-transgender-bathroom-case-donald-trump-anti-discrimination-law-barack-obama-a7615236.html [accessed 7 March 2017].

Erll, Astrid and Ann Rigney, 'Introduction: Cultural Memory and its Dynamics', in *Mediation, Remediation, and the Dynamics of Cultural Memory*, ed. Astrid Erll and Ann Rigney in collaboration with Laura Basu and Paulus Bijl (Berlin: Walter de Gruyter, 2009), pp. 1–13.

Erll, Astrid and Ann Rigney in collaboration with Laura Basu and Paulus Bijl (eds), *Mediation, Remediation and the Dynamics of Cultural Memory* (Berlin: de Gruyter, 2009).

Erskine, David Steuart, 11th earl of Buchan, *The anonymous and fugitive essays of the earl of Buchan, collected from various periodical works* (Edinburgh: n.p., 1812).

'An Experiment', *A Skirt through History*, dir. Philippa Lowthorpe (BBC, 1994), http://explore.bfi.org.uk/4ce2b7d7be08e [accessed 14 April 2017].

Faber, Michel, *The Crimson Petal and the White* (London: Canongate, 2002).

Fassin, Eric, 'Postface: Le vrai genre'. In *Michel Foucault présente Herculine Barbin dite Alexina B., suivi de Un scandale au couvent d'Oscar Panizzi* ([Paris]: Gallimard, 2014), pp. 221–58.

Fay, Jane, 'Anti-trans campaigners are determined to say new gender identity legislation will change everything – it won't', *Independent*, 25 July 2017, http://www.independent.co.uk/voices/gender-identity-law-legislation-trans-transgender-rights-lgbt-legal-confirmation-a7859376.html [accessed 25 July 2017].

Feinberg, Leslie, *Transgender Liberation: A Movement Whose Time Has Come* (New York: World View Forum, 1992).

'A Female Medical Combatant', *Medical Times and Gazette*, 26 August 1865, pp. 227–28.

Fenton, Mrs. Bessie [Elizabeth] Knox, *The Journal of Mrs Fenton: The Narrative of Her Life in India, the Isle of France (Mauritius), and Tasmania During the Years 1826–1830*, with a Preface by Sir Henry Lawrence (London: Edward Arnold, 1901).

Finnerty, Deirdre, 'The transgender Republican trying to change her party', *BBC World Service*, 28 September 2016, http://www.bbc.co.uk/news/magazine-37256151 [accessed 29 September 2016].

Fleming, Nic, 'Revealed: Army surgeon actually a woman', *Telegraph* online, 5 March 2008, http://www.telegraph.co.uk/news/science/science-news/3334909/Revealed-Army-surgeon-actually-a-woman.html [accessed 7 December 2015].

Foster, Roy, '"Something of us will remain": Sebastian Barry and Irish History', in *Out of History: Essays on the Writings of Sebastian Barry*, ed. Christina Hunt Mahony (Dublin: Carysfort Press, 2004), pp. 183–197.

Foucault, Michel [ed.], *Herculine Barbin: Being the Recently Discovered Memoirs of a Nineteenth-Century French Hermaphrodite*, trans Richard McDougall (New York: Vintage, 2010).

Foucault, Michel, 'Introduction' to *Herculine Barbin: Being the Recently Discovered Memoirs of a Nineteenth-Century French Hermaphrodite*, [ed.] Michel Foucault, trans Richard McDougall (New York: Vintage, 2010), pp. vii–xvii.

[Foucault, Michel, ed.,] *Michel Foucault présente Herculine Barbin dite Alexina B., suivi de Un scandale au couvent d'Oscar Panizza* ([Paris]: Gallimard, 2014).

Foucault, Michel, 'Préface: Le vrai sexe', *Michel Foucault présente Herculine Barbin dite Alexina B., suivi de Un scandale au couvent d'Oscar Panizza* ([Paris]: Gallimard, 2014), pp. 9–21.

Fowles, John, *The French Lieutenant's Woman* (London: Panther, 1969).

'Frederic Mohr's Radio Plays', http://www.suttonelms.org.uk/david-mckail.html [accessed 14 April 2017].

Freeman, Elizabeth, 'Queer Belongings: Kinship Theory and Queer Theory', in *A Companion to Lesbian, Gay, Bisexual, Transgender and Queer Studies*, ed. Molly McGarry and George E. Haggarty (Maiden, MA: Blackwell, 2007), Blackwell Reference Online, http://www.blackwellreference.com/subscriber/tocnode.html?id=g9781405113298_chunk_g978140511329816 pp. 295–314 [accessed 14 April 2017].

'From our own correspondent', *Saunders's News-Letter and Daily Advertiser*, 14 August 1865, repr. in Percival R. Kirby, 'The Centenary of the Death of James Barry, M.D., Inspector-General of Hospitals (1795–1865)', *Africana Notes and News*, vol. 16:6 (June 1965), pp. 230–31, Wellcome Library, London, RAMC 455.

Funke, Jana, 'Obscurity and Gender Resistance in Patricia Duncker's *James Miranda Barry*', *European Journal of English Studies*, vol. 16:3 (2012), pp. 15–25.

Furneaux, Holly, *Queer Dickens: Erotics, Families, Masculinities* (Oxford: Oxford University Press, 2009).

Gander, Kashmira, 'British trans man claims he is the first man to have a baby in the UK', *Independent*, 9 July 2017, http://www.independent.co.uk/life-style/health-and-families/trans-man-pregnancy-birth-labour-eggs-donor-uk-british-hayden-cross-scott-parker-gloucester-brighton-a7831571.html [accessed 9 July 2017].

Garber, Marjorie, *Vested Interests: Cross-Dressing and Cultural Anxiety* (1992; London: Penguin, 1993).

Garréta, Anne, *Sphinx*, trans. Emma Ramadan (Dallas, Texas: Deep Vellum Publishing, 2015).

Gaskell, Elizabeth, *North and South* (London: Penguin, 2007).

G.E.C., 'An Amazing Male Impersonation: The Strange Story of James Barry, Esq., M.D.', *Illustrated London News*, 16 March 1929, p.448.

Gelfand, Michael, 'The Somerset Tradition', *S. A. Medical Journal*, 26 June 1965, Wellcome Library, London, RAMC 801/6/5/1, http://wellcomelibrary.org/item/b18495370 [accessed 13 September 2016].

Gender Recognition Act 2004, http://www.legislation.gov.uk/ukpga/2004/7/contents [accessed 20 January 2016].

Geoghegan, Tom, 'Five British heroes overlooked by history', *BBC News Magazine*, 15 November 2009, http://news.bbc.co.uk/1/hi/magazine/8364465.stm [accessed 10 August 2017].

'Germaine Greer gives university lecture despite campaign to silence her', *Guardian* online, 18 November 2015, http://www.theguardian.com/books/2015/nov/18/transgender-activists-protest-germaine-greer-lecture-cardiff-university [accessed 19 November 2015].

'Germaine Greer: Transgender women are "not women"', *BBC News* online, 24 October 2015, http://www.bbc.co.uk/news/uk-34625512 [accessed 5 November 2015].

Getsy, David J, 'Capacity', special issue on 'Posttranssexual: Key Concepts for a Twenty-First Century Transgender Studies', *TSQ: Transgender Studies Quarterly*, vol. 1: 1–2 (2014), pp. 47–49.

Gill, Nicola, 'We are Intersex', *Times Magazine Supplement*, 12 December 2015, pp. 28–36.

Gilmore & Roberts, 'Doctor James', *The Innocent Left*, released by Navigator Records, 2012. [Lyrics by Katriona Gilmore.]

'GLAAD responds to Vanity Fair cover featuring Caitlin Jenner, releases updated top sheets for journalists', GLAAD, 1 June 2015, http://www.glaad.org/blog/glaad-responds-vanity-fair-cover-featuring-caitlyn-jenner-releases-updated-tip-sheet [accessed 16 November 2015].

GLAAD, 'What name and pronoun do I use', http://www.glaad.org/transgender/transfaq [accessed 14 April 2017].

Gleitman, Claire, '"In the dank margins of things": *Whistling Psyche* and the Illness of Empire', in *Out of History: Essays on the Writings of Sebastian Barry*, ed. Christina Hunt Mahony (Dublin: Carysfort Press, 2004), pp. 209–27.

Glendening, John, *Science and Religion in Neo-Victorian Novels: Eye of the Ichthyosaur* (London: Routledge, 2013).

Goldner, Virginia, 'Trans: Gender in Free Fall', in 'Transgender Subjectivities: Theories and Practices', ed. Virginia Goldner, special issue of *Psychoanalytic Dialogues*, vol. 21:2 (2011), pp. 159–71.

Goldner, Virginia, 'Transgender Subjectivities: Introduction to Papers by Goldner, Suchet, Saketopoulou, Hansbury, Salamon & Corbett, and Harris', editorial to 'Transgender Subjectivities: Theories and Practices', ed. Virginia Goldner, special issue of *Psychoanalytic Dialogues*, vol. 21:2 (2011), pp. 153–58.

Goodman, Nelson, *Ways of Worldmaking* (1978; Indianapolis: Hackett Publishing, 1992).

Gordon, H. Laing, M.D. Edin., 'To the Editors of *The Lancet*', 'Notes, Comments, and Answers to Correspondents' section, *Lancet* [letter dated 14 October 1895], vol. 3764, 19 October 1895, p.1021.

Graham, George, General Registrar, letter of 23 August 1865, and reply by [Staff Surgeon Major David Reid] McKinnon on 24 August 1865, Wellcome Library, London, RAMC 373.

Grand, Sarah, *The Heavenly Twins* (1893; London: Heinemann, 1908).

Graziosi, Marco, 'A Blog of Bosh: Edward Lear and Nonsense Literature', https://nonsenselit.wordpress.com/ [accessed 26 August 2017].

Greenblatt, Stephen, *Shakespearean Negotiations: The Circulation of Energy in Renaissance England* (Oxford: Oxford University Press, 2001).

'The Growing Use of Mx as a Gender-inclusive Title in the UK', http://polyin-pictures.com/wp-content/uploads/mxevidencelowres.pdf [accessed 14 April 2017].

Grubgeld, Elizabeth, 'Framing the Body: George Moore's "Albert Nobbs" and the Disappearing Realist Subject', in *George Moore: Across Borders*, ed. Christine Huguet and Fabienne Dabrigeon-Garcier (Amsterdam, Rodopi, 2013), pp. 193–208.

Gruss, Susanne, 'Wilde Crimes: The Art of Murder and Decadent (Homo) Sexuality in Gyles Brandreth's Oscar Wilde Series', 'Neo-Victorian Masculinities', ed. Ann Heilmann and Mark Llewellyn, special issue of *Victoriographies*, vol. 5:2 (2015), pp. 165–182.

Guest, John, 'Sharp Encounter', *Sunday Times*, 9 November 1952, Wellcome Library, London, 'Letters by Nightingale, 1864–1865', Ms 9001/145.

Gujon, É. 'Étude d'un cas d'hermaphrodisme imparfait chez l'homme' [autopsy report of Abel (Herculine) Barbin], *Journal de l'anatomie et de la physiology de l'homme* (1869), pp. 609–39, repr. in 'Dossier', *Michel Foucault présente Herculine Barbin dite Alexina B., suivi de Un scandale au couvent d'Oscar Panizza* ([Paris]: Gallimard, 2014), pp. 151–64.

Gujon, E. 'A study of a case of incomplete hermaphroditism in a man' [autopsy report of Abel (Herculine) Barbin], *Journal de l'anatomie et de la physiology de l'homme* (1869), pp. 609–39, repr. in Michel Foucault, 'The Dossier', *Herculine Barbin*, trans. Richard McDougall (New York: Vintage, 1980), pp. 128–44.

Gutleben, Christian, 'An aesthetic of performativity: Patricia Duncker's art of simulation in James Miranda Barry', *Études Anglaises: revue du monde Anglophone*, vol. 60:2 (2007), pp. 212–25.

Gutleben, Christian *Nostalgic Postmodernism: The Victorian Tradition and the Contemporary British Novel* (Amsterdam: Rodopi, 2001).

Haggerty, George E. and Molly McGarry (eds), *A Companion to Lesbian, Gay, Bisexual, Transgender and Queer Studies* (Malden, MA: Blackwell, 2007).

Halberstam, Jack, 'On Pronouns', 3 September 2012, http://www.jackhalberstam.com/ [accessed 16 November 2015].

Halberstam, Jack, 'Trans* – Gender Transitivity and New Configurations of Body, History, Memory and Kinship', *Parallax*, vol. 22:3 (2016), pp. 366–75.

Halberstam, Jack, *Trans: A Quick and Quirky Account of Gender Variability* (Oakland, CA: University of California Press, 2018)

Halberstam, Judith, *Female Masculinity* (Durham: Duke University Press, 1998).

Halberstam, Judith, *In a Queer Time and Place: Transgender Bodies, Subcultural Lives* (New York: New York University Press, 2005).

Hamilton, Cicely, *A Pageant of Great Women* (1909/1948), repr. in *Literature of the Women's Suffrage Campaign in England*, ed. Carolyn Christensen Nelson (Peterborough, Ontario: Broadview, 2004), pp. 221–32.

Hammond, Mary, 'The Enigma of James Barry' [review of Patricia Duncker's *James Miranda Barry*], *Women: A Cultural Review*, vol. 13:1 (2010), pp. 104–106.

Hargreaves, Reginald, 'Dr James Barry (1795–1865)', *Women-at-Arms: Their Famous Exploits Throughout the Ages* (London: Hutchinson, [1930]), pp. 175–90.

Hargreaves, Reginald, 'Women-at-Arms', *Journal of the Royal United Service Institution*, vol. 101:601 (February 1956), pp. 1–10.

Harris, Mia, 'An insider guide to being transgender in prison', *The Conversation*, 17 May 2017, http://theconversation.com/an-insiders-guide-to-being-transgender-in-prison-74970 [accessed 23 July 2017].

Harvey, Robert, *Liberators: Latin America's Struggle for Independence 1810–1830* (London: John Murray, 2000).

'Heaven and Earth', *Movie Insider*, 5 February 2009, http://www.movieinsider.com/m2261/barry#plot [accessed 15 December 2016].

Heilmann, Ann, '"Neither man nor woman"? Female Transvestism, Object Relations and Mourning in George Moore's "Albert Nobbs"', *Women: a cultural review*, vol. 14:3 (2003), pp. 248–62.

Heilmann, Ann and Mark Llewellyn, *Neo-Victorianism: The Victorians in the Twenty-First Century, 1999–2009* (Basingstoke: Palgrave Macmillan, 2010).

Heinlein, Sabine, 'The transgender body in art: finding visibility "in difficult times like these"', *Guardian* online, 18 November 2016, https://www.theguardian.com/artanddesign/2016/nov/18/transgender-art-trans-hirstory-in-99-objects [accessed 19 November 2016].

Hirschfeld, Magnus, *Transvestites: The Erotic Drive to Cross-Dress*, trans. Michael A. Lombardi-Nash (New York: Prometheus, 1991).

[Hirschfeld, Magnus], 'Transvestitism', in *Sexual Anomalies and Perversions: Physical and Psychological Development and Treatment. A Summary of the Works of the Late Professor Dr. Magnus Hirschfeld*, compiled as a humble memorial by his pupils (London: Torch Publishing Company, 1946), repr. in *Women and Cross-Dressing 1800–1939*, ed. Heike Bauer, 3 vols (London: Routledge, 2006), I, pp. 285–322.

Hirst, Stefanie, 'My son wants to be a girl', *BBC News*, 16 January 2016, http://www.bbc.co.uk/news/uk-35323211 [accessed 17 January 2016].

Ho, Elizabeth, *Neo-Victorianism and the Memory of Empire* (London: Continuum, 2012).

Holmes, Rachel, *Scanty Particulars: The Mysterious, Astonishing and Remarkable Life of Victorian Surgeon James Barry* (London: Penguin, 2002).

Holmes, Rachel, *Scanty Particulars: The Scandalous Life and Astonishing Secret of Queen Victoria's Most Eminent Military Doctor* (New York: Random House, 2002).

Holmes, Rachel, *The Secret Life of Dr James Barry: Victorian England's Most Eminent Surgeon* (Stroud: Tempus, 2007).

Hosie, Rachel, 'Hanne Gaby Odiele: Top intersex model on how doctors tried to change her gender as a child', *Independent*, 24 April 2017, http://www.independent.co.uk/life-style/health-and-families/hanne-gaby-odiele-intersex-model-doctors-gender-change-child-belgian-fashion-lifestyle-a7698796.html [accessed 24 April 2017].

Hosie, Rachel, 'Trans artist helps break down period stigma with bold post', *Independent*, 23 July 2017, http://www.independent.co.uk/life-style/transgender-cass-clemmer-periods-women-photo-poem-menstruation-gender-non-binary-a7855521.html [accessed 25 July 2017].

House of Commons, Women and Equalities Committee, 'Transgender Equality Enquiry' and its findings of 3 November 2015, http://www.parliament.uk/business/committees/committees-a-z/commons-select/women-and-equalities-committee/inquiries/parliament-2015/transgender-equality/ [accessed 14 April 2017].

House of Commons, Women and Equalities Committee, 'Transgender Equality: First Report of Session 2015–16', 14 January 2016, http://www.publications.parliament.uk/pa/cm201516/cmselect/cmwomeq/390/390.pdf [accessed 14 April 2017].

Howe, Julia Ward, *The Hermaphrodite*, ed. Gary Williams (Lincoln: University of Nebraska Press, 2004).

Hoyer, Niels (ed.), *Man into Woman: The First Sex Change. A Portrait of Lili Elbe*, trans. H.J. Stenning (1933; London: Blue Boat, 2004).

Huber, Werner, Martin Middeke and Hubert Zapf (eds), *Self-Reflexivity in Literature* (Würzburg: Königshausen & Neumann, 2005).

Hughes, Kathryn, *Victorians Undone: Tales of the Flesh in the Age of Decorum* (London: 4th Estate, 2017).

Hunks, Van, 'The Mysterious Doctor James Barry: Dr James "Miranda" Barry in South Africa', http://www.vanhunks.com/cape1/barry1.html [accessed 8 November 2015].

Hurwitz, Brian and Ruth Richardson, 'Inspector General James Barry MD: Putting the Woman in her Place', *British Medical Journal*, vol.298: 6669, 4 February 1989, pp. 299–305.

Hutcheon, Linda, *A Poetics of Postmodernism: History, Theory, Fiction* (1988; London: Routledge, 1996).

Hutcheon, Linda, with Siobhan O'Flynn, *A Theory of Adaptation*, second edition (London: Routledge, 2013).

'I'm a non-binary ten-year-old', *BBC News Magazine*, 18 September 2016, http://www.bbc.co.uk/news/magazine-37383914 [accessed 18 September 2016].

Intersex Society of America, 'What is intersex?', http://www.isna.org/faq/what_is_intersex [accessed 29 October 2015].

Jacques, Juliet, 'Five trans role models you should know about', *Guardian* online, 8 June 2012, http://www.theguardian.com/commentisfree/2012/jun/08/five-trans-role-models [accessed 3 November 2015].

Jacques, Juliet, *trans: A Memoir* (London: Verso, 2012).

James, Henry, *The Aspern Papers* (1888), in *The Turn of the Screw and The Aspern Papers* (Ware: Wordsworth Editions, 1993), pp. 129–236.

James, Henry, *The Portrait of a Lady*, ed. Roger Luckhurst (1881; Oxford: Oxford University Press, 2009).

James, Henry, Preface to *The Tragic Muse*, volume 7 of the New York Edition (1908), http://www.henryjames.org.uk/prefaces/page_inframe.htm?page=text07 [accessed 5 November 2015].

'James Miranda Steuart Barry and the Crimean War', Archives@University of Edinburgh, uploaded 6 June 2016, http://libraryblogs.is.ed.ac.uk/edinburghuniversityarchives/2016/06/16/james-miranda-steuart-barry-and-the-crimean-war/ [accessed 5 August 2016].

'James Miranda Stuart Barry (1795–1865) Military Surgeon', *A Gender Variance Who's Who*, 16 January 2008, http://zagria.blogspot.co.uk/2008/01/james-miranda-stuart-barry-1795-1865.html#.Vl5Chr_ziNN [accessed 1 December 2015].

'Jean Binnie', Playwrights Database, http://www.doollee.com/PlaywrightsB/binnie-jean.html [accessed 2 August 2017].

Joyce, Simon, 'The Victorians in the Rearview Mirror', in *Functions of Victorian Culture at the Present Time*, ed. Christine L. Krueger (Athens: Ohio University Press, 2002), pp. 3–17.

Joyce, Simon, *The Victorians in the Rearview Mirror* (Athens: Ohio University Press, 2007).

Juta, Réné, *Cape Currey* (1920; Memphis: General Books, 2010).

Kaplan, Cora, *Victoriana: Histories, Fictions, Criticism* (Edinburgh: Edinburgh University Press, 2007).

Kelly *[sic]*, 'Covers change the story: more hardcover-paperback swaps', *Stacked*, 29 March 2012, http://stackedbooks.org/2012/03/covers-change-story-more-hardcover.html [accessed 6 August 2016].

Kentish, Ben, 'Second World War veteran aged 90 is transitioning to a woman', *Independent*, 30 March 2017, http://www.independent.co.uk/news/uk/

home-news/econd-world-war-veteran-patricia-davies-leicestershire-transition-woman-aged-90-years-old-a7658736.html [accessed 25 July 2017].

Khan, Shehab, 'Transgender man gives birth to baby boy in Oregon', *Independent*, 31 July 2017, http://www.independent.co.uk/news/world/americas/transgender-man-birth-baby-boy-oregon-portland-leo-trystan-reese-biff-chaplow-lgbt-a7868301.html [accessed 31 July 2017].

Kilian, Eveline, *GeschlechtSverkehrt: Theoretische und literarische Perspektiven des gender-bending* (Königstein: Ulrike Helmer Verlag, 2004).

King, Jeannette, *The Victorian Woman Question in Contemporary Feminist Fiction* (Basingstoke: Palgrave Macmillan, 2005).

Kirby, Percival R., 'The Centenary of the Death of James Barry, M.D., Inspector-General of Hospitals (1795–1865): A Re-examination of the Facts relating to his Physical Condition', Read at the Annual General Meeting of the South African Museums Association held at King William's Town on Wednesday, 24 March 1965, *Africana Notes and News*, vol. 16: 6 (June 1965), pp. 223–227, Wellcome Library, RAMC 455.

Kirby, Percival R., 'Dr James Barry, Controversial South African Medical Figure: A Recent Evaluation of his Life and Sex', *South African Medical Journal*, 25 April 1970, pp. 506–16, Wellcome Library, RAMC 658.

Kohlke, Marie-Luise, 'Introduction' to the inaugural issue of *Neo-Victorian Studies*, 1:1 (2008), pp. 1–18.

Kohlke, Marie-Luise, 'Mining the Neo-Victorian Vein: Prospecting for Gold, Buried Treasure and Uncertain Material', in *Neo-Victorian Literature and Culture: Immersions and Revisitations*, ed. Nadine Boehm-Schnitker and Susanne Gruss (London: Routledge, 2014), pp. 21–37.

Kohlke, Marie-Luise, 'Neo-Victorian Biofiction and the Special/Spectral Case of Barbara Chase-Riboud's *Hottentot Venus*', *Australasian Journal of Victorian Studies*, vol. 18:3 (2013), pp. 4–21.

Kohlke, Marie-Luise, 'Sexsation and the Neo-Victorian Novel: Orientalising the Nineteenth Century in Contemporary Fiction', in *Negotiating Sexual Idioms: Image, Text, Performance*, ed. Marie-Luise Kohlke and Luisa Orza (Amsterdam: Rodopi, 2008), pp. 53–77.

Kohlke, Marie-Luise and Christian Gutleben (eds), *Neo-Victorian Tropes of Trauma: The Politics of Bearing After-Witness to Nineteenth-Century Suffering* (Amsterdam: Rodopi, 2010).

Kronenfeld, Ann and Ivan Kronenfeld, *The Secret Life of Dr. James Miranda Barry* (2000; Cambridge, MD: Write Words, ebooksonthenet, 2004).

Kubba, A.K. 'The Life, Work and Gender of Dr James Barry MD (1795–1865)', *Proceedings of the Royal College of Physicians of Edinburgh*, vol. 31 (2001), pp. 352–56.

Lacan, Jacques, 'The Mirror Stage as Formative of the Function of the I as Revealed in Psychoanalytic Experience', *Écrits: A Selection*, trans. Alan Sheridan (London: Tavistock, 1989), pp. 1–8.

LaCapra, Dominick, *Writing History, Writing Trauma* (Baltimore: Johns Hopkins University Press, 2001).

Lackey, Michael, 'Introduction: A narrative space of its own', in *Biographical Fiction: A Reader*, ed. Michael Lackey (New York: Bloomsbury, 2016), pp. 1–15.

Lackey, Michael, 'The Rise of the Biographical Novel and the Fall of the Historical Novel', in 'Biofictions', ed. Michael Lackey, special issue of *a/b: Auto/Biography Studies*, vol. 31:1 (2016), pp. 33–58.

Lackey, Michael (ed.), *Biographical Fiction: A Reader* (New York: Bloomsbury, 2016).

'Language and Pronouns', *Gendered Intelligence*, http://genderedintelligence.co.uk/projects/kip/transidentities/language [accessed 25 March 2017].

Lanser, Susan S., 'Toward (a Queerer and) More (Feminist) Narratology', in *Narrative Theory Unbound: Queer and Feminist Interventions*, ed. Robyn Warhol and Susan S. Lanser (Columbus: Ohio State University Press, 2015), pp. 23–42.

Las Cases, Count [Emmanuel] de, *Mémorial de Sainte Hélène*: *Journal of the Private Life and Conversations of the Emperor Napoleon at Saint Helena*, 4 vols (London: Henry Colburn & Co, 1823), IV.

Laqueur, Thomas, *Making Sex: Body and Gender from the Greeks to Freud* (Cambridge, Massachusetts: Harvard University Press, 1990).

Lawrence, Hannah, 'LGTB group criticizes proposals by Trump administration officials to ban the word "transgender"', *Independent*, 17 December 2017, http://www.independent.co.uk/news/world/americas/trump-centre-disease-control-and-prevention-lgbt-criticism-transgender-latest-department-of-health-a8115246.html [accessed 23 December 2017].

Lee, Hermione, *Body Parts: Essays on Life-Writing* (London: Chatto & Windus, 2005).

The Legacy Project, 'Dr. James Miranda Barry (1789–1855): Transgender British Surgeon', http://www.legacyprojectchicago.org/James_Miranda_Barry/imag000.jpg [accessed 12 August 2017].

Leggett, Bianca, 'Teaching Translit: An Unsettled and Unsettling Genre', in *Teaching 21st Century Genres*, ed. Katy Shaw (Basingstoke: Palgrave, 2016), pp. 149–65.

Leigh, John, *Touché: The Duel in Literature* (Cambridge, MA: Harvard University Press, 2015).

Leitch, Robert, 'The Barry Room: The Tale of a Pioneering Military Surgeon', *U.S. Medicine*, July 2001, http://web.archive.org/web/20070928030206/http://www.usmedicine.com/column.cfm?columnID=53&issueID=28 [accessed 1 December 2015].

Lesnick, Silas, 'Rachel Weisz to Headline Dr. James Barry Biopic', *Movie News*, 12 December 2016, http://www.comingsoon.net/movies/news/794263-james-barry-biopic [accessed 15 December 2016].

Letissier, Georges, 'Nomadic Transgender Identity: Patricia Duncker's *James Miranda Barry* and Wesley Stace's *Misfortune*', *Neo-Victorian Studies*, vol. 9:2 (2017), pp. 15–40.

Lewis, Helen, 'What the row over banning Germaine Greer is really about', *New Statesman* online, 27 October 2015, http://www.newstatesman.com/politics/feminism/2015/10/what-row-over-banning-germaine-greer-really-about [accessed 5 November 2015].

Longford, Elizabeth, 'James Barry', *Eminent Victorian Women* (1981; Stroud: History Press, 2008), pp. 212–33.

Lopaz, Andrea, 'Whistling Psyche' [review of Almeida production, London, 18 May 2004], *Curtain Up*, http://www.curtainup.com/whistlingpsyche.html [accessed 28 October 2015].

Lusin, Caroline, 'Writing Lives and "Worlds": English Biographical Fiction at the Turn of the 21st Century', in *Mediation, Remediation and the Dynamics of Cultural Memory*, ed. Astrid Erll and Ann Rigney in collaboration with Laura Basu and Paulus Bijl (Berlin: de Gruyter, 2009), pp. 265–67.

Lyons, Kate, 'I think Germaine Greer is wrong on trans issues – but banning her isn't the answer', *Guardian* online, 27 October 2015, http://www.theguardian.com/commentisfree/2015/oct/27/germaine-greer-transphobia-cardiff-feminism-inclusive [accessed 5 November 2015].

MacMahon, James Ross, M.D., C.M. IV, 'Dr James Barry: A Study in Deception', *McGill Medical Journal*, vol. 37:1 (February 1968), pp. 25–32; copy held in June Rose collection of papers re James Barry, Wellcome Library, London, RAMC 1264/6.

Mahony, Christina Hunt (ed.), *Out of History: Essays on the Writings of Sebastian Barry* (Dublin: Carysfort Press, 2006).

Mak, Geertje, *Doubting Sex: Inscriptions, bodies and selves in nineteenth-century hermaphrodite case histories* (Manchester: Manchester University Press, 2012).

Malcolm, Janet, *The Silent Woman: Sylvia Plath and Ted Hughes* (London: Papermac, 1995).

Marcus, Stephen, *The Other Victorians: A Study of Sexuality and Pornography in Mid-Nineteenth-Century England* (London: Weidenfeld and Nicolson, 1964).

Margolyes, Miriam and Sonia Fraser, *Dickens's Women* (1989; London: Hesperus Press, 2011).

'Maria Miller and Kellie Maloney on "de-gendering" passports', *BBC News*, 14 January 2016, http://www.bbc.co.uk/news/uk-politics-35311636 [accessed 17 January 2016].

Marvell, George Edwin, 'The Mystery of the Kapok Doctor'. Section on 'Romances of the Cape'. *Cape Times Christmas Annual*, December 1904, pp. 13–19. National Library of South Africa, General Reference Collection 1876–1910.

McDonald, Lynn (ed.), *Florence Nightingale on Women, Medicine, Midwifery and Prostitution* (Waterloo, Ont.: Wilfrid Laurier University Press, 2005).

McKinnon, [Staff Surgeon Major David Reid], letter of 24 August 1865, in reply to letter by George Graham, Registrar General, of 23 August 1865, Wellcome Library, London, RAMC 373.

McMillan, Joyce, 'Barry', *Guardian*, 14 May 1984, National Library of Scotland, Edinburgh, Traverse Theatre Inventory Acc. 9285/8.

M'Crindle, J. C. M., 'Dr James Barry', *Glasgow Herald* (December 1949), Wellcome Library, London, RAMC 238.

Mermin, Dorothy, *The Audience in the Poem: Five Victorian Poets* (New Brunswick: Rutgers University Press, 1983).

Middeke, Martin, 'Introduction: Life-writing, Historical Consciousness, and Postmodernism', in *Biofictions: The Rewriting of Romantic Lives in Contemporary Fiction and Drama*, ed. Martin Middeke and Werner Huber (London: Camden House, 1999), pp. 1–25.

Middeke, Martin and Werner Huber (eds), *Biofictions: The Rewriting of Romantic Lives in Contemporary Fiction and Drama* (London: Camden House, 1999).

Middlemore, [Major-General] G[eorge], 'General Orders, 7 December 1836', Wellcome Library, London, RAMC 1264.

Mikdadi, Faysal, *Return* (n.p., Lulu.com, 2008).

Mill, John Stuart, 'Speech before the House of Commons, 20 May 1867', item 135 in 'Women and the Vote', *Women, the Family, and Freedom: The Debate in Documents*, ed. Susan Groag Bell and Karen M. Offen, 2 vols (Stanford: Stanford University Press, 1983), I, pp. 482–88.

Milsom, Kate, 'James Barry 1789–1865', *No Man's Land* exhibition, Martin Tinney Gallery, Cardiff, 28 February to 24 March 2018, http://www.artwales.com/exhibition-mtg-en.php?locationID=263 [accessed 10 March 2018].

Mindock, Clark, 'Donald Trump bans transgender people from serving in US military due to "disruption" they would cause', *Independent*, 26 July 2017, http://www.independent.co.uk/news/world/americas/us-politics/donald-trump-bans-transgender-people-us-military-army-chelsea-manning-lgbt-rights-gay-president-a7861196.html [accessed 26 July 2017].

Mindock, Clark, 'Second US federal court blocks Trump's transgender military ban', *Independent*, 23 December 2017, http://www.independent.co.uk/news/world/americas/us-politics/donald-trump-transgender-military-ban-latest-second-court-blocks-washington-a8126811.html [accessed 23 December 2017].

Mindock, Clark, 'Senator who lost both legs in Iraq war blasts Trump on transgender military ban', *Independent*, 24 August 2017, http://www.independent.co.uk/news/world/americas/us-politics/trump-transgender-ban-tammy-duckworth-statement-response-us-senator-criticism-a7911526.html [accessed 26 August 2017].

Mitchell, Kate, *History and Cultural Memory in Neo-Victorian Fiction: Victorian Afterimages* (Basingstoke: Palgrave Macmillan, 2010).

'Modern family will feature a transgender child actor in a forthcoming episode', *BBC Newsbeat*, 27 September 2016, http://www.bbc.co.uk/newsbeat/article/37481561/modern-family-will-feature-a-transgender-child-actor-in-a-forthcoming-episode [accessed 27 September 2016].

Moers, Ellen, *The Dandy: Brummell to Beerbohm* (Lincoln: University of Nebraska Press, 1978).

Mohr, Frederic [David McKail], 'Barry'. A dramatization for television of the life of Inspector General of Army Hospitals, MAJOR-GENERAL JAMES MIRANDA BARRY, 1795–1865: The first woman doctor of modern western medicine [Unfinished script, undated]. Scottish Theatre Archive, STA MN57/1, University of Glasgow.

Mohr, Frederic [David McKail], 'Barry: Personal Statements', 1984 play script, National Library of Scotland, Edinburgh, Traverse Theatre Inventory, Acc. 9285/8; also Scottish Theatre Archive, Glasgow, STA Mn 63/7.

Mohr, Frederic, *Barry: Personal Statements*, in *Five Solo Plays* (Edinburgh: [David McKail], [1994]), pp. 43–76.

Moore, C. F., M.D., F.R.C.S., Ireland, 'To the Editors of *The Lancet*', 'Notes, Comments, and Answers to Correspondents' section, *Lancet* [letter dated 14 October 1895], vol. 3764, 19 October 1895, p.1021.

Moore, George, 'Albert Nobbs', *Celibate Lives* (London: William Heinemann, 1927), repr. in Ann Heilmann and Mark Llewellyn (eds), *The Collected Short Stories of George Moore: Gender and Genre*, 5 vols (London: Pickering and Chatto, 2007), V, pp. 189–220.

Morris, Jan, *Conundrum* (London: Faber and Faber, 1974).

Morris, Regan, 'Transgender 13-year-old Zoey having therapy', *BBC News* online, Los Angeles, 12 January 2015, http://www.bbc.co.uk/news/world-us-canada-30783983 [accessed 15 January 2016].

MOTHA (Museum of Transhirstory and Art; Executive Director: Chris E. Vargas), http://www.sfmotha.org/

Moulds, Alison, 'Groundbreakers: James Miranda Barry', FWSA blog, 27 November 2013, http://fwsablog.org.uk/2013/11/27/james-miranda-barry/ [accessed 18 April 2015].

Murray, Jenni, *Votes for Women! The Pioneers and Heroines of Female Suffrage* (London: Oneworld Publications, 2018).

'A Mystery Still', *All the Year Round*, XVII (1866–67), 18 May 1867, pp. 492–95.

Nabokov, Vladimir, *Pale Fire* (New York: Vintage International, 1989).

Nadel, Ira B., 'Narrative and the Popularity of Biography', *Mosaic*, vol. 20: 4 (1987), pp. 131–41.

'Natascha to star as cross dressing doc', *Mirror*, 22 September 2008, updated 3 February 2012, http://www.mirror.co.uk/news/uk-news/natascha-to-star-as-cross-dressing-doc-340064 [accessed 28 October 2015].

Nation, Earl F., M.D., 'James Barry, M.D., Inspector General of Hospitals: Man or Woman?', *Urology*, vol. 31:2 (February 1988), pp. 184–88.

Nayder, Lillian, *The Other Dickens: A Life of Catherine Hogarth* (Ithaca: Cornell University Press, 2011).

'The Need for a Gender-Neutral Pronoun', Gender Neutral Pronoun Blog, https://genderneutralpronoun.wordpress.com/ [accessed 25 March 2017]

Neuhaus, Susan and Sharon Masall-Dare, 'Before Federation: women in military medicine', *Not for Glory: A Century of Service by Medical Women to the Australian Army and its Allies* (Salisbury, Qld: Boolarong Press, 2014), pp. 1–11.

Nightingale, Florence, undated fragment of letter headed 'to Mama by Parthe's desire' [August 1865?], filed with a newspaper clip and transcript by John Guest, 'Sharp Encounter', *Sunday Times*, 9 November 1952, 'Letters by Nightingale, 1864–1865', Wellcome Library, London, Ms 9001/14.5.

Novak, Julia, 'The Notable Woman in Fiction: The Afterlives of Elizabeth Barrett Browning', in 'Biofictions', ed. Michael Lackey, special issue of *a/b: Auto/Biography Studies*, vol. 31:1 (2016), pp. 83–107.

Nünning, Ansgar, 'Fictional Metabiographies and Metaautobiographies: Towards a Definition, Typology and Analysis of Self-Reflexive Hybrid Metagenres', in *Self-Reflexivity in Literature*, ed. Werner Huber, Martin Middeke and Hubert Zapf (Würzburg: Königshausen & Neumann, 2005), pp. 195–209.

Nünning, Ansgar, 'An Intertextual Quest for Thomas Chatterton: the Deconstruction of the Romantic Cult of Originality and the Paradoxes of Life-Writing in Peter Ackroyd's Fictional Metabiography *Chatterton*', in *Biofictions: The Rewriting of Romantic Lives in Contemporary Fiction and Drama*, ed. Martin Middeke and Werner Huber (London: Camden House, 1999), pp. 27–49.

Nünning, Ansgar, 'Making Events – Making Stories – Making Worlds: Ways of Worldmaking from a Narratological Point of View', in *Mediation, Remediation and the Dynamics of Cultural Memory*, ed. Astrid Erll and Ann Rigney in collaboration with Laura Basu and Paulus Bijl (Berlin: de Gruyter, 2009), pp. 191–214.

Oppenheim, Maya, 'Author Chimamanda Ngozi Adichie faces backlash for suggesting transgender women are not real women', *Independent*, 12 March 2017, http://www.independent.co.uk/arts-entertainment/books/news/chimamanda-ngozi-adichie-transgender-women-channel-four-a7625481.html [accessed 14 April 2017].

Oreglia, Giacomo, *The Commedia dell'Arte*, trans. Lovett F. Edwards (London: Methuen, 1968).

Ottoman, E. E., 'Dr. James Barry and the specter of trans and queer history', GLBT History, 24 November 2014, https://acosmistmachine.

com/2015/11/24/dr-james-barry-and-the-specter-of-trans-and-queer-history/ [accessed 12 August 2017].

Ouellette, Sylvie, *Le Secret du docteur Barry* (2012; Paris: Terres de femmes, De Borée, 2013).

Padanna, Ashraf, 'India opens first school for transgender pupils', *BBC News* online, 30 December 2016, http://www.bbc.co.uk/news/world-asia-india-38470192 [accessed 31 December 2016].

Palmer, Beth and Benjamin Poore, 'Introduction' to 'Performing the Neo-Victorian', ed. Beth Palmer and Benjamin Poore, special issue of *Neo-Victorian Studies*, vol. 9:1 (2016), pp. 1–11.

Panizza, Oscar, 'A Scandal at the Convent', trans. Sophie Wilkins ['Ein skandalöser Fall', *Visionen der Dämmerung* (München: G. Müller, 1914)], in Michel Foucault, *Herculine Barbin* (New York: Vintage, 2010), pp. 154–99.

Panizza, Oscar, 'Un scandale au couvent', trans. Jean Bréjoux ['Ein skandalöser Fall', *Visionen der Dämmerung* (München: G. Müller, 1914)], repr. in *Michel Foucault présente Herculine Barbine dite Alexina B., suivi de Un scandale au couvent d'Oscar Panizza* ([Paris]: Gallimard, 2014), pp. 173–220.

Parini, Jay, 'Writing Biographical Fiction: Some Personal Reflections', in 'Biofictions', ed. Michael Lackey, special issue of *a/b: Auto/Biography Studies*, vol. 31:1 (2016), pp. 21–26.

Park, Katharine and Robert A. Nye, 'Destiny is Anatomy – Making Sex: Body and Gender from the Greeks to Freud by Thomas Laqueur', *New Republic*, 18 February 1991, pp. 53–57.

Parker, Andrew and Eve Kosofsky Sedgwick, 'Introduction: Performativity and Performance', in *Performativity and Performance*, ed. Andrew Parker and Eve Kosofsky Sedgwick (London: Routledge, 1995), pp. 1–18.

Pasha-Robinson, Lucy, 'Rachel Dolezal: White woman who identifies as black calls for "racial fluidity" to be accepted', *Independent*, 28 March 2017, http://www.independent.co.uk/news/people/rachel-dolezal-white-woman-black-racial-fluidity-accepted-transracial-naacp-a7653131.html [accessed 29 March 2017].

Pasha-Robinson, Lucy, 'Trans woman receives police payout after being forced to strip naked and being sprayed with mace', *Independent*, 20 June 2017, http://www.independent.co.uk/news/uk/home-news/trans-woman-police-payout-stripped-naked-mace-spray-avon-somerset-constabulary-a7799166.html [accessed 20 June 2017].

Pearsall, Cornelia D.J., 'The dramatic monologue', in *The Cambridge Companion to Victorian Poetry*, ed. Joseph Bristow (Cambridge: Cambridge University Press, 2000), pp. 67–88.

Pells, Rachels, 'Transgender policies in schools "a waste of time and money", claims leading academic', *Independent*, 23 June 2017, http://www.independent.co.uk/news/education/education-news/transgender-policies-school-gender-identity-neutral-toilets-waste-of-time-money-dr-joanna-williams-a7805511.html [accessed 23 June 2017].

Perry, Louise, 'Dr James Barry had no choice but to pretend to be a man', *Guardian* online, 25 July 2017, https://www.theguardian.com/world/2017/jul/25/dr-james-barry-had-no-choice-but-to-pretend-to-be-a-man [accessed 26 July 2017].

Phillips, Howard, 'Home Taught for Abroad: The Training of the Cape Doctor, 1807–1910', in *The Cape Doctor in the Nineteenth Century: A Social History*, ed. Harriet Deacon, Howard Phillips and Elizabeth van Heyningen (Amsterdam: Rodopi, 2004), pp. 105–131.

Poe, Edgar Allan, 'The Purloined Letter' (1845), in *The Portable Poe*, ed. Philip van Doren Stern (Harmondsworth: Penguin, 1977), pp. 439–62.

Poore, Benjamin, *Heritage, Nostalgia and Modern British Theatre: Staging the Victorians* (Basingstoke: Palgrave Macmillan, 2012).

Preez, H. M. du, 'Dr James Barry: the early years revealed', *South African Medical Journal*, vol. 98 (2008), pp. 52–58.

Preez, H. M. du, 'Dr James Barry (1789–1865): the Edinburgh years', *Journal of the Royal College of Physicians of Edinburgh*, vol. 42:3 (2012), pp. 258–65.

Preez, Michael du and Jeremy Dronfield, *Dr James Barry: A Woman Ahead of Her Time* (London: Oneworld Publications, 2016).

Pressly, William L. *The Life and Art of James Barry* (New Haven: Yale University Press, 1981).

Pressly, William L. 'Portrait of a Cork Family: The Two James Barrys', *Cork Historical and Archaeological Society*, vol. 90 (1985), pp. 137–49.

Primorac, Antonija, *Neo-Victorianism on Screen: Postfeminism and Contemporary Adaptations of Victorian Women* (Basingstoke: Palgrave Macmillan, 2018).

Primorac, Antonija and Monika Pietrzak-Franger (eds), 'Neo-Victorianism and Globalisation: Transnational Dissemination of Nineteenth-Century Cultural Texts', special issue of *Neo-Victorian Studies*, vol. 8:1 (2015).

Prosser, Jay, *Second Skins: The Body Narratives of Transsexuality* (New York: Columbia University Press, 1998).

'Protesters gather against Caitleen Jenner outside Chicago House', *AXS Entertainment*, 14 November 2015, http://www.examiner.com/article/protesters-gather-against-caitlyn-jenner-outside-chicago-house [accessed 16 November 2015].

Pulver, Andrew, 'Rachel Weisz to play real-life gender-fluid Victorian doctor', *Guardian*, 13 December 2016, https://www.theguardian.com/film/2016/dec/13/rachel-weisz-stars-james-barry-film-gender-fluid-victorian-doctor [accessed 12 December 2016].

'Rachel Weisz to star in Dr. James Barry biopic', *Female First*, 13 December 2016, http://www.femalefirst.co.uk/movies/movie-news/rachel-weisz-star-james-barry-biopic-1019991.html [accessed 15 December 2016].

Racster, Olga, *Curtain Up! The Story of Cape Theatre* (Cape Town: Juta and Co, 1951).

Racster, Olga and Jessica Grove, *Dr James Barry: A romantic play founded on South African history* (1919), Lord Chamberlain's Office, British Library, LCP 1919/17 I No.2338.

Racster, Olga and Jessica Grove, *Dr James Barry: Her Secret Story* (London: Gerald Howe, 1932). With five illustrations.

Racster, Olga and Jessica Grove, *The Journal of Dr James Barry* (London: Lane, 1932).

Rae, Isobel, *The Strange Story of Dr James Barry: Army Surgeon, Inspector-General of Hospitals, Discovered on Death to be a Woman* (London: Longmans, Green and Co, 1958).

Ramadan, Emma, 'Translator's Note' to Anne Garréta, *Sphinx*, trans. Emma Ramadan (Dallas, Texas: Deep Vellum Publishing, 2015), n.p. [pp. 122–28].

Raymond, Janice G., *The Transsexual Empire: The Making of the She-Male* (1979; New York: Teacher's College Press, 1994).

Reyner, J. R. L., 'Visible Difference', *The Stage and Television Today*, vol. 5613, 10 November 1988, p.16.

Reynolds, Stephen, 'Autobiografiction', *Speaker*, new series, vol. 15: 366, 6 October 1906, p.28, p.30, accessed from Max Saunders's homepage, https://blogs.kcl.ac.uk/maxsaunders/autobiografiction/autobiografiction-scan/ [accessed 27 February 2018].

Richardson, Samuel, *Pamela, Or Virtue Rewarded*, ed. Thomas Keymer and Alice Wakeley (1740; Oxford: Oxford University Press, 2007).

Riordon, Colin, 'Germaine Greer: Having her speak at Cardiff University was the right thing to do', *Times Higher Education*, 3 December 2015, https://www.timeshighereducation.com/comment/germaine-greer-having-her-speak-at-cardiff-university-was-the-right-thing-to-do [accessed 4 December 2015].

Robinson, Alan, *Narrating the Past; Historiography, Memory and the Contemporary Novel* (Basingstoke: Palgrave Macmillan, 2011).

Rodgers, Nigel, *The Dandy: Peacock or Enigma?* (London: Bene Factum Publishing, 2012).

Roen, Katrina, '"Either/Or" and "Both/Neither": Discursive Tensions in Transgender Politics', *Signs*, vol. 27:2 (Winter 2002), pp. 501–22.

Rogers, E[benezer], 'A Female Member of the Army Medical Staff', 'Notes, Comments, and Answers to Correspondents' section, *Lancet* [letter dated 15 October 1895], vol. 3764, 19 October 1895, p.1021.

Rogers, E[benezer], 'A Female Member of the Army Medical Staff', 'Notes, Comments, and Answers to Correspondents' section, *Lancet* [letter dated 21 October 1895], vol. 3765, 26 October 1895, pp. 1086–87.

Rogers, E[benezer], 'A Female Member of the Army Medical Staff', 'Notes, Comments, and Answers to Correspondents' section, *Lancet* [letter dated 28 April 1896], vol. 3792, 2 May 1896, p.264.

Rogers, E[benezer], *Madeline's Mystery.* Edited by the author of Lady Audley's Secret (London: J. and R. Maxwell, [1882]). Harry Ransom Center, The University of Texas at Austin, WOLFF 752.

Rogers, E[benezer], *A Modern Sphinx*, 3 vols (London: John and Robert Maxwell, 1881). British Library Historical Print editions.

Rogers, E[benezer], *A Modern Sphinx: A Novel.* Edition de luxe, with seven illustrations. In one volume (London: n.p. [1896]). British Library General Reference Collection C.194.a.672.

Roland, Charles G., 'Barry, James', in *Dictionary of Canadian Biography*, vol. 9 (University of Toronto / Université Laval, 2003), http://www.biographi.ca/en/bio/barry_james_9E.html [accessed 8 November 2015].

Rooney, Monique, 'Grave endings: the representation of passing', *Australian Humanities Review*, vol. 23 (Sept. 2001), http://australianhumanitiesreview.org/2001/09/01/grave-endings-the-representation-of-passing/ [accessed 22 December 2016].

Rosario, Vernon A., 'The History of Aphallia and the Intersexual Challenge to Sex/Gender', in *A Companion to Lesbian, Gay, Bisexual, Transgender, and Queer Studies*, ed. George E. Haggerty and Molly McGarry (Blackwell Publishing, 2007), pp. 92–111, Blackwell Reference Online, http://www.blackwellreference.com/subscriber/tocnode.html?id=g9781405113298_chunk_g978140511329814 [accessed 16 December 2016].

Rose, Jacqueline, 'Who do you think you are', *London Review of Books*, vol. 38:9, 5 May 2016, http://www.lrb.co.uk/v38/n09/jacqueline-rose/who-do-you-think-you-are [accessed 16 December 2016].

Rose, June, *The Perfect Gentleman: The remarkable life of Dr. James Miranda Barry, the woman who served as an officer in the British Army from 1813 to 1859* (London: Hutchinson, 1977).

Rose, June, *Quest for Dr. James Barry*, prod. Madeau Stewart (BBC radio broadcast, 27 June 1973), Wellcome Library, London, RAMC 1089. [For a synopsis see http://genome.ch.bbc.co.uk/067c12ad2b544f0398e4ea0e806418bc].

Rota, Jess, 'James Barry, unsung hero', *Unsung LGTB Heroes*, repr. from *We Are Family Magazine*, vol. 6 (Summer 2014), https://wearefamilymagazine.co.uk/unsung-lgbt-heroes-james-barry/ [accessed 10 August 2017].

Rutherford, N[athaniel] J[ohn] C[rawford], 'Dr James Barry: Inspector-General of the Army Medical Department', *Journal of the Royal Army Medical Corps*, vol. LXIII (July-Dec. 1939), pp. 106–24, pp. 173–78, pp. 240–48.

Sadoff, Dianne F., *Victorian Vogue: British Novels on Screen* (Minneapolis: University of Minnesota Press, 2010).

Sage, Lorna (ed.), *The Cambridge Guide to Women's Writing in English* (Cambridge: Cambridge University Press, 1999).

Salih, Sarah, *Judith Butler* (London: Routledge, 2002).

Sampathkumar, Mythili, 'The seven words Trump "banned" a health agency from using were projected onto his hotel', *Independent*, 21 December 2017, http://www.independent.co.uk/news/world/americas/us-politics/donald-trump-hotel-cdc-banned-words-lgbt-fetus-science-evidence-a8121311.html [accessed 23 December 2017].

Sampathkumar, Mythili, 'Transgender members of US military speak out against Trump's ban', *Independent*, 26 August 2017, http://www.independent.co.uk/news/transgender-us-military-donald-trump-ban-james-mattis-a7914746.html [accessed 26 August 2017].

Saunders, Max, *Self-Impression: Life-Writing, Autobiografiction, and the Forms of Modern Literature* (Oxford: Oxford University Press, 2010).

Savu, Laura E., *Postmortem Postmodernists: The Afterlife of the Author in Recent Narrative* (Madison: Fairleigh Dickinson University Press, 2009).

Schabert, Ina, 'Fictional Biography, Factual Biography, and their Contamination', *Biography*, vol. 5:1 (Winter 1982), pp. 1–16.

Schabert, Ina, *In Quest of the Other Person: Fiction as Biography* (Tübingen: Francke, 1990).

Scott, Joanna, *Arrogance* (New York: Linden, 1991).

Scott, Joanna, 'On Hoaxes, Humbugs, and Fictional Portraiture', special issue on 'Biofictions', ed. Michael Lackey, *a/b: Auto/Biography Studies,* vol. 31:1 (2016), pp. 27–32.

Sedgwick, Eve Kosofksy, *Between Men: English Literature and Male Homosocial Desire* (New York: Columbia University Press, 1985).

Shakespeare, William, *The Tempest* (Cambridge: Cambridge University Press, 1969).

Shelley, Mary, 'Introduction' (1831), *Frankenstein*, ed. Johanna M. Smith (Boston: Bedford/St. Martin's, 2000), pp. 19–25.

Shepherd-Barr, Kirsten, *Science on Stage: From Doctor Faustus to Copenhagen* (Princeton, NJ: Princeton University Press, 2006).

Showalter, Elaine, *The Civil Wars of Julia Ward Howe: A Biography* (New York: Simon & Schuster, 2016).

Showalter, Elaine, *Sexual Anarchy: Gender and Culture at the Fin de Siècle* (London: Bloomsbury, 1991).

Shugerman, Emily, '"This is discrimination, plain and simple": Trump's ban on transgender military service deemed a "vile attack" on LGTBQ Americans', *Independent*, 26 July 2017, https://www.independent.co.uk/news/world/americas/us-politics/trump-transgender-ban-us-military-nancy-pelosi-lgbt-rights-americans-vile-congress-democrats-a7861611.html [accessed 26 July 2017].

Sini, Rozina, '"We don't care" – the new sign for gender-neutral toilets', *BBC News*, 25 August 2016, http://www.bbc.co.uk/news/world-us-canada-37187370 [accessed 25 August 2016].

Slater, Michael, *Dickens and Women* (London: Dent, 1983).

Smith, Kathleen M., 'Dr. James Barry: Military man – or woman?', *Canadian Medical Association Journal*, vol. 126, 1 April 1982, pp. 854–57.

Smith-Walters, Maisie, 'Hollywood trans roles under fire - again', *BBC News Magazine*, 15 September 2016, http://www.bbc.co.uk/news/magazine-37312338 [accessed 16 September 2016].

Smyth, Ethel, 'The March of the Women', in *Voices & Votes: A literary anthology of the women's suffrage campaign*, ed. Glenda Norquay (Manchester: Manchester University Press, 1995), p.94.

[Snell, Hannah,] *The Female Soldier or the Surprising Life and Adventures of Hannah Snell* (London: R. Walker, 1750), repr. in *Women Adventurers: The Lives of Madame Velazquez, Hannah Snell, Mary Anne Talbot, and Mrs. Christian Davies*, ed. Ménie Muriel Dowie (London: Fisher Unwin, 1893), pp. 197–288.

Solicari, Sonia (ed.), *Victoriana: A Miscellany* (London: Guildhall Art Gallery, 2013).

Stanley, Jo, *Bold in Her Breeches: Women Pirates Across the Ages* (London: Pandora, 1996).

Steinmetz, Katy, 'A Comprehensive Guide to Facebook's New Options for Gender Identity: An expert walks through what they mean, from transgender to pangender', *Time*, 14 February 2014, http://techland.time.com/2014/02/14/a-comprehensive-guide-to-facebooks-new-options-for-gender-identity/ [accessed 23 December 2017].

Stone, Jon, 'People to be allowed to pick their own gender without doctor's diagnosis, under Government plans', *Independent*, 23 July 2017, http://www.independent.co.uk/news/uk/politics/transgender-rules-reform-gender-dysphoria-changes-2004-gender-recognition-self-identify-a7855381.html [accessed 23 July 2017].

'A Strange Story', *Manchester Guardian*, 21 August 1865.

Stryker, Susan, '(De)Subjugated Knowledges: An Introduction to Transgender Studies', in *The Transgender Studies Reader*, ed. Susan Stryker and Stephen Whittle (London: Routledge, 2006), pp. 1–18.

Stryker, Susan and Stephen Whittle (eds), *The Transgender Studies Reader* (London: Routledge, 2006).

'Studying transgender and transvestism archive', Wellcome Library, London, December 2014, http://blog.wellcomelibrary.org/2014/12/studying-transgender-and-transvestism-a-new-archive/ [accessed 15 July 2015].

Talbot, Mary Anne, *The Life and Surprising Adventures of Mary Anne Talbot in the Name of John Taylor* (London: J.G. Barnard, 1809), repr. in Ménie Muriel Dowie (ed.), *Women Adventurers*, pp. 136–96.

'Tara Hudson: "I didn't choose to be this way"', *BBC News* online, 30 October 2015, http://www.bbc.co.uk/news/uk-34683418 [accessed 14 April 2017]

Thackeray, William, *Vanity Fair*, ed. Peter Shillingsburg (1848; New York: Norton, 1994), pp. xi–xvi, pp. 1–696.

Thomas, George, Earl of Albemarle, *Fifty Years of My Life*, 2 vols (London: Macmillan, 1876), II.

Thomas, Julia, 'Illustration and the Victorian Novel', in *The Oxford Handbook of Victorian Literary Culture*, ed. Juliet John (Oxford: Oxford University Press, 2016), pp. 617–36.

Thomas, Julia, *Nineteenth-Century Illustration and the Digital: Studies in Word and Image* (Basingstoke: Palgrave, 2017).

Thornber, Robin, 'Double firsts', *Guardian*, 30 September 1988, p.31.

Thorpe, Vanessa, 'Tragic star to play a legend of medicine', *Observer*, 21 September 2008, http://www.theguardian.com/film/2008/sep/21/medicine.mcelhone [accessed 17 April 2015].

Toíbín, Colm, *The Master* (London: Picador, 2004).

Tomalin, Claire, *Charles Dickens: A Life* (London: Penguin, 2012).

Tomalin, Claire, *The Invisible Woman* (London: Viking, 1990).

Town, Florida Ann, *With a Silent Companion* (1999; Alberta: Red Deer Press, 2000).

'Transgender: A collection of programmes and clips looking at Transgender issues', *BBC Player Radio* (2016), http://www.bbc.co.uk/programmes/p02dt14s [accessed 15 January 2016].

'Transgender' [collection of news items], *Independent*, http://www.independent.co.uk/topic/transgender [accessed 25 July 2017].

'Transgender Americans seek birth certificate rule change', *BBC News Magazine*, 5 January 2012, http://www.bbc.co.uk/news/magazine-16420819 [accessed 14 April 2017].

'Transgender-friendly toilets planned for 2020 Olympics in Tokyo', *Guardian* online, 2 March 2017, https://www.theguardian.com/sport/2017/mar/01/tokyo-2020-olympics-transgender-friendly-toilets [accessed 2 March 2017].

'Transgender Hirstory in 99 Objects' exhibition organized by the Museum of Transgender Hirstory & Art, or MOTHA, ONE National Gay & Lesbian Archives, Los Angeles, 21 March to 11 July 2015, http://www.sfmotha.org/post/113084736715/one [accessed 14 April 2017].

'Transgender pension case to be examined by EU judges', *BBC News* online, 10 August 2016, http://www.bbc.co.uk/news/uk-37033868 [accessed 10 August 2016].

'Transgender Prisoner: I was absolutely terrified', *BBC News* online, 7 December 2015, http://www.bbc.co.uk/news/uk-35029928 [accessed 14 April 2017].

'Transgender prisoner Tara Hudson "feared being raped"', *BBC News* online, 7 December 2015, http://www.bbc.co.uk/news/uk-england-somerset-35030241 [accessed 14 April 2017].

'Transgender woman found dead in cell at HMP Doncaster', *BBC News online*, 5 January 2017, http://www.bbc.co.uk/news/uk-england-south-yorkshire-38518833 [accessed 6 January 2017].

'Transgender woman Tara Hudson moved to female prison', *BBC News* online, 30 October 2015, http://www.bbc.co.uk/news/uk-34683418 [accessed 14 April 2017].

'Transgender woman Vikki Thompson found dead at Armley jail', *BBC News* online, 19 November 2015, http://www.bbc.co.uk/news/uk-england-leeds-34869620 [accessed 14 April 2017]

Transvengers site for young trans people, Wellcome Library, https://wellcomecollection.org/transvengers [accessed 8 July 2016].

Twain, Mark, *Following the Equator: A Journey Around the World* (1897), Project Gutenberg, Ebook ♯2895, http://www.gutenberg.org/files/2895/2895-h/2895-h.htm [accessed 14 April 2017]

'US judge rules against Virginia transgender toilet ban', *BBC News*, 19 April 2016, http://www.bbc.co.uk/news/world-us-canada-36087908 [accessed 4 August 2016].

'US Supreme Court blocks transgender ruling', *BBC News*, 4 August 2016, http://www.bbc.co.uk/news/world-us-canada-36971310 [accessed 4 August 2016].

Vella, Col. E. E. L/RAMC, 'James Barry: Inspector General of Army Hospitals', 'Letters to the Editor' section, *Journal of the Royal Army Medical Corps*, vol. 131 (1985), p.167.

Voigts, Eckhart, 'Bio-Fiction: Neo-Victorian Revisions of Evolution and Genetics', in *Neo-Victorian Literature and Culture: Immersions and Revisitations*, ed. Nadine Boehm-Schnitker and Susanne Gruss (London: Routledge, 2014), pp. 79–92.

Voigts, Eckhart, Barbara Schaff and Monika Pietrzak-Franger (eds), *Reflecting on Darwin* (Farnham: Ashgate, 2014).

Wang, Yang, 'Feminist Germaine Greer still pummelled for "misogynistic views toward transwomen"', *Washington Post* online, 3 November 2015, https://www.washingtonpost.com/news/morning-mix/wp/2015/11/03/feminist-germaine-greer-still-being-pummelled-for-misogynistic-views-toward-transwomen/ [accessed 5 November 2015].

Warhol, Robyn and Susan S. Lanser (eds), *Narrative Theory Unbound: Queer and Feminist Interventions* (Columbus: Ohio State University Press, 2015).

'Watching my son become my daughter', *BBC Magazine*, 1 June 2017, http://www.bbc.co.uk/news/av/magazine-40111723/watching-my-son-become-my-daughter [accessed 1 June 2017].

Waters, Sarah, *Fingersmith* (London: Virago, 2003).

Waters, Sarah, *Tipping the Velvet* (London: Virago, 1998).

Weale, Sally, 'Book explaining gender diversity to primary school children sparks furore', *Guardian* online, 2 January 2017, https://www.theguardian.com/society/2017/jan/02/book-explaining-gender-diversity-to-primary-school-children-sparks-furore [accessed 2 January 2017].

Wheelwright, Julie, *Amazons and Military Maids: Women Who Dressed as Men in Pursuit of Life, Liberty and Happiness* (London: Pandora, 1989).

'Whistling Psyche by Sebastian Barry', Indiegogo, https://www.indiegogo.com/projects/whistling-psyche-by-sebastian-barry#/ [accessed 29 October 2015].

White, Hayden, 'Anomalies of Genre: The Utility of Theory and History for the Study of Literary Genres', *New Literary Theory*, vol. 34:3 (Summer 2003), pp. 597–615.

White, Jeremy B., 'Transgender "curriculum" launched to help tech firms with diversity problems', *Independent*, 2 August 2017, http://www.independent.co.uk/news/world/americas/transgender-curriculum-tech-firms-diversity-silicon-valley-diversity-problem-slack-a7874066.html [accessed 2 August 2017].

Whittle, Stephen, 'Foreword' to *The Transgender Studies Reader*, ed. Susan Stryker and Stephen Whittle (London: Routledge, 2006), pp. xi–xxi.

Whittle, Stephen, *The Transgender Debate: The Crisis Surrounding Gender Identity* (Reading: South Street Press, 2000).

Wilson, Alice, 'The Enigma of Dr James Barry', *Health, Law & Ethics*, downloaded from *LJSM*, vol.1, 30 April 2010, pp. 243–45, http://issuu.com/lsjm/docs/hle [accessed 2 November 2015].

Williams, Gary, 'Speaking with the Voices of Others', Introduction to Julia Ward Howe, *The Hermaphrodite*, ed. Gary Williams (Lincoln: University of Nebraska Press, 2004), pp. ix–xliv.

Wintle, Justin (ed.), *Makers of Nineteenth Century Culture 1800–1914* (London: Routledge & Kegan Paul, 1982).

Woolf, Virginia, 'Mr. Bennett and Mrs. Brown' (1924), repr. in *The Gender of Modernism: A Critical Anthology*, ed. Bonnie Kime Scott (Bloomington: Indiana University Press, 1990), pp. 634–41.

Woolf, Virginia, *Orlando* (1928; London: Penguin, 1993).

Woolf, Virginia, *A Room of One's Own*, in *A Room of One's Own/Three Guineas*, ed. Michèle Barrett (London: Penguin, 1993), pp. 1–114.

The Works of James Barry, Esq.: Historical Painter, 2 vols (London: Cadell and Davies, 1809).

Young, Sarah, 'Transgender dad and partner announce they are expecting first biological child', *Independent*, 1 June 2017, http://www.independent.co.uk/

life-style/transgender-dad-gay-partner-first-biological-child-trystan-reese-biff-chaplow-oregon-a7767271.html [accessed 1 June 2017].

Young, Robert, J.C., *Colonial Desire: Hybridity in Theory, Culture and Race* (London: Routledge, 1995).

Zwigtman, Floortje, *Adrian Mayfield: Auf Leben und Tod [Spigeljongen]* (Baarn: De Fontein, 2011).

Zwigtman, Floortje, *Adrian Mayfield: Versuch einer Liebe [Tegenspel]* (Baarn: De Fontein, 2007).

Zwigtman, Floortje, *Ich, Adrian Mayfield [Schijnbwegingen]* (Baarn: De Fontein, 2005).

Index[1]

[1] Note: Page numbers followed by 'n' refer to notes; Numbers in bold refer to illustrations.

A. Heilmann, *Neo-/Victorian Biographilia and James Miranda Barry*, https://doi.org/10.1007/978-3-319-71386-1

C

S

The manufacturer's authorised representative in the EU is Springer Nature Customer Service Centre GmbH, Europaplatz 3, 69115 Heidelberg, Germany. If you have any concerns regarding our products, please contact ProductSafety@springernature.com

Printed and bound by CPI Group (UK) Ltd, Croydon, CR0 4YY
07/05/2026
02104559-0001